The Relevance of Nutrition for Pediatric Allergy and Immunity

The Relevance of Nutrition for Pediatric Allergy and Immunity

Editors

R.J. Joost van Neerven
Janneke Ruinemans-Koerts

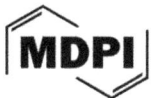 Basel • Beijing • Wuhan • Barcelona • Belgrade • Novi Sad • Cluj • Manchester

Editors
R.J. Joost van Neerven
Wageningen University &
Research
Wageningen, The Netherlands

Janneke Ruinemans-Koerts
Wageningen University &
Research
Wageningen, The Netherlands

Editorial Office
MDPI
St. Alban-Anlage 66
4052 Basel, Switzerland

This is a reprint of articles from the Special Issue published online in the open access journal *Nutrients* (ISSN 2072-6643) (available at: https://www.mdpi.com/journal/nutrients/special_issues/Nutrition_Allergy_Immunity).

For citation purposes, cite each article independently as indicated on the article page online and as indicated below:

Lastname, A.A.; Lastname, B.B. Article Title. *Journal Name* **Year**, *Volume Number*, Page Range.

ISBN 978-3-0365-9516-0 (Hbk)
ISBN 978-3-0365-9517-7 (PDF)
doi.org/10.3390/books978-3-0365-9517-7

© 2023 by the authors. Articles in this book are Open Access and distributed under the Creative Commons Attribution (CC BY) license. The book as a whole is distributed by MDPI under the terms and conditions of the Creative Commons Attribution-NonCommercial-NoDerivs (CC BY-NC-ND) license.

Contents

Preface vii

R. J. Joost van Neerven and Janneke Ruinemans-Koerts
The Relevance of Nutrition for Pediatric Allergy and Immunity
Reprinted from: *Nutrients* 2023, 15, 1881, doi:10.3390/nu15081881 1

John O. Warner and Jill Amanda Warner
The Foetal Origins of Allergy and Potential Nutritional Interventions to Prevent Disease
Reprinted from: *Nutrients* 2022, 14, 1590, doi:10.3390/nu14081590 5

Brit Trogen, Samantha Jacobs and Anna Nowak-Wegrzyn
Early Introduction of Allergenic Foods and the Prevention of Food Allergy
Reprinted from: *Nutrients* 2022, 14, 2565, doi:10.3390/nu14132565 19

**Antonia Zoe Quake, Taryn Audrey Liu, Rachel D'Souza, Katherine G. Jackson,
Margaret Woch, Afua Tetteh, et al.**
Early Introduction of Multi-Allergen Mixture for Prevention of Food Allergy: Pilot Study
Reprinted from: *Nutrients* 2022, 14, 737, doi:10.3390/nu14040737 29

**Laurien Ulfman, Angela Tsuang, Aline B. Sprikkelman, Anne Goh
and R. J. Joost van Neerven**
Relevance of Early Introduction of Cow's Milk Proteins for Prevention of Cow's Milk Allergy
Reprinted from: *Nutrients* 2022, 14, 2659, doi:10.3390/nu14132659 51

**Malin Barman, Mia Stråvik, Karin Broberg, Anna Sandin, Agnes E. Wold
and Ann-Sofie Sandberg**
Proportions of Polyunsaturated Fatty Acids in Umbilical Cord Blood at Birth Are Related to
Atopic Eczema Development in the First Year of Life
Reprinted from: *Nutrients* 2021, 13, 3779, doi:10.3390/nu13113779 69

**Yvan Vandenplas, Janusz Książyk, Manuel Sanchez Luna, Natalia Migacheva,
Jean-Charles Picaud, Luca A. Ramenghi, et al.**
Partial Hydrolyzed Protein as a Protein Source for Infant Feeding: Do or Don't?
Reprinted from: *Nutrients* 2022, 14, 1720, doi:10.3390/nu14091720 87

Alexander S. Colquitt, Elizabeth A. Miles and Philip C. Calder
Do Probiotics in Pregnancy Reduce Allergies and Asthma in Infancy and Childhood? A
Systematic Review
Reprinted from: *Nutrients* 2022, 14, 1852, doi:10.3390/nu14091852 93

Hanna Danielewicz
Breastfeeding and Allergy Effect Modified by Genetic, Environmental, Dietary, and
Immunological Factors
Reprinted from: *Nutrients* 2022, 14, 3011, doi:10.3390/nu14153011 105

**Raphaela Freidl, Victoria Garib, Birgit Linhart, Elisabeth M. Haberl, Isabelle Mader,
Zsolt Szépfalusi, et al.**
Extensively Hydrolyzed Hypoallergenic Infant Formula with Retained T Cell Reactivity
Reprinted from: *Nutrients* 2023, 15, 111, doi:10.3390/nu15010111 117

Chi-Nien Chen, Yu-Chen Lin, Shau-Ru Ho, Chun-Min Fu, An-Kuo Chou and Yao-Hsu Yang
Association of Exclusive Breastfeeding with Asthma Risk among Preschool Children: An
Analysis of National Health and Nutrition Examination Survey Data, 1999 to 2014
Reprinted from: *Nutrients* 2022, 14, 4250, doi:10.3390/nu14204250 137

Patricia Macchiaverni, Ulrike Gehring, Akila Rekima, Alet H. Wijga and Valerie Verhasselt
House Dust Mite Exposure through Human Milk and Dust: What Matters for Child Allergy Risk?
Reprinted from: *Nutrients* **2022**, *14*, 2095, doi:10.3390/nu14102095 147

Mojtaba Porbahaie, Huub F. J. Savelkoul, Cornelis A. M. de Haan, Malgorzata Teodorowicz and R. J. Joost van Neerven
Direct Binding of Bovine IgG-Containing Immune Complexes to Human Monocytes and Their Putative Role in Innate Immune Training
Reprinted from: *Nutrients* **2022**, *14*, 4452, doi:10.3390/nu14214452 157

Soraya Regina Abu Jamra, Camila Gomes Komatsu, Fernando Barbosa, Jr., Persio Roxo-Junior and Anderson Marliere Navarro
Proposal to Screen for Zinc and Selenium in Patients with IgA Deficiency
Reprinted from: *Nutrients* **2023**, *15*, 2145, doi:10.3390/nu15092145 175

Victoria Garib, Daria Trifonova, Raphaela Freidl, Birgit Linhart, Thomas Schlederer, Nikolaos Douladiris, et al.
Milk Allergen Micro-Array (MAMA) for Refined Detection of Cow's-Milk-Specific IgE Sensitization
Reprinted from: *Nutrients* **2023**, *15*, 2401, doi:10.3390/nu15102401 187

Antonia Zoe Quake, Taryn Audrey Liu, Rachel D'Souza, Katherine G. Jackson, Margaret Woch, Afua Tetteh, et al.
Correction: Quake et al. Early Introduction of Multi-Allergen Mixture for Prevention of Food Allergy: Pilot Study. *Nutrients* 2022, *14*, 737
Reprinted from: *Nutrients* **2023**, *15*, 135, doi:10.3390/nu15010135 205

Preface

Dear Reader,

The Special Issue of *Nutrients* entitled "The Relevance of Nutrition for Pediatric Allergy and Immunity" aims to provide an overview of the role of nutrition in early life to support immune development, hopefully leading to the prevention of infections and the development of allergies in very young children and infants. Although much is still unknown, the evidence is presented about the positive effects of nutrition on the immune system will hopefully stimulate further research in this field.

Many scientists from around the world contributed to this Special Issue. We would like to thank everyone for their contributions and for helping to make it a success. Similarly, we would like to thank the team at *Nutrients* for making the printed version available, as it is also an indication of the impact of this collection of original papers and reviews.

We hope you enjoy reading this Special Issue.

Warm regards,

R.J. Joost van Neerven and Janneke Ruinemans-Koerts
Editors

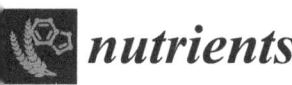

Editorial

The Relevance of Nutrition for Pediatric Allergy and Immunity

R. J. Joost van Neerven [1,2,*] and Janneke Ruinemans-Koerts [1,3]

1. Cell Biology and Immunology, Wageningen University & Research, 6708 WD Wageningen, The Netherlands
2. FrieslandCampina, 3818 LE Amersfoort, The Netherlands
3. Laboratory of Clinical Chemistry and Hematology, Rijnstate Hospital, 6815 AD Arnhem, The Netherlands
* Correspondence: joost.vanneerven@wur.nl

1. Introduction

The development of the immune system in early life is essential to shape an immune system. The first three years (or 1000 days) of life seem to be crucial for the development of the immune system, which provides resistance to infection and cancer, and this is related to learning to tolerate non-infectious proteins it is exposed to, such as dietary proteins and other proteins, and infants should thus not develop allergies to foods and inhaled proteins. However, even though infants still have frequent respiratory and gastrointestinal infections, child mortality has been reduced significantly. Contrary to this, the prevalence of asthma, rhinitis, and food allergy has increased tremendously in recent decades. Understanding how the function and development of the immune system can be influenced in early life will hopefully help to improve protection against infection and the development of allergies in early life.

2. Special Issue

This Special Issue of Nutrients, entitled "The relevance of Nutrition for Pediatric Allergy and Immunity", is an attempt to provide an overview of the current knowledge of the influence of different nutritional components both in mother and child on the prevention of infections and allergy development in children. The influence of dietary components can be provided directly to the infant by breastfeeding or early life nutrition, or indirectly, by the maternal diet (thus influencing fetal development, as well as breastmilk composition).

The influence of the immune system of pregnant women on their unborn child is regarded as the most critical phase in *the development of the fetal immune* system. To set the scene for this special issue, Warner and Warner describe the changes in the maternal immune system for protection of pregnancy and its effect on the immune system of the unborn child in early life [1]. After birth, the immune system of the neonate adapts under influence of the normal human microbiome, which is affected by many factors, such as maternal health and diet, exposure to antibiotics, mode of delivery, and breast or cow's milk formula feeding. Nowadays, dietary composition differs largely from decades ago. Additionally, the current deficiency of specific nutrients, which affect the immune system, are associated with the increase in the prevalence of allergies. However, intervention studies, by employing single nutrient supplementation, have achieved limited proof. Two reports here describe the effect of *maternal dietary supplementation* on allergic outcomes in infants. Colquitt and colleagues performed a systematic review on such an intervention, e.g., probiotics during pregnancy [2]. They concluded that studies showed inconsistent results, from no effect to a lower incidence in children at high risk. Barman and colleagues reported, in an observational study, that higher proportions of n-6 and lower proportions of n-3 polyunsaturated fatty acids (PUFA) in the maternal diet were significantly associated with atopic eczema development in the first year of age [3]. The authors stated that their results might be influenced by the risk of residual confounding, and thus causality could not be confirmed. On the other hand, as stated by Warner and Warner [1], it might be the soup of nutrients, which is more important than an individual nutrient because observational studies with overall dietary practices, such as the Mediterranean and other healthy diets, have been associated with a reduced prevalence of allergies.

Much research has been performed on the positive effects of *breastfeeding* in general, but its effects on the reduction of the development of allergies is underexposed. Chi-Nien Chen and colleagues found, in a study with 6000 children, that exclusive breastfeeding for four to six months was associated with a decreased risk of asthma in children three to six years old, although the effect appeared to diminish at older age [4]. However, in a narrative review by Danielewicz, it becomes clear that outcomes of these kinds of population-based studies are influenced by factors, such as human milk oligosaccharide composition, as well as environmental (allergen exposure, caesarean section), dietary (short fatty acids and introduction of solid food), and immunological factors [5]. As an illustration of this, Macchiaverni and colleagues showed an increased risk of having high levels of IgE and a trend of increased asthma risk in children breastfed by mothers with detectable Der p 1 in human milk, while such an association was not found for Der p 1 in infant mattresses [6].

There exists much evidence for the prevention of food allergies in infants at high risk by *early introduction* of potential allergens, such as peanuts, tree nuts, and eggs, as summarized by Trogen and colleagues [7]. However, further studies are necessary regarding their effects in low-risk patients. As there are multiple potential allergens, which have to be introduced, and which take much time and adherence of parents and patients, the study from the group of Quake is hopeful, as they showed that early introduction of simultaneous mixtures of multiple allergenic foods may be safe and efficacious for preventing food allergy [8]. Although much evidence of the effect of early introduction of peanut and tree nuts on allergy development, less is known about the introduction of cow's milk, as many children already receive cow's-milk-based formula much earlier in life. In relation to cow's milk allergy, Ulfman and colleagues discussed, in a narrative review, that studies have shown that breastfeeding from birth with early introduction of cow's milk supplementation within the first month of life and continued daily consumption of small amounts without hampering breastfeeding may reduce the risk of developing cow's milk allergy [9]. However, when the introduction of cow's milk is interrupted by periods of avoidance, the risk of developing cow's milk allergy seems to increase.

The use of (partial) *hydrolysed milk formula* to prevent cow's milk allergy is still being debated, as depicted by Vandenplas and colleagues [10]. Although in vitro and animal studies indicate benefit, there is insufficient evidence to recommend their universal use. Furthermore, hydrolyzed milk formula differs in its degree of hydrolysis and composition (e.g., supplementation with pre- and probiotics), and so much more research has to be performed on their safety and effectivity, but also how they can induce tolerance induction, as shown by Freidl's et al. [11]. Knowledge on which milk components are key factors in inducing the immune system to a tolerogenic state will enhance the development and application of hydrolyzed milk formula for both treatment and prevention of cow's milk allergy. Regarding this, the milk allergen micro-array (MAMA), described in this special issue by Garib et al. [12], may be an interesting novel tool to map IgE reactivity to many milk components simultaneously, using a *component resolved diagnostic* approach.

Finally, the potential impact of *early life nutrition and infection* was touched upon by Porbahaie et al. [13], who studied the effect of immune complexes consisting of bovine milk-derived IgG and the RSV pre-F protein. They demonstrated that such immune complexes may induce innate trained immunity, which improves the ability of the innate immune system in relation to TLR stimulation. As such, it may lead to increased innate immune reactivity and immune protection upon infection. Although this work focused on the functional effect of these immune complexes, consuming pasteurized milk during nasal RSV infection may bring these components together and thus influence innate immune reactivity to infectious challenges.

3. Concluding Remarks

In this Special Issue, several effects of dietary components on the development of allergy have been described. Not all relevant aspects and dietary approaches have been covered (e.g., microbiota targeted interventions via prebiotics and milk oligosaccharides, although probiotics were discussed), and the main focus turned out to be on allergy, rather than on infection, in this Special Issue. It is important to stress that breastfeeding for the first six months of life is very important for immune development, and it is associated with protection against infections, and it is also dependent on compositions related to allergies. Therefore, exclusive breastfeeding is recommended by WHO for the first six months of life, and other nutrition during this period should only be given if breastfeeding is not possible.

In conclusion, it is clear that dietary modulation of immune function in early life is an important, relevant topic, as well as an important approach, which can help to support immune health in the fist 1000 days of life.

Author Contributions: Both authors contributed to the design and writing of this editorial. All authors have read and agreed to the published version of the manuscript.

Conflicts of Interest: R.J.J.v.N. is employed by FrieslandCampina.

References

1. Warner, J.O.; Warner, J.A. The Foetal Origins of Allergy and Potential Nutritional Interventions to Prevent Disease. *Nutrients* **2022**, *14*, 1590. [CrossRef] [PubMed]
2. Colquitt, A.S.; Miles, E.A.; Calder, P.C. Do Probiotics in Pregnancy Reduce Allergies and Asthma in Infancy and Childhood? A Systematic Review. *Nutrients* **2022**, *14*, 1852. [CrossRef] [PubMed]
3. Barman, M.; Stråvik, M.; Broberg, K.; Sandin, A.; Wold, A.E.; Sandberg, A.-S. Proportions of Polyunsaturated Fatty Acids in Umbilical Cord Blood at Birth Are Related to Atopic Eczema Development in the First Year of Life. *Nutrients* **2021**, *13*, 3779. [CrossRef] [PubMed]
4. Chen, C.-N.; Lin, Y.-C.; Ho, S.-R.; Fu, C.-M.; Chou, A.-K.; Yang, Y.-H. Association of Exclusive Breastfeeding with Asthma Risk among Preschool Children: An Analysis of National Health and Nutrition Examination Survey Data, 1999 to 2014. *Nutrients* **2022**, *14*, 4250. [CrossRef] [PubMed]
5. Danielewicz, H. Breastfeeding and Allergy Effect Modified by Genetic, Environmental, Dietary, and Immunological Factors. *Nutrients* **2022**, *14*, 3011. [CrossRef] [PubMed]
6. Macchiaverni, P.; Gehring, U.; Rekima, A.; Wijga, A.H.; Verhasselt, V. House Dust Mite Exposure through Human Milk and Dust: What Matters for Child Allergy Risk? *Nutrients* **2022**, *14*, 2095. [CrossRef] [PubMed]
7. Trogen, B.; Jacobs, S.; Nowak-Wegrzyn, A. Early Introduction of Allergenic Foods and the Prevention of Food Allergy. *Nutrients* **2022**, *14*, 2565. [CrossRef] [PubMed]
8. Quake, A.Z.; Liu, T.A.; D'Souza, R.; Jackson, K.G.; Woch, M.; Tetteh, A.; Sampath, V.; Nadeau, K.C.; Sindher, S.; Chinthrajah, R.S.; et al. Early Introduction of Multi-Allergen Mixture for Prevention of Food Allergy: Pilot Study. *Nutrients* **2022**, *14*, 737. [CrossRef] [PubMed]
9. Ulfman, L.; Tsuang, A.; Sprikkelman, A.B.; Goh, A.; van Neerven, R.J.J. Relevance of Early Introduction of Cow's Milk Proteins for Prevention of Cow's Milk Allergy. *Nutrients* **2022**, *14*, 2659. [CrossRef] [PubMed]
10. Vandenplas, Y.; Książyk, J.; Luna, M.S.; Migacheva, N.; Picaud, J.-C.; Ramenghi, L.A.; Singhal, A.; Wabitsch, M. Partial Hydrolyzed Protein as a Protein Source for Infant Feeding: Do or Don't? *Nutrients* **2022**, *14*, 1720. [CrossRef] [PubMed]
11. Freidl, R.; Garib, V.; Linhart, B.; Haberl, E.M.; Mader, I.; Szépfalusi, Z.; Schmidthaler, K.; Douladiris, N.; Pampura, A.; Varlamov, E.; et al. Extensively Hydrolyzed Hypoallergenic Infant Formula with Retained T Cell Reactivity. *Nutrients* **2022**, *15*, 111. [CrossRef] [PubMed]
12. Garib, V.; Trifonova, D.; Freidl, R.; Linhart, B.; Schlederer, T.; Douladiris, N.; Pampura, A.; Dolotova, D.; Lepeshkova, T.; Gotua, M.; et al. Milk allergen micro-array (MAMA) for refined diagnosis of cow's milk-specific IgE sensitization. *Nutrients* **2023**, *in press*.
13. Porbahaie, M.; Savelkoul, H.F.J.; de Haan, C.A.M.; Teodorowicz, M.; van Neerven, R.J.J. Direct Binding of Bovine IgG-Containing Immune Complexes to Human Monocytes and Their Putative Role in Innate Immune Training. *Nutrients* **2022**, *14*, 4452. [CrossRef] [PubMed]

Review

The Foetal Origins of Allergy and Potential Nutritional Interventions to Prevent Disease

John O. Warner [1,2,*] and Jill Amanda Warner [2]

[1] National Heart and Lung Institute, Imperial College, London SW3 6LY, UK
[2] Paediatric Allergy, Red Cross Memorial Children's Hospital, University of Cape Town, Cape Town 7700, South Africa; dr.jill.warner@gmail.com
* Correspondence: j.o.warner@imperial.ac.uk

Abstract: The first nine months from conception to birth involves greater changes than at any other time in life, affecting organogenesis, endocrine, metabolic and immune programming. It has led to the concept that the "first 1000 days" from conception to the second birthday are critical in establishing long term health or susceptibility to disease. Immune ontogeny is predominantly complete within that time and is influenced by the maternal genome, health, diet and environment pre-conception and during pregnancy and lactation. Components of the immunological protection of the pregnancy is the generation of Th-2 and T-regulatory cytokines with the consequence that neonatal adaptive responses are also biased towards Th-2 (allergy promoting) and T-regulatory (tolerance promoting) responses. Normally after birth Th-1 activity increases while Th-2 down-regulates and the evolving normal human microbiome likely plays a key role. This in turn will have been affected by maternal health, diet, exposure to antibiotics, mode of delivery, and breast or cow milk formula feeding. Complex gene/environment interactions affect outcomes. Many individual nutrients affect immune mechanisms and variations in levels have been associated with susceptibility to allergic disease. However, intervention trials employing single nutrient supplementation to prevent allergic disease have not achieved the expected outcomes suggested by observational studies. Investigation of overall dietary practices including fresh fruit and vegetables, fish, olive oil, lower meat intake and home cooked foods as seen in the Mediterranean and other healthy diets have been associated with reduced prevalence of allergic disease. This suggests that the "soup" of overall nutrition is more important than individual nutrients and requires further investigation both during pregnancy and after the infant has been weaned. Amongst all the potential factors affecting allergy outcomes, modification of maternal and infant nutrition and the microbiome are easier to employ than changing other aspects of the environment but require large controlled trials before recommending changes to current practice.

Keywords: allergic sensitization; foetal immune ontogeny; gene/environment interactions; asthma; eczema; food allergy; maternal diet; PUFAs; vitamin D; Mediterranean diet; microbiome

1. Introduction

During delivery the neonate leaves the controlled and sterile environment of the uterus to be exposed to potentially overwhelming physical challenges. Development through pregnancy can be viewed as a preparation for extra-uterine existence with maternal gene/environment interactions influencing organ development and the programming of foetal immune, metabolic and endocrine responses. This concept arises from the hypothesis that the origins of health or risks of most diseases are a consequence of minor perturbations during organogenesis and periods of rapid cell division. It has evolved into the science known as "The Developmental Origins of Health And Disease (DOHAD)" or in common parlance the first 1000 days from conception to the second birthday [1]. A mismatch between the intra- and extra-uterine environment is more likely to result in adverse outcomes, because programming has not prepared the neonate for different exposures.

Birth-cohort and migration studies have highlighted this phenomenon in relation to changing susceptibility to cardio-vascular disease, metabolic syndrome and non-communicable immune mediated diseases [2] (Figure 1). Studies have shown that first-generation people migrating from countries with a low prevalence of allergic disease had a lower prevalence of allergy than second generation immigrants. The younger the child on arrival in a new high allergy prevalence country and the longer duration resident in that country directly correlates with changes in the subsequent incidence of allergic disease. Many factors interact to affect outcomes, but all relate to changes in life style and environmental exposures [3].

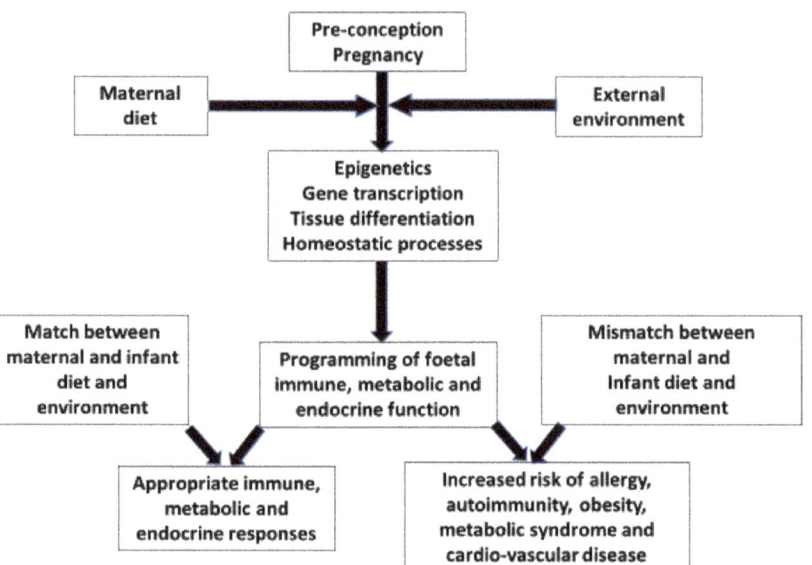

Figure 1. The evolutionary hypothesis based on Crespi BJ Front. Endocrinol. 2020 [2]. The preconception and pregnancy maternal gene/environment interactions are the mechanisms by which the foetus is prepared for extra-uterine life. If there is a mismatch between the maternal environment in her earlier life and that of her new-born, programming will be inappropriate for the infants' environment. This will lead to endocrine, metabolic and immune responses which are ill-equipped to handle environmental exposures with increased risks of cardio-vascular disease, metabolic syndrome and non-communicable inflammatory diseases. Arrows indicate the direction of effect.

The immunological mechanisms underlying allergic disease are the expression of T-lymphocyte-mediated responses to common environmental allergens that are biased towards T lymphocytes with helper-2 (Th-2) activity. Th-2 lymphocytes release peptide regulatory factors (cytokines) such as interleukins (IL) 4, IL-5, IL-9 and IL-13, which trigger the production of immunoglobulin-E (IgE), the allergy promoting antibody, and activate inflammatory cells such as eosinophils. Counter regulation is achieved by T-helper-1 (Th-1) lymphocytes generating cytokines such as interferon-gamma (IFN-gamma) which down-regulates Th-2 activity, while IL-4 suppresses Th-1 function. A group of T-lymphocyte regulators (T-regs) suppress both Th-1 and Th-2 activity by either cell–cell contact or the generation of IL-10 and transforming growth factor (TGF) beta [4]. Based on this paradigm it is likely that either over-expression of Th-2 activity or a failure of control by Th-1 or T-regulatory function will result in a higher probability of the development of allergy and allergic inflammation. Indeed, assaying these counter regulatory factors have been used as biomarkers of allergic disease activity and response to treatment such as to allergen immunotherapy [5]. As Th-1 activity is a feature of response to infection it is of note that the demographic trends in allergic and auto-immune disease prevalence have increased significantly, commensurate with decreases in severe infectious diseases. The basis of the so-called hygiene hypothesis arose from this mechanistic insight. However, it is the overall microbial exposure rather than active infection which affects outcomes and much focus, of late, has been directed to the influence of the human microbio-genome (metagenomics) [6,7].

The pattern of response of T-lymphocytes is dictated by the nature of the signaling from antigen presenting cells (APCs). They, in turn are affected by the nature of the antigen exposure and the presence or absence of co-stimulatory signals. Mucosal epithelial cells are the usual first contact points with antigens, which if recognised as conferring potential danger, by, for instance, having enzymic activity, cytokines known as alarmins (IL-25, 33 and Thymic Stromal Lymphopoietin-TSLP) are released by epithelial cells. The alarmins stimulate innate lymphocytic cells with a type-2 phenotype, which amongst a range of cytokines, release IL-4 and 5. This creates the environment to bias the adaptive response to increased Th-2 activity thereby promoting IgE production and eosinophil activation. This is the normal immune response to parasite infestation but is also characteristic of allergy [8]. APCs generate IL-12, -15, -18 and -23 which predominantly stimulate Th-1 responses while IL-10 from APCs and regulatory T-cells inhibit IL-12 and therefore favour Th-2 activity. Relatively minor perturbations of the balance between Th-1 and Th-2 activity, during primary sensitisation, is likely to have significant effects on outcomes, because the mutual counter regulation of each, orchestrated by IFN-gamma and IL-4 respectively enhances the long-lasting commitment to either Th-1 or Th-2 responses [9].

This review focusses on events during foetal life that influence susceptibility to allergic sensitisation and/or allergic disease. In evaluating the outputs from observational and interventional studies it is important to discriminate between immunological processes leading to allergic sensitisation from those that evolve into the diseases associated with allergy such as eczema, asthma, rhinitis and food allergy. As the modification of maternal and infant diets is easier to achieve than changing other aspects of the early-life environment, the final section focuses on nutrition.

2. Immunology of Pregnancy and Neonatal Immune Responses

The neonatal immune system should be able to recognise diverse antigens to identify and destroy pathogens while maintaining tolerance to self, to food, and other harmless environmental exposures. Pregnancy is immunologically equivalent to an organ transplant because the foetus expresses both paternal and maternal antigens to which maternal Th-1 tissue rejecting responses would be expected. Where this occurs, it causes intra-uterine growth retardation or early miscarriage in both murine models and human pregnancies. Counter-balancing this response is in part due to a Th-2 and T-regulatory cytokine profile produced by decidual tissues which down-regulate maternal Th-1 responses (Figure 2) [10]. While several studies support this concept, others are less clear. However, clinical evidence comes from the common observation that Th-1 autoimmune diseases improve during pregnancy [11]. Additional modulation of the maternal Th1 response is affected by the expression of a monomorphic tissue type (HLA-G) on extra-villous trophoblasts at the foeto–maternal interface [12]. Antigen-presenting cells in lymphoid accumulations in the foetal gut express markers of maturation and co-stimulatory molecules from 14–16 weeks' gestation. They are seen in close apposition with T cells within lymphoid accumulations in the small intestine, which exhibit the capping of receptors, suggesting that primary sensitization has occurred [13].

Newborn infants have allergen reactive T-cells which are characterised by greater production of Th-2 rather than Th-1 cytokines. Normally, the post-natal environment modulates responses with an increase in Th-1 and reduction in Th-2 activity. Infants destined to develop allergic disease have a different pattern with sustained Th-2 activity. There are differences in allergen induced cytokine production at birth in infants who have subsequently developed allergic disease. There is a generally reduced capacity in such infants to generate both IFN-gamma the archetypal Th-1 cytokine and IL-13 a characteristic

Th-2 cytokine [14,15]. IL-13 immune reactivity can be detected in the placenta between 16 to 27 weeks' gestation but not thereafter. From 27 weeks onwards until 34 weeks, IL-13 can be found spontaneously released from foetal mononuclear cells, but then it is only released on cell stimulation [16]. Thus, there must be a very subtle regulation of production of this and likely other cytokines with an interaction between the mother, the placenta and the foetus. Factors that influence the post-natal evolution of the allergic immune response include the route, dose and timing of allergen exposure in association with a disturbed human microbiome (dysbiosis), which forms the basis of the hygiene hypothesis [6]. Many environmental factors which have been linked with rising trends of allergic diseases have embraced the concept of an alteration in the balance of immune responses between those which are associated with an allergic pattern, those associated with protection against infection, and those which regulate all responses (Figure 3).

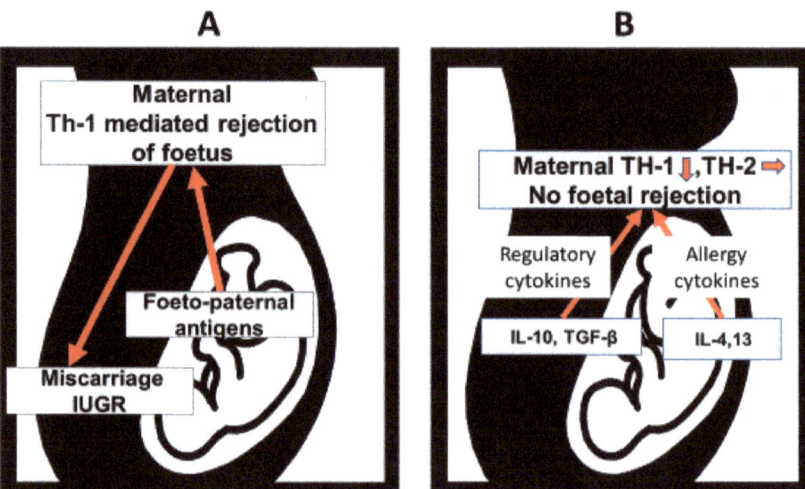

Figure 2. A schematic representation of components of the immunological interactions between mother and foetus. As the foetus and decidual tissues express paternal as well as maternal antigens, a maternal Th-1 tissue rejecting response might be expected, which would compromise the pregnancy with either intra-uterine growth retardation (IUGR) or early miscarriage (**A**). Part of the mechanism to protect the pregnancy is a regulatory and allergy promoting cytokine milieu at the foeto-maternal interface which protects the foetus from maternal Th-1 rejection of foeto-paternal antigens (**B**). The arrows indicate the direction of effect.

The neonate has a relatively immature innate immune response to pathogen challenge as a consequence of low circulating complement levels, impaired neutrophil function, natural killer cell function and macrophage activation [17,18]. Adaptive responses are also attenuated and predominantly tolerogenic, thereby reducing the generation of inappropriate responses to harmless antigens during the development of antigen-specific memory. Despite the neonatal immature cellular responses, the foetus can mount an antigen-specific T-cell response to intra-uterine viral infection as early as at 28 weeks' gestation [18]. Antigen-specific T-cell proliferation has been demonstrated to egg and house-dust mite allergens from 22 weeks' gestation [19]. Neonates' relatively inadequate response to infection is partly explained by Th-2 and T-reg cytokines impairing Th-1 responses [17,18].

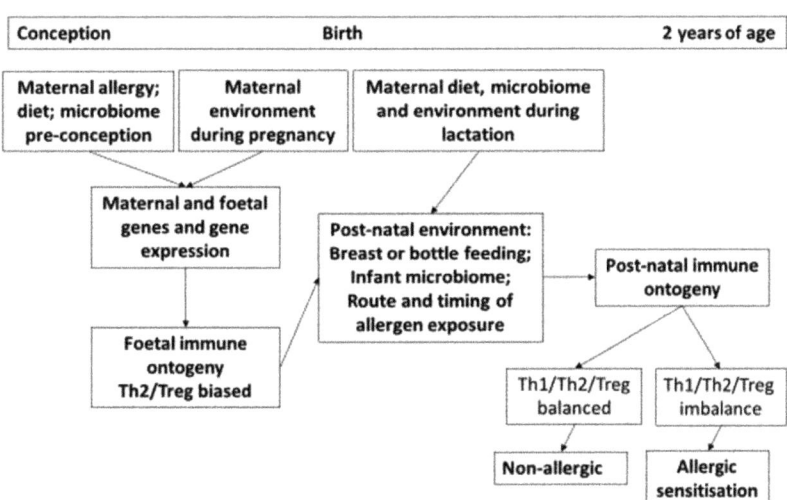

Figure 3. The first 1000 days representing the early life origins of allergic sensitisation. Ante-natal factors include maternal genome, epigenome, metagenome, diet and environment. In the post-natal period, the evolving infant microbiome, diet, route and timing of allergen exposure are critical to balancing the otherwise Th-2 allergy biased neonatal immune response. Failure to down-regulate the neonatal Th-2 biased response is associated with a higher risk of allergic sensitization. The arrows indicate the direction of effect.

3. Foetal Sensitization to Allergens

Amniotic fluid contains antigens/allergens to which the mother has been exposed together with desidual tissue derived Th-2 cytokines, which are swallowed by the foetus. This is a potential route toTh-2 biased sensitisation in the small intestine [20,21]. A relatively Th-2 biased immune response is well established in murine models but less clear from human studies [22,23]. However, the concept is supported by the positive association between maternal exposure to house dust mite and cat allergen exposure during pregnancy and neonatal cord blood IgE levels [24]. This study also showed a negative correlation between ante-natal endotoxin exposure and neonatal IgE. Endotoxin would be expected to enhance Th-1 responses and suppress Th-2 and therefore restrict IgE production [24]. Furthermore, successive studies have shown that human neonates destined to become allergic have different peripheral blood mononuclear cell (PBMC) responses to allergens [25]. Cord blood PBMCs from neonates born into farming families have high T-regulatory function and lower Th-2 activity in response to house dust mite stimulation. The effect was increased with progressive higher maternal exposure to farm animals and stables [26]. This likely explains the finding of reduced allergy and allergic diseases in the offspring of farming families [27]. However, an alternative factor reducing risks is maternal ingestion of unpasteurized milk which will affect the maternal and infant microbiome and is clearly more likely in faming families and those living in rural environments [28]. In murine models, high house-mite allergen exposure in pregnancy is associated with increased house mite induced bronchial reactivity in offspring [29]. However, house-mite avoidance measures commonly also reduce endotoxin exposures, thereby reducing T-reg and Th-1 activity as suggested by farming studies [26–28]. In murine models it is possible to control for all confounding factors which may increase the effect of allergen exposure, but in human observational and interventional studies there are many confounders likely to modify outcomes. It is therefore not surprising that pregnancy house-dust mite avoidance trials have produced no overall effect on allergy, childhood wheezing or asthma [30,31]. Similar, negative outcomes have occurred with trials of pregnancy avoidance of common food allergens. Indeed, avoidance may compromise nutrition [32]. As complete avoidance is rarely achievable and may have adverse effects, high exposure may be a more practical preventive strategy, but controlled trials are required before changing the present advice to continue as normal, but at least there is no justification to avoid any potential allergen for primary prevention. There is likely to be a bell-shaped curve of risk of sensitisation in relation to levels of allergen exposure in pregnancy. Very low levels are insufficient to induce sensitisation while very high levels induce tolerance through a range of mechanisms.

Amniotic fluid also contains IgE antibodies at 10% of maternal circulating levels by 16 weeks' gestation. IgE receptors are present on cells within the lamina propria of the foetal gut. Therefore, there is the potential for the high-affinity pick-up of antigens by APCs. This is a phenomenon known as antigen focusing. With IgE on low and high affinity IgE receptors, sensitization occurs to 100–1000-fold lower concentrations of allergens than would occur without IgE [33]. While the likely route of primary sensitisation to allergens in pregnancy is via the foetal gut during the second trimester, there is also exposure to allergen directly into the foetal circulation in the third trimester. This is a consequence of the active transport of the IgG antibodies across the placenta complexed with antigens and allergens. Higher IgG antibody levels to specific allergens, due to high maternal exposure, diminish the likelihood of subsequent sensitisation to those allergens. This had been demonstrated for egg, cat and dog allergens [34,35]. Rye-grass allergen immunotherapy continued during pregnancy, which increases IgG antibodies, and has been associated with less subsequent rye-grass allergy in the offspring [36]. Birch and timothy grass pollen exposure via the mother during the first six months of pregnancy increased risks of allergic sensitisation in the infant while later exposure resulted in tolerance in one study [37]. However, a more recent large study showed that higher pollen exposure in late pregnancy was associated with a higher risk of hospital admission for wheezing in infants over the first year of life, while high exposure in the first trimester reduced risks though only in smoking mothers [38]. There was potential for confounding in these studies in relation to maternal vitamin D levels, other potential confounders and post-natal pollutant exposures. [37,38]. There are clearly complex relationships between the timing of exposure to allergens in pregnancy, the concentration, the nature (complexed with IgG or free), co-existent nutritional and other environmental variations all of which have subtly different influences on allergy outcomes.

4. Foetal Gene/Environment Interactions

Single nucleotide gene polymorphisms (SNPs) have variously been associated with allergy and/or asthma, and/or eczema, and/or rhinitis, but account for only a small proportion of variability in the phenotype. It has been suggested that it will be more fruitful to focus on gene/environment interactions, epigenetics, and pharmaco-genetics [39]. Twin and family studies have shown that allergy is hereditable, and a many SNPs have been associated with allergy, though not necessarily allergic disease. Numerous mechanistically credible SNPs have been associated with increased risks of allergic sensitization and/or disease, but Variability of phenotyping has compromised the merging of data. Initially, studies utilizing the candidate gene approach focused on the cytokine gene cluster on the long arm of chromosome 5 (5q31–33). This contains the genes for many Th-2 cytokines and an endotoxin receptor, CD-14, which is credible in relation to clinical observations and immunological insights. More recent genome-wide association studies (GWAS) have highlighted many more associations which have begun to separate influences on allergic sensitisation from those which increase risks of specific allergic diseases because the evolution of allergic sensitisation to specific diseases such as eczema or asthma is not inevitable [40]. Indeed, allergic sensitisation sometimes exists in the absence of any disease, and both eczema and asthma occur in the absence of allergic sensitisation. GWAS have highlighted distinct SNPs only expressed on genes in epithelial but not immune cells which increase the risks of eczema (filaggrin SNPs) or asthma (A Dysintegrin And Metalloprotease33—ADAM-33) with or without allergy [41].

However, genetic influences on outcomes contribute relatively small effects because the impact of the polymorphisms will only be apparent at critical stages during development and/or the presence of environmental stressors. For example, ADAM-33 is expressed during airway branching morpho-genesis and SNPs may have their greatest impact very early in foetal life because airway formation is complete by the middle of the second trimester of pregnancy [42]. The metabolism of paracetamol (acetaminophen) results in the depletion of anti-oxidant activity, and maternal SNPs in the antioxidant glutathione-S methyl transferase P1 gene only manifests as wheezing in five-year-old offspring if the mother had high usage of paracetamol during pregnancy [43]. Some gene SNPs identified by GWAS affect both airway form and function and immune responsiveness. This is the case for Orosomucoid like 3 (ORMDL3) gene SNPs resulting in over-expression in airway smooth muscle and epithelial cells [44]. Filaggrin SNPs are associated with an increased risk of asthma and food allergy as well as eczema. It is likely that excessive epithelial permeability facilitates sensitisation to allergens through the skin, particularly in the presence of skin inflammation [45] (Figure 4).

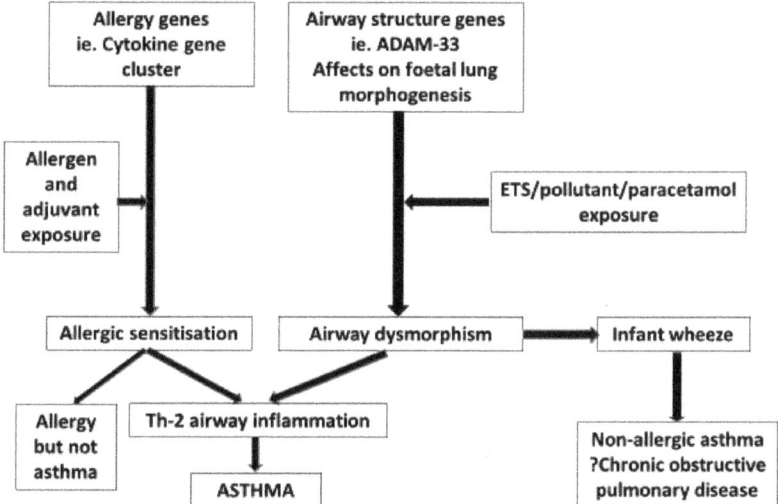

Figure 4. An algorithm of the distinct effects of gene/environment interactions increasing risks of airway dymorphisms and/or allergic sensitisation. When combined they lead to the development of allergic asthma. Isolated airway dysmorphisms increase the risks of infant wheeze and also chronic obstructive pulmonary disease. Arrows indicate the direction of effect.

The other way in which environment impacts on gene expression is through modification of molecules attached to DNA sequences or the histones around which chromosomes wind. This is the relatively new discipline of epigenetics which not only directly affects phenotype but is also hereditable. Cigarette smoking induces many epigenetic changes and grand-maternal smoking increases risks of asthma in grand-children independent of maternal smoking [46]. Levels of DNA (CpG motif) methylation if increased (hyper-methylation) silences gene expression. Hypo-methylation of the GATA-3 gene in cord blood has been associated with a higher risk of doctor diagnosed asthma at three years of age [47]. Folic acid is a potent methyl donor increasing hyper-methylation and there have been some weak associations between intake of this vitamin in late pregnancy and increased risks of respiratory illness in early childhood [48]. Folic acid supplementation in late pregnancy may increase susceptibility of the infant to respiratory illness, but supplementation pre-conception and in the first half of pregnancy is important to prevent neural tube defects.

5. Foetal Nutrition and Allergic Disease

The maternal diet will affect the mother's gut microbiome and therefore the infant's inoculum during delivery. However, the maternal microbiome and other confounders have hitherto not been comprehensively analyzed in relation to studies of the impact of pregnancy nutriention on allergy outcomes. This means that outcomes must be interpreted with caution.

Foetal growth and nutrition have an impact on the ontogeny of immune responses. There is an unexpected association between large head circumference at birth and levels of total IgE at birth in childhood and adulthood [49]. It has been hypothesised that a large head circumference at birth is representative of an early rapid foetal growth trajectory because of good nutrient supply in early pregnancy. The foetus is subsequently programmed to maintain a rapid growth trajectory necessitating a high nutrient demand. If this is not met in the later stages of pregnancy there is continuing head growth at the expense of relatively poorer nutrient delivery to the body with consequent adverse effects on immune and lung development. Rapid immediate post-natal weight gain is often a consequence of late intra-uterine growth faltering and is associated with poorer infant lung function [50]. The combination of compromised immune responses and lung function leads to a higher risk of infant wheezing and allergic asthma. High birthweight has been associated with increased risks of subsequently positive allergy skin tests but not necessarily asthma [51]. While allergy has been associated with high foetal abdominal girth growth velocity, infant wheeze was associated with low abdominal growth velocity [52]. These observations are consistent with the concept that allergy is a consequence of affluence and good nutrition while airway disease follows gene/environment aberrations including impaired nutrition, which compromises airway development.

The key question is whether there are any specific nutrients of importance in promoting appropriate immune responsiveness. Reduced intake of fresh fruit and vegetables has been associated with a higher rate of allergic sensitisation in many studies [53]. A high intake of fish in pregnancy has been associated with less subsequent allergy in the offspring [54]. Conversely, a high maternal free sugar intake in pregnancy has been associated with a higher risk of allergy and asthma [55]. A meta-analysis of studies investigating maternal pregnancy intake of vitamins and trace elements suggested a protective effect of vitamins D and E, and zinc against the development of wheezing illnesses in offspring, but inconclusive effects on the prevalence of asthma and other allergic conditions [56]. This emphasizes the distinction between obstructive airway diseases resulting in wheeze and allergic asthma. Conflicting outcomes have been noted for pregnancy intake of numerous other trace elements, many associated with anti-oxidant activity, but heterogeneity of outcome phenotyping precludes meaningful conclusions and association studies do not distinguish cause from consequence [57]. Trials of supplementation in pregnancy are required to establish causal relationships.

Maternal obesity has been associated with higher risks of wheezing illnesses and asthma but not other allergic disorders in children. There are credible mechanistic explanations because mediators, known as adipokines, that are released by adipocytes are pro-inflammatory. They will have effects at the materno-foetal interface leading to foetal immune and neuro-endocrine dysregulation. Obesity also likely has epigenetic effects with enhanced pro-inflammatory gene expression [58]. There are, however, confounding factors affecting outcomes which have not been accounted for in association studies. Overall dietary patterns may be different in obese mothers which could affect constituents implicated as influencing allergy outcomes as discussed above. Maternal obesity increases the risk of caesarean section delivery which in turn results in higher risks of infant asthma and food allergy, probably due to gut dysbiosis [59,60]. A study of elective caesarean section without medical indication showed an association with both infant asthma and allergic rhinitis. Breast feeding, which provides pre-biotic oligosaccharides, abrogated the effect suggesting that gut dysbiosis was indeed the cause [61]. Pregnancy antibiotics also modify the neonatal microbiome, and infants born to mothers who received antibiotics during pregnancy had increased prevalences of eczema and food allergy [62].

Several studies have focused on lipids as being important in immune ontogeny. Indeed, fatty acids have a crucial role as a source of energy, as the principle component of cell membranes, and as precursors for the synthesis of prostaglandins and leukotrienes. Minor variations in levels could have a profound effect on immune responses. Fish oils have a high level of omega-3 polyunsaturated fatty acids (n-3 PUFAs) and Western diets have a diminished intake of n-3 PUFAs with corresponding increases in n-6 PUFAs. This change has been associated with increasing rates of allergic disease and asthma [63]. Low cord blood n-3:n-6 ratios have been correlated with increased subsequent infant eczema and are related to higher maternal meat eating rather than fish eating [64]. Several randomised controlled studies have employed the administration of a fish oil dietary supplement to mothers through pregnancy and lactation with monitoring of outcomes in the offspring, particularly in high risk cohorts, with conflicting outcomes. Even recent systematic reviews have produced differing results. One found no effect on eczema, wheeze, food allergy or allergic rhinitis, but moderate level evidence of a reduction in egg and peanut allergy in high risk cohorts [65]. This review also showed that probiotic supplementation during the last month of pregnancy and lactation to six months may reduce eczema [65]. However, another systematic review suggested that high dose fish oil supplementation reduced asthma [66]. As a proof of concept that the pregnancy fish oil supplementation and microbiome manipulation has some effects, further studies would be worthwhile

Vitamin D receptors (VDR) have been identified on many immune active cells and vitamin D has important immunoregulatory functions. Most notable are effects on T-regs through TGF-beta expression and signaling. Polymorphisms in the VDR have been linked to an increased risk of asthma [67]. While some studies have associated low vitamin D levels with enhanced inflammation in patients with asthma, others have shown no or negative effects. A systematic review suggests that there is currently no evidence to support supplementation trials in pregnancy [68]. The complexity of VDR function in relation to varying levels of vitamin D exposure and their effects on inflammatory processes requires considerably more elaboration before any clinical implications can be addressed. It is possible that there is a U-shaped curve of vitamin D levels and susceptibility to inflammation with both very high and low levels, increasing risks. Indeed, one study has shown this in relation to IgE levels [69]. We have yet to establish optimal levels for immunological health, which may be different from those for bone health.

Most studies of maternal dietary factors affecting allergic disease outcomes in offspring have attempted to identify beneficial influences. There are a few recent studies suggesting adverse effects of some nutrients such as refined sugar and pro-inflammatory factors [55,57]. A high intake of red meat increases levels of circulating advanced-glycation end products (AGEs), which are similar to molecules expressed on bacteria. They are recognized by a pattern recognition receptor known as (RAGE) which is particularly expressed in the airway epithelium and activates innate pro-inflammatory responses which are appropriate to handle infection, but a "false alarm" if related to dietary AGEs. Current child high dietary AGE intake has been associated with a high prevalence of asthma [70,71]. However, effects of high AGE intake by pregnant mothers in the one published study to date did not affect child outcomes [72]. A ten-year transgenerational cohort study utilised an early pregnancy dietary inflammatory index (predominantly a high fat intake) and healthy eating index (similar to a Mediterranean diet) to assess the effects on asthma development in children over a nine-year follow-up. A low quality pro-inflammatory diet increased asthma risk, while the health diet was protective [71]. What is unclear is whether the impact on outcomes is exclusively due to either a healthy or unhealthy diet or a balance between each. However, the study of total diet rather than individual nutrients may be more likely to show worthwhile effects.

Associations between omega-3 PUFAs, vitamins D, E and zinc at best show only weak beneficial effects, while intervention trials have produced conflicting results with variable outcomes, phenotyping and confounding being critical issues. As is apparent from all pregnancy gene/environment interactions, the relationships are complex, being influenced by timing, dose, and combinations of exposures which are not normally analysed in observational or intervention studies. Some studies of the so-called Mediterranean diet (Med-Diet) with its high intake of fish, olive oil, fresh vegetables and fruits with low intake of chicken and red-meat (i.e., higher n-3:n-6 ratios) have suggested reductions in some but not all allergic phenotypes. A systematic review indicated that maternal adherence to the Med-Diet reduced offspring wheeze/asthma in the first year of life but not thereafter, and had minor effects on allergy but none on eczema [73]. A more recent birth cohort observational study suggested that the Med-Diet in pregnancy improved offspring small-airway function but not the prevalence of any allergic disease [74]. This would explain the reduction in infant wheeze suggested by the previous review [66]. As the Med-Diet in pregnancy has been shown to be safe and beneficial to both mothers' and infants' health, further research into mechanisms and controlled trials are indicated [75]. Principle component analysis of dietary diversity from the UK contingent of the "Prevalence of Infant Food Allergy (PIFA)" study revealed that infants having a more diverse intake of fresh fruit, vegetables and home prepared food had a significantly lower prevalence of food allergy by two years of age, as confirmed by controlled challenge [76]. While the focus of this study was on the diet of infants, it is very likely that the pattern of eating would have been similar for mothers during pregnancy. Therefore, the critical timing for the introduction of a diverse healthy diet remains to be established (Table 1).

Table 1. Tabulation of the most promising interventions to prevent allergic disease based on published observational and interventional studies focusing on the first 1000 days. Published evidence referenced in brackets. However, before recommending any interventions it will not only be necessary to demonstrate worthwhile benefit but also to be mindful of potential adverse effects. For instance, paracetamol is the only mild to moderate analgesic recommended for use in pregnancy, while antibiotics for bacterial infection in pregnancy and caesarean section are sometimes essential for medical reasons. Based on all the published evidence, a "healthy diet" would appear to be the best and most practicable option, pre-conception, during pregnancy and lactation.

Timing	Target	Intervention
Pre-conception	Maternal obesity [58]	Weight loss No maternal or grand-mother smoking [46]
Pre-conception	Maternal nutrition	Healthy balanced diet [76]
Pregnancy	Maternal nutrition	More fish less meat Fresh fruit and vegetables [75] Optimal vitamins D, E and zinc [67–70] No allergen avoidance [29–32]
Pregnancy	Medications to avoid if possible	Antibiotics [62] Paracetamol [43]
Pregnancy	Maternal microbiome [6]	Pre-/pro-/syn-biotics [6]
Delivery	Avoid if possible	Caesarean section [59–61] Bottle feeding [15]
Neonatal period	Infant microbiome [6]	Breast feeding [15] Pre-/pro-/syn-biotics [6]

6. Conclusions

Complex interactions at the materno-placental-foetal interface have a profound influence on the infants' immune maturation and the likelihood of developing allergic sensitisation and disease. Gene/environment interactions and timing of exposures through pregnancy add further degrees of complexity. Understanding the early life origins of allergy will only be possible by embracing this complexity. Studies will now need to investigate combinations of dietary, pollutant, medication and microbial exposures during pregnancy in relation to genomics, epigenomics, metagenomics and metabolomics in relation to infant/child outcomes. Controlled trials of a "healthy diet" during pregnancy are likely to yield better outcomes than focusing on single nutrients which hitherto have produced disappointing results. The manipulation of the neonates' evolving microbiome is suggested as another focus for controlled prevention trials.

Funding: This research received no external funding.

Institutional Review Board Statement: Not applicable.

Informed Consent Statement: Not applicable.

Data Availability Statement: Not applicable.

Conflicts of Interest: J.O.W. has received bursaries for serving on scientific advisory boards and delivering lectures at sponsored meetings for Danone/Nutricia, Friesland Campina and Airsonett.

References

1. Susuki, K. The developing world of DOHaD. *J. Dev. Orig. Health Dis.* **2018**, *9*, 266–269. [CrossRef] [PubMed]
2. Crespi, B.J. Why and How Imprinted Genes Drive Fetal Programming. *Front. Endocrinol.* **2020**, *10*, 940. [CrossRef] [PubMed]
3. Tham, E.H.; Loo, E.X.L.; Zhu, Y.; Shek, L.P.C. Effects of migration on allergic diseases. *Int. Arch. Allergy Immunol.* **2019**, *178*, 128–140. [CrossRef] [PubMed]
4. Tsitoura, D.C.; Tassios, Y. Immunomodulation: The future cure for allergic diseases. *Ann. N. Y. Acad. Sci.* **2006**, *1088*, 100–115. [CrossRef]
5. Breiteneder, H.; Peng, Y.Q.; Agache, I.; Diamant, Z.; Eiwegger, T.; Fokkens, W.J.; Traidl-Hoffmann, C.; Nadeau, K.; O'Hehir, R.E.; O'Mahony, L.; et al. Biomarkers for diagnosis and prediction of therapy responses in allergic diseases and asthma. *Allergy* **2020**, *75*, 3039–3068. [CrossRef]
6. Peroni, D.G.; Nuzzi, G.; Trambusti, I.; Di Cicco, M.E.; Comberiati, P. Microbiome Composition and Its Impact on the Development of Allergic Diseases. *Front. Immunol.* **2020**, *11*, 700. [CrossRef]
7. Garn, H.; Potaczek, D.P.; Pfefferle, P.I. The Hygiene Hypothesis and New Perspectives—Current Challenges Meeting an Old Postulate. *Front. Immunol.* **2021**, *12*, 847. [CrossRef]
8. Gurram, R.K.; Zhu, J. Orchestration between ILC2s and Th2 cells in shaping type 2 immune responses. *Cell. Mol. Immunol.* **2019**, *16*, 225–235. [CrossRef]
9. Wambre, E.; Bajzik, V.; DeLong, J.H.; O'Brien, K.; Nguyen, Q.A.; Speake, C.; Gersuk, V.H.; DeBerg, H.A.; Whalen, E.; Ni, C.; et al. A phenotypically and functionally distinct human TH2 cell subpopulation is associated with allergic disorders. *Sci. Transl. Med.* **2017**, *9*, eaam9171. [CrossRef]
10. Prescott, S.L.; Macaubas, C.; Holt, B.J.; Smallacombe, T.B.; Loh, R.; Sly, P.D.; Holt, P.G. Transplacental Priming of the Human Immune System to Environmental Allergens: Universal Skewing of Initial T Cell Responses Toward the Th2 Cytokine Profile. *J. Immunol.* **1998**, *160*, 4730–4737.
11. Abu-Raya, B.; Michalski, C.; Sadarangani, M.; Lavoie, P.M. Maternal Immunological Adaptation During Normal Pregnancy. *Front. Immunol.* **2020**, *11*, 575197. [CrossRef] [PubMed]
12. Xu, X.; Zhou, Y.; Wei, H. Roles of HLA-G in the Maternal-Fetal Immune Microenvironment. *Front. Immunol.* **2020**, *11*, 592010. [CrossRef] [PubMed]
13. Jones, C.A.; Vance, G.H.; Power, L.L.; Pender, S.L.; MacDonald, T.T.; Warner, J.O. Costimulatory molecules in the developing human gastrointestinal tract: A pathway for fetal allergen priming. *J. Allergy Clin. Immunol.* **2001**, *108*, 235–241. [CrossRef] [PubMed]
14. Belderbos, M.; Levy, O.; Bont, L. Neonatal innate immunity in allergy development. *Curr. Opin. Pediatr.* **2009**, *21*, 762–769. [CrossRef] [PubMed]
15. Zepeda-Ortega, B.; Goh, A.; Xepapadaki, P.; Sprikkelman, A.; Nicolaou, N.; Hernandez, R.E.H.; Latiff, A.H.A.; Yat, M.T.; Diab, M.; Hussaini, B.A.; et al. Strategies and Future Opportunities for the Prevention, Diagnosis, and Management of Cow Milk Allergy. *Front. Immunol.* **2021**, *12*, 1877. [CrossRef]
16. Williams, T.J.; Jones, C.A.; Miles, E.A.; Warner, J.O.; Warner, J.A. Fetal and neonatal IL-13 production during pregnancy and at birth and subsequent development of atopic symptoms. *J. Allergy Clin. Immunol.* **2000**, *105*, 951–959. [CrossRef]
17. Tsafaras, G.P.; Ntontsi, P.; Xanthou, G. Advantages and limitations of the neonatal immune system. *Front. Pediatr.* **2020**, *8*, 5. [CrossRef]
18. Basha, S.; Surendran, N.; Pichichero, M. Immune responses in neonates. *Expert Rev. Clin. Immunol.* **2014**, *10*, 1171–1184. [CrossRef]
19. Jones, A.C.; Miles, E.A.; Warner, J.O.; Colwell, B.M.; Bryant, T.N.; Warner, J.A. Fetal peripheral blood mononuclear cell proliferative responses to mitogenic and allergenic stimuli during gestation. *Pediatr. Allergy Immunol.* **1996**, *7*, 109–116. [CrossRef]
20. Holloway, J.A.; Warner, J.O.; Vance, G.H.; Diaper, N.D.; Warner, J.A.; Jones, C.A. Detection of house-dust-mite allergen in amniotic fluid and umbilical-cord blood. *Lancet* **2000**, *356*, 1900–1902. [CrossRef]
21. Power, L.L.; Popplewell, E.J.; Holloway, J.A.; Diaper, N.D.; Warner, J.O.; Jones, C.A. Immunoregulatory molecules during pregnancy and at birth. *J. Reprod. Immunol.* **2002**, *56*, 19–28. [CrossRef]

22. Zaghouani, H.; Hoeman, C.M.; Adkins, B. Neonatal immunity: Faulty T-helpers and the shortcomings of dendritic cells. *Trends Immunol.* **2009**, *30*, 585–591. [CrossRef] [PubMed]
23. Semmes, E.C.; Chen, J.-L.; Goswami, R.; Burt, T.D.; Permar, S.R.; Fouda, G.G. Understanding Early-Life Adaptive Immunity to Guide Interventions for Pediatric Health. *Front. Immunol.* **2021**, *11*, 3544. [CrossRef] [PubMed]
24. Heinrich, J.; Bolte, G.; Holscher, B.; Douwes, J.; Lehmann, I.; Fahlbusch, B.; Bischof, W.; Weiss, M.; Borte, M.; Wichmann, H.-E. Allergens and endotoxin on mothers' mattresses and total immunoglobulin E in cord blood of neonates. *Eur. Respir. J.* **2002**, *20*, 617–623. [CrossRef] [PubMed]
25. Warner, J.O. The foetal origins of allergy. *Curr. Allergy Clin. Immunol.* **2017**, *30*, 60–68.
26. Schaub, B.; Liu, J.; Höppler, S.; Schleich, I.; Huehn, J.; Olek, S.; Wieczorek, G.; Illi, S.; von Mutius, E. Maternal farm exposure modulates neonatal immune mechanisms through regulatory T cells. *J. Allergy Clin. Immunol.* **2009**, *123*, 774–782. [CrossRef]
27. Campbell, B.E.; Lodge, C.J.; Lowe, A.J.; Burgess, J.A.; Matheson, M.C.; Dharmage, S.C. Exposure to 'farming'and objective markers of atopy: A systematic review and meta-analysis. *Clin. Exp. Allergy* **2015**, *45*, 744–757. [CrossRef]
28. Perkin, M.R.; Strachan, D.P. Which aspects of the farming lifestyle explain the inverse association with childhood allergy? *J. Allergy Clin. Immunol.* **2006**, *117*, 1374–1781. [CrossRef]
29. Richgels, P.K.; Yamani, A.; Chougnet, C.A.; Lewkowich, I.P. Maternal house dust mite exposure during pregnancy enhances severity of house dust mite–induced asthma in murine offspring. *J. Allergy Clin. Immunol.* **2017**, *140*, 1404–1415. [CrossRef]
30. Torrent, M.; Sunyer, J.; Garcia, R.; Harris, J.; Iturriaga, M.V.; Puig, C.; Vall, O.; Antó, J.M.; Taylor, A.J.N.; Cullinan, P. Early-Life Allergen Exposure and Atopy, Asthma, and Wheeze up to 6 Years of Age. *Am. J. Respir. Crit. Care Med.* **2007**, *176*, 446–453. [CrossRef]
31. Liccardi, G.; Cazzola, M.; Canonica, G.W.; Passalacqua, G.; D'Amato, G. New insights in allergen avoidance measures for mite and pet sensitized patients. A critical appraisal. *Respir. Med.* **2005**, *99*, 1363–1376. [CrossRef] [PubMed]
32. Kramer, M.S.; Kakuma, R. Maternal dietary antigen avoidance during pregnancy or lactation, or both, for preventing or treating atopic disease in the child. *Evid. Based Child Health A Cochrane Rev. J.* **2014**, *9*, 447–483. [CrossRef] [PubMed]
33. Thornton, C.A.; Holloway, J.A.; Popplewell, E.J.; Shute, J.K.; Boughton, J.; Warner, J.O. Fetal exposure to intact immunoglobulin E occurs via the gastrointestinal tract. *Clin. Exp. Allergy* **2003**, *33*, 306–311. [CrossRef] [PubMed]
34. Vance, G.H.S.; Grimshaw, K.E.C.; Briggs, R.; Lewis, S.A.; Mullee, M.A.; Thornton, C.A.; Warner, J.O. Serum ovalbumin-specific IgG responses during pregnancy reflects maternal intake of dietary egg and relate to the development of allergy in infancy. *Clin. Exp. Allergy* **2004**, *34*, 1855–1861. [CrossRef]
35. Jenmalm, M.C.; Björkstén, B. Cord blood levels of immunoglobulin G subclass antibodies to food and inhalant allergens in relation to maternal atopy and the development of atopic disease during the first 8 years of life. *Clin. Exp. Allergy* **2000**, *30*, 34–40. [CrossRef]
36. Glovsky, M.M.; Ghekiere, L.; Rejzek, E. Effect of maternal immunotherapy on immediate skin test reactivity, specific rye I IgG and IgE antibody, and total IgE of the children. *Ann. Allergy* **1991**, *67*, 21–24.
37. Van Duren-Schmidt, K.; Pichler, J.; Ebner, C.; Bartmann, P.; Förster, E.; Urbanek, R.; Szépfalusi, Z. Prenatal Contact with Inhalant Allergens. *Pediatr. Res.* **1997**, *41*, 128–131. [CrossRef]
38. Lowe, A.J.; Olsson, D.; Bråbäck, L.; Forsberg, B. Pollen exposure in pregnancy and infancy and risk of asthma hospitalisation-a register based cohort study. *Allergy Asthma Clin. Immunol.* **2012**, *8*, 17. [CrossRef]
39. Collins, S.A.; Lockett, G.A.; Holloway, J.W. The genetics of allergic diseases and asthma. In *Pediatric Allergy Principles and Practice*, 3rd ed.; Leung, Y.M., Sampson, H.A., Geha, R.S., Szefler, S.J., Eds.; Elsevier: Amsterdam, The Netherlands, 2016; pp. 18–30.
40. Ortiz, R.A.; Barnes, K.C. Genetics of Allergic Diseases. *Immunol. Allergy Clin. N. Am.* **2015**, *35*, 19–44. [CrossRef]
41. Moffatt, M.F.; Gut, I.G.; Demenais, F.; Strachan, D.P.; Bouzigon, E.; Heath, S.; von Mutius, E.; Farrall, M.; Lathrop, M.; Cookson, W.O. A large-scale, consortium-based genomewide association study of asthma. *N. Engl. J. Med.* **2010**, *363*, 1211–1221. [CrossRef]
42. Davies, E.R.; Kelly, J.F.; Howarth, P.H.; Wilson, D.I.; Holgate, S.T.; Davies, D.E.; Whitsett, J.A.; Haitchi, H.M. Soluble ADAM33 initiates airway remodeling to promote susceptibility for allergic asthma in early life. *JCI Insight.* **2016**, *1*, e87632. [CrossRef] [PubMed]
43. Perzanowski, M.S.; Miller, R.L.; Tang, D.; Ali, D.; Garfinkel, R.S.; Chew, G.L.; Goldstein, I.F.; Perera, F.P.; Barr, R.G. Prenatal acetaminophen exposure and risk of wheeze at age 5 years in an urban low-income cohort. *Thorax* **2010**, *65*, 118–123. [CrossRef] [PubMed]
44. Luthers, C.R.; Dunn, T.M.; Snow, A.L. ORMDL3 and Asthma: Linking Sphingolipid Regulation to Altered T Cell Function. *Front. Immunol.* **2020**, *11*, 3120. [CrossRef] [PubMed]
45. McLean, W. Filaggrin failure-from ichthyosis vulgaris to atopic eczema and beyond. *Br. J. Dermatol.* **2016**, *175*, 4–7. [CrossRef] [PubMed]
46. Lodge, C.J.; Brabak, L.; Lowe, A.J.; Dharmage, S.C.; Olsson, D.; Forsberg, B. Grandmaternal smoking increases asthma risk in grandchildren: A nationwide Swedish cohort. *Clin. Exp. Allergy* **2018**, *48*, 167–174. [CrossRef]
47. Barton, S.J.; Ngo, S.; Costello, P.; Garratt, E.; El-Heis, S.; Antoun, E.; Clarke-Harris, R.; Murray, R.; Bhatt, T.; Burdge, G.; et al. DNA methylation of Th2 lineage determination genes at birth is associated with allergic outcomes in childhood. *Clin. Exp. Allergy* **2017**, *47*, 1599–1608. [CrossRef]

48. Veeranki, S.P.; Gebretsadik, T.; Mitchel, E.F.; Tylavsky, F.A.; Hartert, T.V.; Cooper, W.O.; Dupont, W.D.; Dorris, S.L.; Hartman, T.J.; Carroll, K.N. Maternal folic acid supplementation during pregnancy and early childhood asthma. *Epidemiology* **2015**, *26*, 934. [CrossRef]
49. Godfrey, K.; Barker, D.J.P.; Osmond, C. Disproportionate fetal growth and raised IgE concentration in adult life. *Clin. Exp. Allergy* **1994**, *24*, 641–648. [CrossRef]
50. Lucas, J.S.; Inskip, H.M.; Godfrey, K.M.; Foreman, C.T.; Warner, J.O.; Gregson, R.K.; Clough, J.B. Small size at birth and greater postnatal weight gain: Relationships to diminished infant lung function. *Am. J. Respir. Crit. Care Med.* **2004**, *170*, 534–540. [CrossRef]
51. Tedner, S.G.; Örtqvist, A.K.; Almqvist, C. Fetal growth and risk of childhood asthma and allergic disease. *Clin. Exp. Allergy* **2012**, *42*, 1430–1447. [CrossRef]
52. Pike, K.C.; Crozier, S.R.; Lucas, J.S.; Inskip, H.M.; Robinson, S.; Roberts, G.; Godfrey, K.M. Southampton Women's Survey Study Group. Patterns of fetal and infant growth are related to atopy and wheezing disorders at age 3 years. *Thorax* **2010**, *65*, 1099–1106. [CrossRef] [PubMed]
53. Erkkola, M.; Nwaru, B.I.; Kaila, M.; Kronberg-Kippilä, C.; Ilonen, J.; Simell, O.; Veijola, R.; Knip, M.; Virtanen, S. Risk of asthma and allergic outcomes in the offspring in relation to maternal food consumption during pregnancy: A Finnish birth cohort study. *Pediatr. Allergy Immunol.* **2012**, *23*, 186–194. [CrossRef] [PubMed]
54. Calvani, M.; Alessandri, C.; Sopo, S.M.; Panetta, V.; Pingitore, G.; Tripodi, S.; Zappala, D.; Zicari, A.M.; the Lazio Association of Pediatric Allergology (APAL) Study Group. Consumption of fish, butter and margarine during pregnancy and development of allergic sensitizations in the offspring: Role of maternal atopy. *Pediatr. Allergy Immunol.* **2006**, *17*, 94–102. [CrossRef] [PubMed]
55. Bédard, A.; Northstone, K.; Henderson, A.J.; Shaheen, S.O. Maternal intake of sugar during pregnancy and childhood respiratory and atopic outcomes. *Eur. Respir. J.* **2017**, *50*, 1700073. [CrossRef] [PubMed]
56. Beckhaus, A.A.; Garcia-Marcos, L.; Forno, E.; Pacheco-Gonzalez, R.M.; Celedon, J.C.; Castro-Rodriguez, J.A. Maternal nutrition during pregnancy and risk of asthma, wheeze, and atopic diseases during childhood: A systematic review and meta-analysis. *Allergy* **2015**, *70*, 1588–1604. [CrossRef]
57. Bédard, A.; Li, Z.; Ait-hadad, W.; Camargo, C.A., Jr.; Leynaert, B.; Pison, C.; Dumas, O.; Varraso, R. The Role of Nutritional Factors in Asthma: Challenges and Opportunities for Epidemiological Research. *Int. J. Environ. Res. Public Health.* **2021**, *18*, 3013. [CrossRef]
58. Rizzo, G.S.; Sen, S. Maternal obesity and immune dysregulation in mother and infant: A review of the evidence. *Paediatr. Respir. Rev.* **2015**, *16*, 251–257. [CrossRef]
59. Darabi, B.; Rahmati, S.; Hafeziahmadi, M.R.; Badfar, G.; Azami, M. The association between caesarean section and childhood asthma: An updated systematic review and meta-analysis. *Allergy Asthma Clin. Immunol.* **2019**, *15*, 1–13. [CrossRef]
60. Mitselou, N.; Hallberg, J.; Stephansson, O.; Almqvist, C.; Melén, E.; Ludvigsson, J.F. Cesarean delivery, preterm birth, and risk of food allergy: Nationwide Swedish cohort study of more than 1 million children. *J. Allergy Clin. Immunol.* **2018**, *142*, 1510–1514. [CrossRef]
61. Chu, S.; Zhang, Y.; Jiang, Y.; Sun, W.; Zhu, Q.; Wang, B.; Jiang, F.; Zhang, J. Cesarean section without medical indication and risks of childhood allergic disorder, attenuated by breastfeeding. *Sci. Rep.* **2017**, *7*, 9762. [CrossRef]
62. Metzler, S.; Frei, R.; Schmaußer-Hechfellner, E.; von Mutius, E.; Pekkanen, J.; Karvonen, A.M.; Kirjavainen, P.V.; Dalphin, J.C.; Divaret-Chauveau, A.; Riedler, J.; et al. Association between antibiotic treatment during pregnancy and infancy and the development of allergic diseases. *Pediatr. Allergy Immunol.* **2019**, *30*, 423–433. [CrossRef] [PubMed]
63. Miles, E.A.; Calder, P.C. Can Early Omega-3 Fatty Acid Exposure Reduce Risk of Childhood Allergic Disease? *Nutrients* **2017**, *9*, 784. [CrossRef]
64. Barman, M.; Stråvik, M.; Broberg, K.; Sandin, A.; Wold, A.E.; Sandberg, A.-S. Proportions of Polyunsaturated Fatty Acids in Umbilical Cord Blood at Birth Are Related to Atopic Eczema Development in the First Year of Life. *Nutrients* **2021**, *13*, 3779. [CrossRef]
65. Larsen, V.G.; Ierodiakonou, D.; Jarrold, K.; Cunha, S.; Chivinge, J.; Robinson, Z.; Geoghegan, N.; Ruparelia, A.; Devani, P.; Trivella, M.; et al. Diet during pregnancy and infancy and risk of allergic or autoimmune disease: A systematic review and meta-analysis. *PLoS Med.* **2018**, *15*, e1002507. [CrossRef]
66. Wu, S.; Li, C. Influence of Maternal Fish Oil Supplementation on the Risk of Asthma or Wheeze in Children: A Meta-Analysis of Randomized Controlled Trials. *Front. Pediatr.* **2022**, *10*, 817110. [CrossRef]
67. Wöbke, T.K.; Sorg, B.L.; Steinhilber, D. Vitamin D in inflammatory diseases. *Front. Physiol.* **2014**, *5*, 244. [CrossRef]
68. Tareke, A.A.; Hadgu, A.A.; Ayana, A.M.; Zerfu, T.A. Prenatal vitamin D supplementation and child respiratory health: A systematic review and meta-analysis of randomized controlled trials. *World Allergy Organ. J.* **2020**, *13*, 100486. [CrossRef]
69. Hypponen, E.; Berry, D.J.; Wjst, M.; Power, C. Serum 25-hydroxyvitamin D and IgE-a significant but nonlinear relationship. *Allergy* **2009**, *64*, 613–620. [CrossRef]
70. Chen, L.W.; Lyons, B.; Navarro, P.; Shivappa, N.; Mehegan, J.; Murrin, C.M.; Hébert, J.R.; Kelleher, C.C.; Phillips, C.M. Maternal dietary inflammatory potential and quality are associated with offspring asthma risk over 10-year follow-up: The Lifeways Cross-Generation Cohort Study. *Am. J. Clin. Nutr.* **2020**, *111*, 440–447. [CrossRef]

71. Wang, J.G.; Liu, B.; Kroll, F.; Hanson, C.; Vicencio, A.; Coca, S.; Uribarri, J.; Bose, S. Increased advanced glycation end product and meat consumption is associated with childhood wheeze: Analysis of the National Health and Nutrition Examination Survey. *Thorax* **2021**, *76*, 292–294. [CrossRef]
72. Venter, C.; Pickett, K.; Starling, A.; Maslin, K.; Smith, P.K.; Palumbo, M.P.; O'Mahony, L.; Ben Abdallah, M.; Dabelea, D. Advanced glycation end product intake during pregnancy and offspring allergy outcomes: A Prospective cohort study. *Clin. Exp. Allergy* **2021**, *51*, 1459–1470. [CrossRef] [PubMed]
73. Castro-Rodriguez, J.A.; Garcia-Marcos, L. What Are the Effects of a Mediterranean Diet on Allergies and Asthma in Children? *Front. Pediatr.* **2017**, *5*, 72. [CrossRef] [PubMed]
74. Bédard, A.; Northstone, K.; Henderson, A.J.; Shaheen, S.O. Mediterranean diet during pregnancy and childhood respiratory and atopic outcomes: Birth cohort study. *Eur. Respir. J.* **2020**, *55*, 1901215. [CrossRef] [PubMed]
75. Amati, F.; Hassounah, S.; Swaka, A. The Impact of Mediterranean Dietary Patterns During Pregnancy on Maternal and Offspring Health. *Nutrients* **2019**, *11*, 1098. [CrossRef] [PubMed]
76. Grimshaw, K.E.; Maskell, J.; Oliver, E.M.; Morris, R.C.; Foote, K.D.; Mills, E.C.; Margetts, B.M.; Roberts, G. Diet and food allergy development during infancy: Birth cohort study findings using prospective food diary data. *J. Allergy Clin. Immunol.* **2014**, *133*, 511–519. [CrossRef] [PubMed]

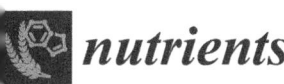

Review

Early Introduction of Allergenic Foods and the Prevention of Food Allergy

Brit Trogen [1,*], Samantha Jacobs [1] and Anna Nowak-Wegrzyn [2,3]

1. Department of Pediatrics, NYU Grossman School of Medicine, Hassenfeld Children's Hospital, New York, NY 10016, USA; samantha.jacobs@nyulangone.org
2. Allergy and Immunology, Department of Pediatrics, NYU Grossman School of Medicine, Hassenfeld Children's Hospital, New York, NY 10016, USA; anna.nowak-wegrzyn@nyulangone.org
3. Department of Pediatrics, Gastroenterology and Nutrition, Collegium Medicum, University of Warmia and Mazury, 10-719 Olsztyn, Poland
* Correspondence: brit.trogen@nyulangone.org

Abstract: The increasing prevalence of food allergies is a growing public health problem. For children considered high risk of developing food allergy (particularly due to the presence of other food allergies or severe eczema), the evidence for the early introduction of allergenic foods, and in particular peanut and egg, is robust. In such cases, the consensus is clear that not only should such foods not be delayed, but that they should be introduced at approximately 4 to 6 months of age in order to minimize the risk of food allergy development. The early introduction of allergenic foods appears to be an effective strategy for minimizing the public health burden of food allergy, though further studies on the generalizability of this approach in low-risk populations is needed.

Keywords: allergy; food allergy; atopic dermatitis; eczema; atopy; prevention; sensitization; oral tolerance; early food introduction

1. Introduction

Although clear epidemiologic data are lacking, food allergies are believed to affect up to 10% of individuals in Westernized countries [1]. The prevalence of food allergy overall, and of peanut allergy in particular, appears to be steadily increasing, including in developing countries [1,2]. Food allergies can result in significant morbidity and psychosocial burden (including the risk of nutritional deficiencies and life-threatening anaphylaxis), as well as high costs for the healthcare system and for families of food-allergic children [3,4]. As a result, food allergies can have a significant negative impact on quality of life [5]. Given the significant morbidity associated with these conditions and their inability to be cured, preventing the development of food allergies before they begin is essential.

Substantial research has aimed to identify primary prevention strategies for food allergy. Many interventions that have been attempted in pregnant or breastfeeding women and infants appear to have little to no benefit in preventing food allergy, including dietary avoidance of food allergens, vitamin supplements, fish oil, probiotics, prebiotics, and synbiotics—however, it should be noted that the evidence remains uncertain in many cases [6]. Optimal skin care and aggressive early treatment of atopic dermatitis using emollients, while thought to enhance skin barrier function, has also failed to show significant impact in the later development of food allergy, though some have argued that studies have not targeted high-risk infants or the use of optimal emollient methods [6–9]. In this setting, early introduction of allergenic foods in infancy has emerged as one of the more promising strategies to decrease food allergy development.

2. Evolution of the Guidelines for Food Allergy Prevention

Until 2008, clinical practice guidelines from the American Academy of Pediatrics (AAP) and other professional societies recommended delaying the introduction of allergenic foods,

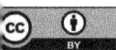

such as peanut, until 3 years of age. This recommendation was based on the theory that the lack of exposure to allergenic foods during early infancy—which was posited to be a developmental window of high susceptibility—would prevent later development of allergy. Though well-intentioned, it is now clear that these guidelines may have contributed to, rather than prevented, the development of food allergies in children. The dual exposure hypothesis offers one possible explanation as to why this approach failed, proposing that allergen exposure through skin may lead to IgE sensitization unless oral tolerance is first induced through the gastrointestinal tract [10]. Children with eczema are known to be at higher risk of developing peanut and egg allergy, possibly due to the increased likelihood of sensitization, due to skin barrier disruption, see Figure 1 [1]. Both clinical observation and animal studies also support the "outside-in" model of epicutaneous food allergen sensitization, suggesting that later introduction of allergens in the diet may occur too late, after allergens have already been introduced via the skin or respiratory tract [9]. In response to these findings, many food allergy prevention guidelines now recommend the early introduction of allergenic foods, such as peanut and egg, as part of complementary feeding in infancy, see Table 1 [2].

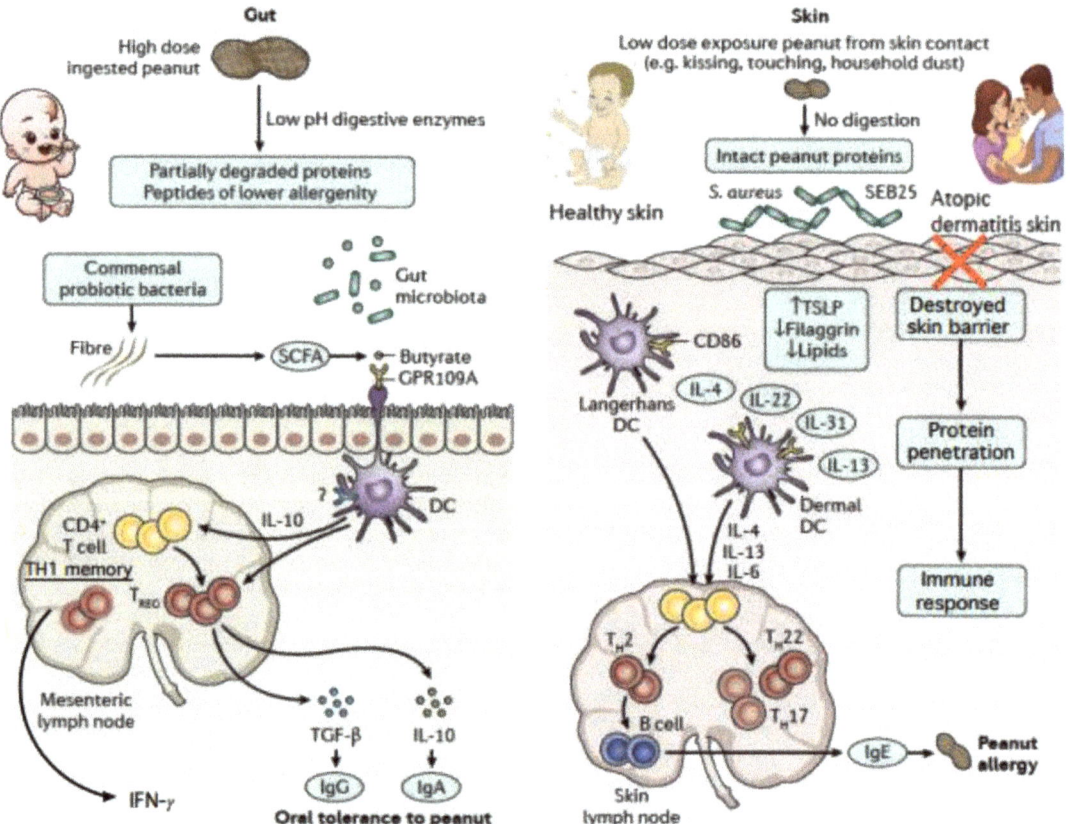

Figure 1. Exposure to foods via ingestion results in oral tolerance in contrast to cutaneous or inhalational exposures that promote IgE-sensitization [11].

Table 1. A summary of international consensus guidelines on early introduction of allergenic foods.

Professional Body	Publication Year	Recommendations
American Academy of Pediatrics (AAP) [12]	2019	• High-risk infants (presence of severe eczema and/or egg allergy) should be introduced to peanut as early as 4–6 months of age, following successful feeding of other solid food(s) to ensure the infant is developmentally ready. Allergy testing is strongly advised prior to peanut introduction for this group. • Infants with mild-to-moderate eczema should be introduced to peanut around 6 months of age, in accordance with family preferences and cultural practices, to reduce the risk of peanut allergy • Infants without eczema or food allergy who are not at increased risk: peanut should be introduced freely into the diet together with other solid foods and in accordance with family preferences and cultural practices.
Asia Pacific Association of Pediatric Allergy, Respirology & Immunology (APAPARI) [13]	2017	• Healthy infants: Introduce complementary foods at 6 months of age. • At-risk infants (family history of atopy): No delay in introduction of allergenic foods. To be introduced in a sensible manner once weaning has commenced. • High-risk infants with severe eczema: Allergy testing to egg (and peanut in countries with high peanut allergy prevalence). Supervised oral challenges in sensitized infants, followed by introduction of the allergenic food into the infant's regular diet if challenge negative. Introduction of all allergenic foods should not be delayed. Aggressive control of eczema.
Australian Society of Clinical Immunology and Allergy (ASCIA) [14]	2020	• At around six months, but not before four months, start to introduce a variety of solid foods, starting with iron rich foods, while continuing breastfeeding. • All infants should be given allergenic solid foods including peanut butter, cooked egg, dairy, and wheat products in the first year of life. This includes infants at high risk of allergy.
Canadian Paediatric Society (CPS) [15]	2021	• For high-risk infants, encourage the introduction of allergenic foods (e.g., cooked (not raw) egg, peanut) early, at about 6 months and not before 4 months of age, in a safe and developmentally appropriate way, at home. In infants at low risk for food allergy, allergenic foods can also be introduced at around 6 months of age. • When allergenic foods have been introduced, make sure that ongoing ingestion of age-appropriate serving sizes is regular (i.e., a few times a week), to maintain tolerance.
European Academy of Allergy and Immunology (EAACI) [16]	2020	• The EAACI Task Force suggests introducing well-cooked hen's egg, but not raw egg or uncooked pasteurized egg, into the infant diet as part of complementary feeding to prevent egg allergy in infants. • In populations where there is a high prevalence of peanut allergy, the EAACI Task Force suggests introducing peanuts into the infant diet in an age-appropriate form as part of complementary feeding in order to prevent peanut allergy in infants and young children. • The EAACI Task Force suggests avoiding supplementing with cow's milk formula in breastfed infants in the first week of life to prevent cow's milk allergy in infants and young children (low quality evidence).
German Society for Allergology and Clinical Immunology (DGAKI) [17]	2014	• The current recommendation in Germany to introduce solid foods to infants over the age of 4 months is reasonable given increasing nutritional requirements. The introduction of solid foods should not be delayed as a means of allergy prevention. • There is no evidence to suggest that dietary restriction in the form of avoiding potent food allergens in the first year of life has a preventive effect. Such a measure is therefore not recommended. • There is currently no reliable evidence that the introduction of potent food allergens during the first 4 months of life has a preventive effect. • There is evidence that a child's consumption of fish during the first year of life has a protective effect against the development of atopic diseases. Fish should be introduced in solid foods.

Table 1. Cont.

Professional Body	Publication Year	Recommendations
National Institute of Allergy and Infectious Diseases (NIAID) [18]	2017	• For infants with severe eczema, egg allergy, or both: Strongly consider evaluation by sIgE measurement and/or SPT and, if necessary, an OFC. Based on test results, introduce peanut-containing foods as early as 4 to 6 months of age to reduce the risk of peanut allergy. • For infants with mild-to-moderate eczema: introduce age-appropriate peanut-containing food around 6 months of age. • For infants without eczema or any food allergy: introduce age-appropriate peanut-containing foods freely together with other solid foods and in accordance with family preferences and cultural practices.

2.1. Peanut

The landmark Learning Early About Peanut (LEAP) study published in 2015 was the first to suggest that the early introduction of allergenic foods decreases the incidence of food allergy, leading to a paradigm shift away from early food avoidance [19]. LEAP demonstrated that the introduction of peanut in high-risk infants between the ages of 4–6 months decreased the prevalence of IgE-mediated peanut allergy at 5 years of age by over 80% when compared to introduction after 12 months of age [19]. High-risk infants in this study were defined as those with severe eczema and/or egg allergy.

In a follow-up study entitled the Persistence of Oral Tolerance to Peanut (LEAP-On), children who consumed peanuts from infancy through to age five followed by one year of peanut avoidance were 74% less likely to have peanut allergy than children who had consistently avoided peanuts up until age six, suggesting that the tolerance induced by early introduction can persist even in the absence of repeated exposures. Later analysis of the LEAP study cohort showed that early introduction of peanut did not negatively impact growth, nutrition, or duration of breastfeeding [20]. In addition, early introduction of peanut was found to be allergen-specific, and had no impact on the development or resolution of other allergic diseases, including asthma and atopic dermatitis [21]. Subsequent studies also identified additional independent risk factors for the development of peanut allergy in the context of peanut avoidance, including genetic susceptibility (via the MALT1 gene and HLA alleles) and *Staphylococcus aureus* colonization [22–24]. These findings are suggestive of the multiple environmental, genetic, epigenetic, and social factors at play in the development of food allergy.

2.2. Egg

Trials examining the early introduction of eggs as a means of reducing egg allergy have yielded mixed results. In 2017, the Prevention of Egg Allergy with Tiny Amount Intake Trial (PETIT) randomized 147 infants with atopic dermatitis to consume either heated egg powder or placebo, in addition to undergoing the aggressive treatment of atopic dermatitis [25]. When compared to the avoidance of egg for the first year of life, those infants who consumed egg powder from 6 to 12 months of age had a significant reduction in the development of egg allergy (8% of the egg group, compared with 38% of the placebo group), resulting in the trial being stopped early to avoid harm to the placebo group [25].

In contrast to these positive findings, the Solids Timing for Allergy Research (STAR) trial randomized high-risk infants with moderate-to-severe eczema to receive either whole egg powder or rice powder daily from 4 to 8 months of age, followed by cooked egg from 8 months onward [26]. Although there was a non-significant trend towards reduced egg allergy in the egg ingestion group, this trial was terminated early due to the high rates of allergic reactions in the egg powder group. It was also noted that 36% of infants in this study had high levels of egg-specific IgE at 4 months of age even in the absence of known egg exposure, suggesting that pre-existing sensitization may be common in this high-risk group [26].

In the 2017 Beating Egg Allergy Trial (BEAT), 319 infants with at least one first-degree relative with an allergic disease were randomized to receive whole-egg powder or placebo from 4 to 8 months of age, after which diets were liberalized in both groups [27]. At 12 months of age, the absolute risk reduction the development of a positive egg white skin prick test was 9.8%, though there was no statistically significant decrease in the proportion of children with a probable egg allergy.

In the Hen's Egg Allergy Prevention (HEAP) study, 383 infants aged 4 to 6 months with confirmed negative skin prick tests prior to trial initiation were randomized to receive either egg white powder (equivalent to raw egg whites) or placebo three times a week until 12 months of age [28]. No statistically significant reduction in rates of egg allergy was observed in this trial. Rather, this study was concerning due to the fact that of infants initially excluded from the trial due to positive skin prick testing, two-thirds developed anaphylaxis when subsequently introduced to egg via oral challenge to raw egg white powder. Given that such test results are rarely available in real-world settings, these findings raise concern for the universal implementation of early egg introduction using raw egg white powder.

2.3. Milk

Several studies suggest that early exposure to cow's milk may prevent later development of cow's milk protein allergy. In 2010, an observational study of over 13,000 Israeli infants from a population-based birth cohort found that early and regular exposure to cow's milk-based formula (beginning in the first two weeks of life) was associated with significantly decreased rates of milk allergy by age 3–5 years in comparison to those introduced to formula after 3 months of age [29].

In the HealthNuts Study, an observational longitudinal study of 5276 infants, early exposure to cow's milk in the first 3 months of life was associated with the decreased risk of cow's milk sensitization (measured via skin prick testing) and parent-reported cow's milk allergy at one year of age [30]. No significant differences were noted in risk of other food allergies.

The timing of milk introduction appears especially important given the widespread use of supplementary cow's milk-based formula in the first days and weeks of life. In a 2016 case-control study of 185 infants, the early introduction of cow's milk formula was associated with a lower incidence of IgE-mediated cow's milk allergy in comparison to infants who received delayed (after one month of age) or no formula [31]. However, in the Atopy Induced by Breastfeeding or Cow's Milk Formula (ABC) study, temporary cow's milk formula supplementation in the first 3 days of life with subsequent removal from the infant diet was associated with an increased risk of milk allergy and anaphylaxis in early childhood [6]. When consumed on a regular basis, cow's milk formula did not appear to increase the risk of milk allergy in this study [6].

2.4. Multiple Foods

Some trials have examined the early introduction of multiple allergenic foods simultaneously. In the 2016 Enquiring About Tolerance (EAT) Study, 1303 infants were randomized to the introduction of six allergenic foods (peanut, cooked egg, cow's milk, sesame, whitefish, and wheat) at either 3 months (early introduction) or 6 months of age (standard) [32]. Although the study was limited by high rates of non-adherence to dietary protocols, a significant reduction in the prevalence of peanut and egg allergy was observed in the subset of the early introduction group that consumed at least 2 g of each food protein per week [32]. In the primary analysis, a 20% reduction in food allergy overall was also observed in the early introduction group, though these results were not statistically significant [32]. An additional analysis found that introduction of gluten between the ages 4 and 6 months was associated with reduced prevalence of celiac disease [33]. A secondary intention-to-treat analysis of this trial conducted in 2019 found that early introduction was effective in preventing food allergies among a subset of infants considered high risk for allergy development: those with food sensitization at enrollment, and those with visible eczema at enrollment [34]. Of note, the early introduction of solids was also not associated with the decreased rates of breastfeeding in this study, but did result in small but significant improvements in infant sleep duration and quality [35,36].

In a similar vein, the SEED trial was a randomized controlled trial in which 163 infants aged 3–4 months with atopic dermatitis were randomized to receive either mixed allergenic food powder (containing egg, milk, wheat, soybean, buckwheat, and peanuts) or placebo powder [37]. The amount of powder was gradually increased over the trial and continued for 12 weeks. Following this intervention, a significant difference was noted in the incidence of food allergy episodes (RR 0.301, 95% CI 0.116–0.784, $p = 0.0066$) and egg allergies at 18 months of age [37]. The Tolerance Induction Through Early Feeding to Prevent Food Allergy in Infants with Eczema (TEFFA) study is a randomized controlled trial that will build on these findings by examining whether the early introduction of hen's egg, cow's milk, peanut, and hazelnut can reduce the risk of developing food allergies in the first year of life in children with atopic dermatitis [38].

3. Study Generalizability

A question remains regarding the efficacy of the early introduction of allergenic foods for preventing food allergy in a general population with no underlying risk factors for allergy. Some have argued that the evidence supporting the efficacy of early food introduction in the general (i.e., not high-risk) population is less compelling given that the intention-to-treat analysis of both HEAP and EAT failed to show a statistically significant decrease in food allergies in a general population [39]. Although per-protocol analysis in EAT did show a statistically significant reduction in food allergy, the potential for bias to be influencing these results cannot be discounted. In a 2020 systematic review, the lack of uniformity in study methodology and patient population was cited as a limitation in both the generalizability of study conclusions as well as accurate subgroup analysis [6].

4. Barriers to Adherence

Multiple barriers may prevent the successful implementation of food allergy prevention programs based on early food introduction [40]. Issues with respect to patient education, access to health services, child cooperation, parental fears or perceived low self-efficacy, and practical difficulties adhering to complicated or long-term treatment plans have been identified as interfering with early food introduction programs [41]. In the EAT study, nonwhite ethnicity, increased maternal age, and infants with feeding difficulties and early onset eczema were all associated with decreased protocol adherence [32,42].

Addressing health disparities based on race and ethnicity is especially important given that Black children are at greater risk of developing food allergies in comparison to other racial groups, and that allergies are increasing in prevalence in this population [43]. Black food-allergic patients are also more likely to experience heightened psychosocial burdens and negative health outcomes related to food allergies [43]. Understanding and addressing these racial and ethnic disparities must be prioritized in future guidelines and public health programs aimed at preventing food allergy. Like food allergen exposure itself, patient and community involvement should occur early and be sustained throughout the development of such programs if they are to be effective [40].

5. Other Directions in Food Allergy Prevention

A number of other strategies are under active investigation for the prevention of food allergy. At this time, there are 14 active clinical trials listed on clinicaltrials.gov investigating probiotics, diet enriched in *Prevotella* spp. and butyrate, vaginal seeding, Mediterranean diet in pregnancy, vitamin D supplementation, and intensive restoration of skin barrier function in atopic dermatitis [44]. An overview of the potential alternative targets for food allergy prevention is also illustrated in Figure 2.

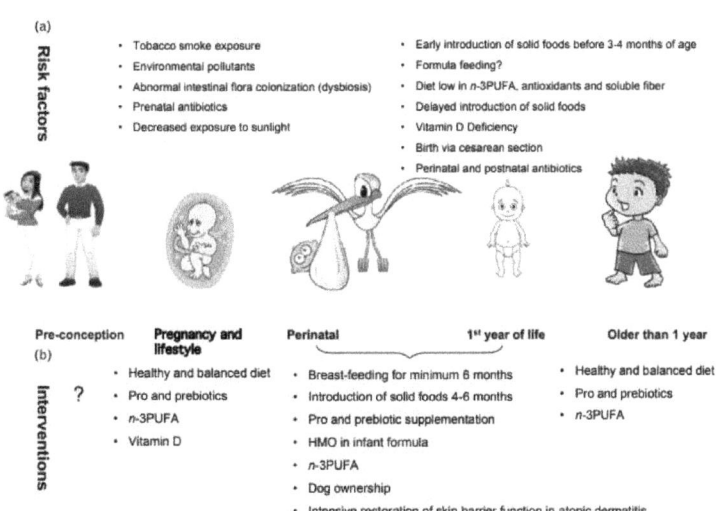

Figure 2. Other directions currently being investigated for food allergy prevention; (**a**) risk factors; (**b**) interventions. Modified with permission from Prescott and Nowak-Węgrzyn [45]. Legend: n-3PUFA: n-3 Polyunsaturated Fatty Acids, which can include eicosapentaenoic acid (EPA) and docosahexaenoic acid (DHA) can provide multiple health benefits including anti-inflammatory effects [46]. HMO: Human milk oligosaccharides, a naturally present constituent of human milk that can modulate the immune system [47].

6. Conclusions

The increasing prevalence of food allergies around the world is a growing global public health problem. Recent research suggests that while cutaneous or inhalational exposures of allergens may promote IgE-sensitization, ingestion of allergenic foods can result in oral tolerance [46]. As a result, many health organizations have updated their guidelines away from allergen avoidance in early infancy in favor of early exposure. The early introduction of allergenic foods appears to be an effective strategy for minimizing the population burden of food allergy, though further studies on the generalizability of this approach in low-risk populations are needed. For children considered at high risk of developing food allergy (particularly due to the presence of other food allergies or severe eczema), the evidence for the early introduction of allergenic foods, and in particular peanut and egg, is robust. In such cases, the consensus is clear that not only should such foods not be delayed, but that they should be introduced at approximately 4 to 6 months of age in order to minimize the risk of food allergy development. The many clinical trials currently underway examining food allergy prevention will further strengthen our understanding of the complex process of food allergy development.

In line with the dual exposure hypothesis, high-dose exposure to ingested food protein promotes development of oral tolerance, whereas low-dose exposure through inflamed skin (disrupted epithelial barrier) or via inhalation is more likely to prime for IgE-sensitization to food proteins. Modified from Nowak-Wegrzyn, Szajewska, and Lack [11].

Author Contributions: Conceptualization, A.N.-W., B.T. and S.J.; methodology, A.N.-W., B.T. and S.J.; resources, A.N.-W., B.T. and S.J.; data curation, A.N.-W., B.T. and S.J.; writing—original draft preparation, A.N.-W., B.T. and S.J.; writing—review and editing, A.N.-W., B.T. and S.J.; visualization, A.N.-W., B.T. and S.J.; supervision, A.N.-W. All authors have read and agreed to the published version of the manuscript.

Funding: This research received no external funding.

Conflicts of Interest: The authors declare no conflict of interest.

References

1. Sicherer, S.H.; Sampson, H.A. Food Allergy: A Review and Update on Epidemiology, Pathogenesis, Diagnosis, Prevention, and Management. *J. Allergy Clin. Immunol.* **2018**, *141*, 41–58. [CrossRef] [PubMed]
2. Vale, S.L.; Lobb, M.; Netting, M.J.; Murray, K.; Clifford, R.; Campbell, D.E.; Salter, S.M. A Systematic Review of Infant Feeding Food Allergy Prevention Guidelines—Can We AGREE? *World Allergy Organ. J.* **2021**, *14*. [CrossRef] [PubMed]
3. Protudjer, J.L.P.; Jansson, S.-A.; Heibert Arnlind, M.; Bengtsson, U.; Kallström-Bengtsson, I.; Marklund, B.; Middelveld, R.; Rentzos, G.; Sundqvist, A.-C.; Åkerström, J.; et al. Household Costs Associated with Objectively Diagnosed Allergy to Staple Foods in Children and Adolescents. *J. Allergy Clin. Immunol. Pract.* **2015**, *3*, 68–75. [CrossRef] [PubMed]
4. Gupta, R.; Holdford, D.; Bilaver, L.; Dyer, A.; Holl, J.L.; Meltzer, D. The Economic Impact of Childhood Food Allergy in the United States. *JAMA Pediatr.* **2013**, *167*, 1026–1031. [CrossRef]
5. Sicherer, S.H.; Noone, S.A.; Muñoz-Furlong, A. The Impact of Childhood Food Allergy on Quality of Life. *Ann. Allergy Asthma Immunol.* **2001**, *87*, 461–464. [CrossRef]
6. de Silva, D.; Halken, S.; Singh, C.; Muraro, A.; Angier, E.; Arasi, S.; Arshad, H.; Beyer, K.; Boyle, R.; du Toit, G.; et al. Preventing Food Allergy in Infancy and Childhood: Systematic Review of Randomised Controlled Trials. *Pediatr. Allergy Immunol.* **2020**, *31*, 813–826. [CrossRef]
7. Kelleher, M.M.; Cro, S.; Cornelius, V.; Carlsen, K.C.L.; Skjerven, H.O.; Rehbinder, E.M.; Lowe, A.J.; Dissanayake, E.; Shimojo, N.; Yonezawa, K.; et al. Skin Care Interventions in Infants for Preventing Eczema and Food Allergy. *Cochrane Database Syst. Rev.* **2021**, *2*, CD013534. [CrossRef]
8. Skin Care and Synbiotics for Prevention of Atopic Dermatitis or Food Allergy in Newborn Infants: A 2 × 2 Factorial, Randomized, Non-Treatment Controlled Trial—PubMed. Available online: https://pubmed.ncbi.nlm.nih.gov/31394530/ (accessed on 27 April 2022).
9. Brough, H.A.; Lanser, B.J.; Sindher, S.B.; Teng, J.M.C.; Leung, D.Y.M.; Venter, C.; Chan, S.M.; Santos, A.F.; Bahnson, H.T.; Guttman-Yassky, E.; et al. Early Intervention and Prevention of Allergic Diseases. *Allergy* **2022**, *77*, 416–441. [CrossRef]
10. Lack, G. Epidemiologic Risks for Food Allergy. *J. Allergy Clin. Immunol.* **2008**, *121*, 1331–1336. [CrossRef]
11. Nowak-Wegrzyn, A.; Szajewska, H.; Lack, G. Food Allergy and the Gut. *Nat. Rev. Gastroenterol. Hepatol.* **2017**, *14*, 241–257. [CrossRef]
12. Greer, F.R.; Sicherer, S.H.; Burks, A.W.; Committee on Nutrition; Section on Allergy and Immunology; Abrams, S.A.; Fuchs, G.J.; Kim, J.H.; Lindsey, C.W.; Magge, S.N.; et al. The Effects of Early Nutritional Interventions on the Development of Atopic Disease in Infants and Children: The Role of Maternal Dietary Restriction, Breastfeeding, Hydrolyzed Formulas, and Timing of Introduction of Allergenic Complementary Foods. *Pediatrics* **2019**, *143*, e20190281. [CrossRef] [PubMed]
13. Tham, E.H.; Shek, L.P.-C.; Van Bever, H.P.; Vichyanond, P.; Ebisawa, M.; Wong, G.W.; Lee, B.W.; the Asia Pacific Association of Pediatric Allergy, R. & I. (APAPARI). Early Introduction of Allergenic Foods for the Prevention of Food Allergy from an Asian Perspective—An Asia Pacific Association of Pediatric Allergy, Respirology & Immunology (APAPARI) Consensus Statement. *Pediatr. Allergy Immunol.* **2018**, *29*, 18–27. [CrossRef]
14. ASCIA Guidelines for Infant Feeding and Allergy Prevention—Australasian Society of Clinical Immunology and Allergy (ASCIA). Available online: https://www.allergy.org.au/hp/papers/infant-feeding-and-allergy-prevention (accessed on 27 April 2022).
15. Dietary Exposures and Allergy Prevention in High-Risk Infants | Canadian Paediatric Society. Available online: https://cps.ca/documents/position/dietary-exposures-and-allergy-prevention (accessed on 27 April 2022).
16. Halken, S.; Muraro, A.; de Silva, D.; Khaleva, E.; Angier, E.; Arasi, S.; Arshad, H.; Bahnson, H.T.; Beyer, K.; Boyle, R.; et al. EAACI Guideline: Preventing the Development of Food Allergy in Infants and Young Children (2020 Update). *Pediatr. Allergy Immunol.* **2021**, *32*, 843–858. [CrossRef] [PubMed]
17. Schäfer, T.; Bauer, C.-P.; Beyer, K.; Bufe, A.; Friedrichs, F.; Gieler, U.; Gronke, G.; Hamelmann, E.; Hellermann, M.; Kleinheinz, A.; et al. S3-Guideline on Allergy Prevention: 2014 Update: Guideline of the German Society for Allergology and Clinical Immunology (DGAKI) and the German Society for Pediatric and Adolescent Medicine (DGKJ). *Allergo J. Int.* **2014**, *23*, 186–199. [CrossRef]
18. Togias, A.; Cooper, S.F.; Acebal, M.L.; Assa'ad, A.; Baker, J.R.; Beck, L.A.; Block, J.; Byrd-Bredbenner, C.; Chan, E.S.; Eichenfield, L.F.; et al. Addendum guidelines for the prevention of peanut allergy in the United States: Report of the National Institute of Allergy and Infectious Diseases–sponsored expert panel. *World Allergy Organ. J.* **2017**, *10*, 1–18. [CrossRef]
19. Du Toit, G.; Roberts, G.; Sayre, P.H.; Bahnson, H.T.; Radulovic, S.; Santos, A.F.; Brough, H.A.; Phippard, D.; Basting, M.; Feeney, M.; et al. Randomized Trial of Peanut Consumption in Infants at Risk for Peanut Allergy. *N. Engl. J. Med.* **2015**, *372*, 803–813. [CrossRef] [PubMed]
20. Feeney, M.; Du Toit, G.; Roberts, G.; Sayre, P.H.; Lawson, K.; Bahnson, H.T.; Sever, M.L.; Radulovic, S.; Plaut, M.; Lack, G.; et al. Impact of Peanut Consumption in the LEAP Study: Feasibility, Growth, and Nutrition. *J. Allergy Clin. Immunol.* **2016**, *138*, 1108–1118. [CrossRef] [PubMed]
21. du Toit, G.; Sayre, P.H.; Roberts, G.; Lawson, K.; Sever, M.L.; Bahnson, H.T.; Fisher, H.R.; Feeney, M.; Radulovic, S.; Basting, M.; et al. Allergen Specificity of Early Peanut Consumption and Effect on Development of Allergic Disease in the Learning Early About Peanut Allergy Study Cohort. *J. Allergy Clin. Immunol.* **2018**, *141*, 1343–1353. [CrossRef]

22. Winters, A.; Bahnson, H.T.; Ruczinski, I.; Boorgula, M.P.; Malley, C.; Keramati, A.R.; Chavan, S.; Larson, D.; Cerosaletti, K.; Sayre, P.H.; et al. The MALT1 Locus and Peanut Avoidance in the Risk for Peanut Allergy. *J. Allergy Clin. Immunol.* **2019**, *143*, 2326–2329. [CrossRef]
23. Kanchan, K.; Grinek, S.; Bahnson, H.T.; Ruczinski, I.; Shankar, G.; Larson, D.; Du Toit, G.; Barnes, K.C.; Sampson, H.A.; Suarez-Farinas, M.; et al. HLA Alleles and Sustained Peanut Consumption Promote IgG4 Responses in Subjects Protected from Peanut Allergy. *J. Clin. Investig.* **2022**, *132*, e152070. [CrossRef]
24. Tsilochristou, O.; du Toit, G.; Sayre, P.H.; Roberts, G.; Lawson, K.; Sever, M.L.; Bahnson, H.T.; Radulovic, S.; Basting, M.; Plaut, M.; et al. Association of Staphylococcus Aureus Colonization with Food Allergy Occurs Independently of Eczema Severity. *J. Allergy Clin. Immunol.* **2019**, *144*, 494–503. [CrossRef] [PubMed]
25. Natsume, O.; Kabashima, S.; Nakazato, J.; Yamamoto-Hanada, K.; Narita, M.; Kondo, M.; Saito, M.; Kishino, A.; Takimoto, T.; Inoue, E.; et al. Two-Step Egg Introduction for Prevention of Egg Allergy in High-Risk Infants with Eczema (PETIT): A Randomised, Double-Blind, Placebo-Controlled Trial. *Lancet* **2017**, *389*, 276–286. [CrossRef]
26. Palmer, D.J.; Metcalfe, J.; Makrides, M.; Gold, M.S.; Quinn, P.; West, C.E.; Loh, R.; Prescott, S.L. Early Regular Egg Exposure in Infants with Eczema: A Randomized Controlled Trial. *J. Allergy Clin. Immunol.* **2013**, *132*, 387–392.e1. [CrossRef] [PubMed]
27. Wei-Liang Tan, J.; Valerio, C.; Barnes, E.H.; Turner, P.J.; Van Asperen, P.A.; Kakakios, A.M.; Campbell, D.E.; Beating Egg Allergy Trial (BEAT) Study Group. A Randomized Trial of Egg Introduction from 4 Months of Age in Infants at Risk for Egg Allergy. *J. Allergy Clin. Immunol.* **2017**, *139*, 1621–1628.e8. [CrossRef] [PubMed]
28. Bellach, J.; Schwarz, V.; Ahrens, B.; Trendelenburg, V.; Aksünger, Ö.; Kalb, B.; Niggemann, B.; Keil, T.; Beyer, K. Randomized Placebo-Controlled Trial of Hen's Egg Consumption for Primary Prevention in Infants. *J. Allergy Clin. Immunol.* **2017**, *139*, 1591–1599.e2. [CrossRef]
29. Katz, Y.; Rajuan, N.; Goldberg, M.R.; Eisenberg, E.; Heyman, E.; Cohen, A.; Leshno, M. Early Exposure to Cow's Milk Protein Is Protective against IgE-Mediated Cow's Milk Protein Allergy. *J. Allergy Clin. Immunol.* **2010**, *126*, 77–82.e1. [CrossRef]
30. Peters, R.L.; Koplin, J.J.; Dharmage, S.C.; Tang, M.L.K.; McWilliam, V.L.; Gurrin, L.C.; Neeland, M.R.; Lowe, A.J.; Ponsonby, A.-L.; Allen, K.J. Early Exposure to Cow's Milk Protein Is Associated with a Reduced Risk of Cow's Milk Allergic Outcomes. *J. Allergy Clin. Immunol. Pract.* **2019**, *7*, 462–470.e1. [CrossRef]
31. Onizawa, Y.; Noguchi, E.; Okada, M.; Sumazaki, R.; Hayashi, D. The Association of the Delayed Introduction of Cow's Milk with IgE-Mediated Cow's Milk Allergies. *J. Allergy Clin. Immunol. Pract.* **2016**, *4*, 481–488.e2. [CrossRef]
32. Perkin, M.R.; Logan, K.; Tseng, A.; Raji, B.; Ayis, S.; Peacock, J.; Brough, H.; Marrs, T.; Radulovic, S.; Craven, J.; et al. Randomized Trial of Introduction of Allergenic Foods in Breast-Fed Infants. *N. Engl. J. Med.* **2016**, *374*, 1733–1743. [CrossRef]
33. Logan, K.; Perkin, M.R.; Marrs, T.; Radulovic, S.; Craven, J.; Flohr, C.; Bahnson, H.T.; Lack, G. Early Gluten Introduction and Celiac Disease in the EAT Study. *JAMA Pediatr.* **2020**, *174*, 1041–1047. [CrossRef]
34. Perkin, M.R.; Logan, K.; Bahnson, H.T.; Marrs, T.; Radulovic, S.; Craven, J.; Flohr, C.; Mills, E.N.; Versteeg, S.A.; van Ree, R.; et al. Efficacy of the Enquiring About Tolerance (EAT) Study among Infants at High Risk of Developing Food Allergy. *J. Allergy Clin. Immunol.* **2019**, *144*, 1606–1614.e2. [CrossRef] [PubMed]
35. Turner, P.J.; Perkin, M.R. RCT Evidence Suggests That Solids Introduction before Age 6 Months Does Not Adversely Impact Duration of Breastfeeding. *Matern Child. Nutr.* **2020**, *16*, e13029. [CrossRef] [PubMed]
36. Perkin, M.R.; Bahnson, H.T.; Logan, K.; Marrs, T.; Radulovic, S.; Craven, J.; Flohr, C.; Lack, G. Association of Early Introduction of Solids With Infant Sleep. *JAMA Pediatr.* **2018**, *172*, e180739. [CrossRef] [PubMed]
37. Nishimura, T.; Fukazawa, M.; Fukuoka, K.; Okasora, T.; Yamada, S.; Kyo, S.; Homan, M.; Miura, T.; Nomura, Y.; Tsuchida, S.; et al. Early Introduction of Very Small Amounts of Multiple Foods to Infants: A Randomized Trial. *Allergol. Int.* **2022**. [CrossRef]
38. Kalb, B.; Meixner, L.; Trendelenburg, V.; Unterleider, N.; Dobbertin-Welsch, J.; Heller, S.; Dölle-Bierke, S.; Roll, S.; Lau, S.; Lee, Y.-A.; et al. Tolerance Induction through Early Feeding to Prevent Food Allergy in Infants with Eczema (TEFFA): Rationale, Study Design, and Methods of a Randomized Controlled Trial. *Trials* **2022**, *23*, 210. [CrossRef] [PubMed]
39. Krawiec, M.; Fisher, H.R.; Du Toit, G.; Bahnson, H.T.; Lack, G. Overview of Oral Tolerance Induction for Prevention of Food Allergy-Where Are We Now? *Allergy* **2021**, *76*, 2684–2698. [CrossRef] [PubMed]
40. Fisher, H.R.; Du Toit, G.; Bahnson, H.T.; Lack, G. The Challenges of Preventing Food Allergy: Lessons Learned from LEAP and EAT. *Ann. Allergy Asthma Immunol.* **2018**, *121*, 313–319. [CrossRef]
41. Voorheis, P.; Bell, S.; Cornelsen, L.; Quaife, M.; Logan, K.; Marrs, T.; Radulovic, S.; Craven, J.; Flohr, C.; Lack, G.; et al. Challenges Experienced with Early Introduction and Sustained Consumption of Allergenic Foods in the Enquiring About Tolerance (EAT) Study: A Qualitative Analysis. *J. Allergy Clin. Immunol.* **2019**, *144*, 1615–1623. [CrossRef]
42. Perkin, M.R.; Bahnson, H.T.; Logan, K.; Marrs, T.; Radulovic, S.; Knibb, R.; Craven, J.; Flohr, C.; Mills, E.N.; Versteeg, S.A.; et al. Factors Influencing Adherence in a Trial of Early Introduction of Allergenic Food. *J. Allergy Clin. Immunol.* **2019**, *144*, 1595–1605. [CrossRef]
43. Warren, C.; Turner, P.J.; Chinthrajah, R.S.; Gupta, R. Advancing Food Allergy through Epidemiology: Understanding and Addressing Disparities in Food Allergy Management and Outcomes. *J. Allergy Clin. Immunol. Pract.* **2021**, *9*, 110–118. [CrossRef]
44. Home—ClinicalTrials.gov. Available online: https://clinicaltrials.gov/ (accessed on 2 May 2022).
45. Prescott, S.; Nowak-Wegrzyn, A. Strategies to Prevent or Reduce Allergic Disease. *Ann. Nutr. Metab.* **2011**, *59* (Suppl. S1), 28–42. [CrossRef]

46. Siriwardhana, N.; Kalupahana, N.S.; Moustaid-Moussa, N. Health benefits of n-3 polyunsaturated fatty acids: Eicosapentaenoic acid and docosahexaenoic acid. *Adv. Food Nutr. Res.* **2012**, *65*, 211–222. [CrossRef] [PubMed]
47. Wiciński, M.; Sawicka, E.; Gębalski, J.; Kubiak, K.; Malinowski, B. Human Milk Oligosaccharides: Health Benefits, Potential Applications in Infant Formulas, and Pharmacology. *Nutrients* **2020**, *12*, 266. [CrossRef] [PubMed]

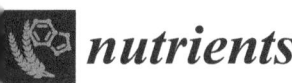 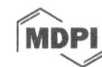

Article

Early Introduction of Multi-Allergen Mixture for Prevention of Food Allergy: Pilot Study

Antonia Zoe Quake, Taryn Audrey Liu, Rachel D'Souza, Katherine G. Jackson, Margaret Woch, Afua Tetteh, Vanitha Sampath, Kari C. Nadeau *, Sayantani Sindher, R. Sharon Chinthrajah and Shu Cao

Department of Medicine, Division of Pulmonary, Allergy and Critical Care Medicine,
Sean N. Parker Center for Allergy and Asthma Research at Stanford University, Stanford, CA 94305, USA;
zoeq@stanford.edu (A.Z.Q.); tliu2236@gmail.com (T.A.L.); rdsouza@zis.ch (R.D.);
kjawesomeness3@gmail.com (K.G.J.); mwoch@stanford.edu (M.W.); okobea@gmail.com (A.T.);
vsampath@stanford.edu (V.S.); tina.sindher@stanford.edu (S.S.); schinths@stanford.edu (R.S.C.);
shucao@stanford.edu (S.C.)
* Correspondence: knadeau@stanford.edu

Abstract: The incidence and prevalence of food allergy (FA) is increasing. While several studies have established the safety and efficacy of early introduction of single allergens in infants for the prevention of FA, the exact dose, frequency, and number of allergens that can be safely introduced to infants, particularly in those at high or low risk of atopy, are still unclear. This 1-year pilot study evaluated the safety of the early introduction of single foods (milk, egg, or peanut) vs. two foods (milk/egg, egg/peanut, milk/peanut) vs. multiple foods (milk/egg/peanut/cashew/almond/shrimp/walnut/wheat/salmon/hazelnut at low, medium, or high doses) vs. no early introduction in 180 infants between 4–6 months of age. At the end of the study, they were evaluated for plasma biomarkers associated with food reactivity via standardized blood tests. Two to four years after the start of the study, participants were evaluated by standardized food challenges. The serving sizes for the single, double, and low dose mixtures were 300 mg total protein per day. The serving sizes for the medium and high dose mixtures were 900 mg and 3000 mg total protein, respectively. Equal parts of each protein were used for double or mixture foods. All infants were breastfed until at least six months of age. The results demonstrate that infants at either high or low risk for atopy were able to tolerate the early introduction of multiple allergenic foods with no increases in any safety issues, including eczema, FA, or food protein induced enterocolitis. The mixtures of foods at either low, medium, or high doses demonstrated trends for improvement in food challenge reactivity and plasma biomarkers compared to single and double food introductions. The results of this study suggest that the early introduction of foods, particularly simultaneous mixtures of many allergenic foods, may be safe and efficacious for preventing FA and can occur safely. These results need to be confirmed by larger randomized controlled studies.

Keywords: multi-allergen; early introduction; food allergy; safety; efficacy; prevention

Citation: Quake, A.Z.; Liu, T.A.; D'Souza, R.; Jackson, K.G.; Woch, M.; Tetteh, A.; Sampath, V.; Nadeau, K.C.; Sindher, S.; Chinthrajah, R.S.; et al. Early Introduction of Multi-Allergen Mixture for Prevention of Food Allergy: Pilot Study. *Nutrients* **2022**, *14*, 737. https://doi.org/10.3390/nu14040737

Academic Editors: RJ Joost Van Neerven and Janneke Ruinemans-Koerts

Received: 26 January 2022
Accepted: 4 February 2022
Published: 9 February 2022
Corrected: 28 December 2022

Publisher's Note: MDPI stays neutral with regard to jurisdictional claims in published maps and institutional affiliations.

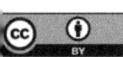

Copyright: © 2022 by the authors. Licensee MDPI, Basel, Switzerland. This article is an open access article distributed under the terms and conditions of the Creative Commons Attribution (CC BY) license (https://creativecommons.org/licenses/by/4.0/).

1. Introduction

The incidence and prevalence of food allergy (FA) has increased significantly in recent years [1–3]. Today, an estimated 7.6% of U.S. children and nearly 11% of adults have reported FAs to at least one food [4,5]. Reactions can be mild, moderate, severe, or life-threatening, with clinical symptoms varying considerably between individuals and over one's lifetime [6]. Although a number of foods are known to be allergenic, cow's milk, hen's egg, peanuts, soy, wheat, tree nuts, fish, and shellfish account for 90% of all FAs [7]. Accidental ingestion rates for peanut, egg, and milk range from 14 to 33% [8], 19–50%, and 17–36%, respectively [9].

There is an urgent and unmet need to prevent and treat FAs. Despite limited data, older guidelines recommended delaying exposure to cow's milk until 12 months, hen's egg until 24 months, and peanut, tree nut, and fish until three years [10] to prevent FA. In 2015, results of a large randomized controlled study, the Learning Early About Peanut (LEAP) study, challenged these early guidelines and concluded that early introduction of peanuts significantly reduced the likelihood of developing peanut allergy and, conversely, delayed introduction significantly increased the likelihood of developing peanut allergy in infants. The study also indicated that delayed introduction may lead to impaired immune responses [11]. The benefits of early introduction of allergenic foods for prevention of FA are now supported by a number of randomized controlled trials, particularly for peanut, egg and milk. A meta-analysis found strong evidence of positive benefits of early introduction of allergenic foods [12].

Allergen diversity in infants has also been found to play a role in preventing FA. In 2014, the PASTURE study found that increased diversity of complementary allergenic foods introduced in the first year of life was inversely associated with doctor-diagnosed FA up to 6 years of age, food sensitization, and increased expression of a T regulatory cell marker [13]. Diet diversity was also evaluated in a large prospective study using standardized questionnaires. The study showed that the introduction of each additional allergenic food at 6 and 12 months of age reduced the odds of developing FA over the first 10 years of life by 10.8% and 33.2%, respectively [14]. Systemic reviews suggest that allergen diversity in infancy may be associated with reduced allergy outcomes (including FA) [15,16].

Among children with FA, up to 40% are allergic to multiple foods [5]. This suggests that there is a need to include multiple allergenic foods into the diets of these infants for prevention of FA, as research shows that it is allergen-specific [17]. At the current time, only a few studies have looked at the introduction of multiple allergenic foods for the prevention of FA. In the Enquiring About Tolerance (EAT) study, infants were randomized at three months and sequentially introduced to six allergenic foods (including cow's milk, peanut, hard-boiled egg, sesame, cod and wheat) vs. to a standard group where infants avoided allergenic foods. Per protocol analysis indicated that the early introduction group had a 67% relative risk reduction of any FA compared to the standard group [18]. While the EAT study showed that it was safe and effective to introduce multiple allergens, the amounts of allergens used were impractical as per the USDA guidelines for daily caloric intake in infants (528, 619, and 806 calories daily for infants of four, six, and 12 months of age, respectively) [19]. Infants in the EAT study were asked to consume the equivalent of 4 g of each allergenic protein per week, which amounted to two small 40- to 60-g portions of cow's milk yogurt, three rounded teaspoons of peanut butter, 1 small hard-boiled egg, three rounded teaspoons of sesame paste, 25 g of whitefish, and two wheat-based cereal biscuits. There were 10 participants whose families reported food protein induced enterocolitis syndrome (FPIES)-like reactions, seven in the early-introduction group and three in the standard-introduction group. The difference between the two groups was not statistically significant ($p = 0.34$). Holl et al. conducted a blinded randomized placebo-controlled study to determine whether early introduction of multiple allergens simultaneously is acceptable to caregivers and tolerable to any healthy infant. In this study, the 16 most common allergenic foods (peanut, soy, almond, cashew, hazelnut, pecan, pistachio, walnut, wheat, oat, milk, egg, cod, shrimp, salmon, and sesame) were premixed and fed to infants between the ages of 5–11 months, for a total of 480 mg of proteins per day for 28 days. This study had a high completion rate indicating acceptability, and showed no significant difference in safety between the active vs. the placebo group ($p = 0.76$). There were no increases in adverse events and there were no increases in reported IgE-type allergic reactions in the active vs. the placebo group [20]. In fact, the placebo group had allergic reactions likely due to the delayed introduction of allergenic foods.

As evidence increasingly suggested that allergen diversity and early intervention may decrease FA [11,21], infant feeding guidelines were revised, and currently recommend full introduction of diverse allergenic foods at 4 to 6 months [22–24]. However, the early and consistent introduction of not just single allergens, but multiple allergens can be difficult to administer in infants. Further research on the number of allergens, amount of allergenic proteins, and length of time allergens need to be consumed is needed to optimize tolerability while providing a convenient and practical method for the early introduction of proteins to infants. Therefore, in the current pilot descriptive study, we conducted a one-year-feeding randomized clinical trial to evaluate the safety of simultaneously introducing a multi-allergen mix vs. double mix vs. single foods vs. no early introduction in infants with high and low risk of allergy. In addition to clinical evaluations of ingestion tolerance via oral food challenges, biomarkers were also measured (allergen-specific IgE and IgG$_4$).

2. Materials and Methods

Study Design: The pilot study was conducted at the Sean N. Parker Center for Allergy and Asthma Research at Stanford University under an approved Stanford IRB study protocol (8629). This was a descriptive study that was designed to be a pilot study for the preliminary assessment of the safety of a 10-allergen protein mixture. Parents or legal guardians consented for their infants to participate in the study for one year and were given instructions for how to give the daily servings of the food proteins (in powder or flour form).

Flours and powder preparation: The flours and powders for each food were prepared in a Good Manufacturing Practice facility at the Sean N Parker Center for Allergy and Asthma Research at Stanford University. Each flour and powder were obtained by manufacturers that had to meet specifications of low yeast, no salmonella and no *E. coli* content. Each flour and powder was examined for protein integrity by standard SDS protein gel electrophoresis and by protein concentration methods using the standard BioRad assay.

Samples from each lot of allergen and placebo substance received were analyzed upon receipt to confirm that the identity of the material and to ensure that microbial levels fall within acceptable limits prior to use in the manufacture of the drug product. A summary of baseline analyses and their methodology can be found in Table 1. Upon meeting all acceptance criteria, the lot was accepted for use in the study. To prepare the 10-food protein mixture, flours and/or powders were weighed in the GMP facility using standard operating procedures and per mg protein amount, added in a 1:1:1:1:1:1:1:1:1:1 ratio. SDS PAGE gels were also run on the mixtures to ensure all proteins were present at equal ratios.

Table 1. Summary of Analyses with Reference Methodology.

Category	Analysis	Reference Method
Protein Characterization	SDS-PAGE	Bio-Rad Laboratories or Thermofisher Scientific—Pierce Protein Methodology
Protein Quantitation	Kjeldahl Titration	AOAC 991.20
Bioburden	Total Aerobic Microbial Count—Pour Plate	USP/NF <61> or FDA BAM
	Total Yeast and Mold Count—Pour Plate	USP/NF <61> or FDA BAM
	Escherichia coli—Direct Inoculation	USP/NF <62> or FDA BAM
	Salmonella species—Direct Inoculation	USP/NF <62> or FDA BAM
	Listeria species—Absent/Present	AOAC-RI 061702
	Listeria monocytogenes—Absent/Present	AOAC-RI 061701
	Listeria species Confirmation (Genus 48 h)	FDA BAM Chapter 10
	Aflatoxin Panel	AOAC 2005.8 or Modified AOAC 999.07

SDS-PAGE—Sodium dodecyl sulfate polyacrylamide gel electrophoresis; USP/NF—United States Pharmacopeia/National Formulary; AOAC-RI—Association of Official Analytical Chemists—Research Institute; FDA BAM—Food and Drug Administration Bacteriological Analytical Manual.

2.1. Substance Identity & Protein Composition

Excluding placebo (oat powder), the active ingredients within each allergen-specific food powder are the combined proteins or singular proteins. For each allergen, the presence and intensity of a readily observable allergenic protein/subunit specific to each allergen substance was confirmed via sodium dodecyl sulfate polyacrylamide gel electrophoresis (SDS-PAGE) after Coomassie Blue staining (Table 2).

Table 2. Summary of Total Protein and Marker Protein Acceptance Criteria.

Allergen	Marker Protein	Published Weight (kDa)	Observed Reference Data		Initial Acceptance Criteria, Inclusive		
			Weight (kDa)	Intensity (10 µg Load)	Weight (kDa)	Intensity (10 µg Load)	Total Protein
Almond	Pru du 6 (Amandin)	40	38.5–41.7	1,142,948–4,526,868	34.7–45.9	800,064–5,884,928	10–70%
Cashew	Ana o 2 (Anacardein)	33	26.5–34.1	752,512–6,028,437	23.9–37.5	526,758–7,836,968	10–55%
Egg	Gal d 2 (Ovalbumin)	43–45	39.0–44.6	6,627,824–14,047,568	35.1–49.1	4,639,477–18,261,838	50–95%
Hazelnut	Cor a 9 (Corylin)	35–40	31.7–34.8	1,963,532–6,958,956	28.5–38.3	1,374,472–9,046,643	10–65%
Milk	Bos d 5 (β-Lactoglobulin)	18–18.3	14.7–16.9	1,007,988–4,842,720	13.2–18.6	705,592–6,295,536	10–65%
Peanut	Ara h 3 (Glycinin)	37	35.0–40.4	1,125,819–3,025,396	31.5–44.4	788,073–3,933,015	15–75%
Salmon	Sal s 2 (β-enolase)	47.3	41.2–47.4	147,088–529,396	37.1–52.1	102,962–688,215	35–99%
Shrimp	Pen a 1 (Tropomyosin)	36	38.7–38.8	953,381–1,453,936	34.8–42.7	667,367–1,890,117	60–99%
Walnut	Jug r 4 (11S globulin)	30–40	29.6–36.2	1,211,022–6,709,672	26.6–39.8	847,715–8,722,574	10–75%
Wheat	Tri a 26 (Glutenin)	88	75.9–94.6	209,988–1,396,822	68.3–104.1	146,992–1,815,869	10–95%

Manufacturers were as follows for each powder or flour. Milk: Now REAL foods, Illinois; almond: Honeyville Farms, CA, USA; egg: Honeywell Farms, CA, USA; cashew: nuts.com, NJ; hazelnut and walnut: Holmquist Orchards, CA, USA; oat (placebo) and wheat: Arrowhead Mills, NY, USA; shrimp and salmon: Invico, WA, USA. Peanut: Golden Peanut Company, Alpharetta, GA, USA.

Enrollment and Eligibility: Both high risk infants and low risk infants were enrolled and stratified 1:1. High risk was defined as one first degree relative with FA/atopic dermatitis or two first degree relatives with atopic disease [25]. Exclusion criteria included infants with chronic diseases or known genetic diseases or with known FA. The study was conducted with IRB approval with enrollment between June 2017 and July 2019 and infants between two months and 12 months of age were enrolled (NCT04828603). Participants were randomized (but not blinded) equally: singles (egg, milk, or peanut; n = 15 each), doubles in equal parts by mg protein (peanut plus milk, peanut plus egg, or milk plus egg, n = 15 each), or a 10-allergen mixture (almonds, cashew, egg, hazelnut, milk, peanut, salmon, shrimp, walnut, wheat) and an age- and sex-matched control group (n = 45) which avoided all potentially allergenic foods for the first year of the study. The serving sizes for the 10-allergen mixture were low, medium, or high (i.e., 300 mg per day, n = 15, 900 mg per day, n = 15; 3000 mg per day, n = 15, in equal 1:1 parts of the 10 proteins, respectively). Participants were fed the first serving in the clinic and observed for 2 h post-ingestion. Upon leaving, parents were instructed to observe the participants at-home for the next 4 h and report any adverse events within 24-h post-ingestion. Participants were in the active phase of the study for one year with regular daily servings of their food in their assigned group. The parent or guardian of each participant was asked to fill out a food diary over a seven day period at the end of the one year study to assess the child's ability to eat table foods from the same foods as in the 10-protein mixture. If a child ate that food as a table food in the week following the end of the one year study period, they was defined as being able to eat that table food. At baseline and at one year, participants underwent a blood draw. Allergen-specific IgE and IgG4 were measured using a standard ImmunoCAP assay (Phadia, Uppsala, Sweden). Oral food challenges (up to 8 g of total protein from the 10-food allergen mixture) were conducted between 2–4 years after the start of the study in a facility with trained personnel with staged, monitored standard methods. Questionnaires were provided at baseline and one year and at the time of the food challenge.

2.2. Statistical Analysis

The study was a pilot descriptive study to test the preliminary safety of a mixture of 10 food allergen proteins in otherwise healthy infants with no current food allergies. The study was not designed to be a phase 2 or phase 3 study, and was not powered to detect a difference in safety between subgroups. Efficacy was measured as an exploratory endpoint and was tested through a standard food challenge and reported here. In addition, bioindicators such as plasma markers were evaluated as exploratory measures and reported here.

The changes of allergen-specific IgE, IgG4, and IgG4 to IgE ratio from baseline to 1 year are depicted as box plots. The Wilcoxon signed rank test was performed to determine whether the change was significant from baseline to 1 year. The Benjamini-Hochberg (BH) procedure was used to control the false discovery rate (FDR) for multiple comparisons among all multi-allergen groups for each marker. Q value was used to denote the adjusted *p* value. The food challenge outcome at one year was illustrated using a bar chart, and the success rate of participants passing the food challenge between groups were compared using a chi-squared test. *p* values were adjusted using BH procedures and denoted as Q values. All tests were two-sided and conducted at the 0·05 level of significance. All analyses were conducted using R software v4.0.3. Descriptive statistics for questionnaire results and demographic information were documented in tables.

3. Results

One hundred and eighty healthy infants aged 2 months to 12 months were recruited at a single site. Participants were randomized and stratified so that 50% of participants were at high risk for FA, and 50% of participants were not at risk of FA. Each of the active groups were further randomized into specific allergen groups as depicted in the consort diagram (Figure 1). No participant dropped out early from the study. Infants consumed daily proteins for an average of 12.1 $\pm$ 3.2 months. There was a 95% adherence rate for each infant. The control group avoided the same 10 food proteins for the first 12 months. All children were breastfed to at least six months of age. All participants had available values (or there were no missing values found) for all tested allergen-specific IgE, IgG4, and food challenge outcomes.

Patient demographics are shown in Table 3. In this cohort, 149 (83%) reported having atopic dermatitis. Fifty-one percent were of high risk, and this was evenly spread throughout all the cohorts. Fifty-one percent% were female. The median age at the start of the study was six months. Eleven percent of participants were Hispanic, 20% were Asian, 51% Caucasian, 14% African American, and 4% Pacific Islander.

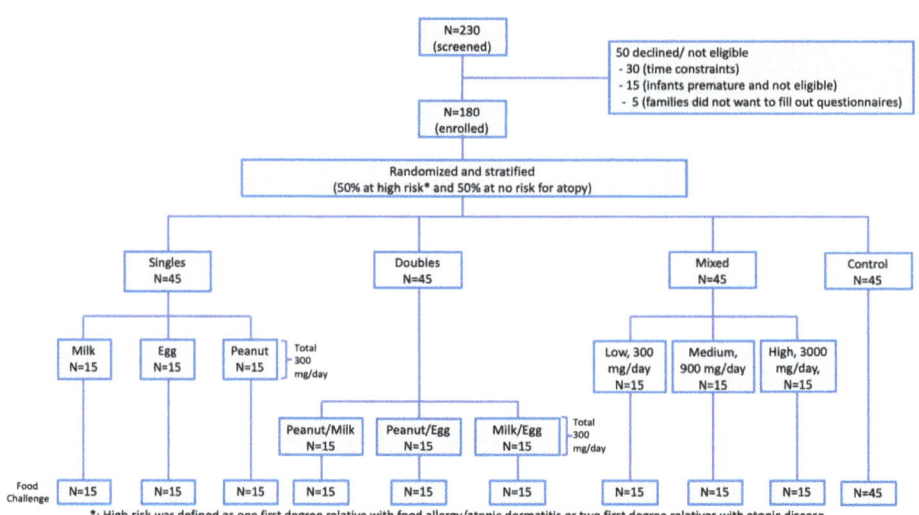

Figure 1. Consort diagram. 180 participants were randomized into three active and one control group. The active phase of the study was for one year and there were no dropouts. Single foods (milk, egg, or peanut); two foods (milk/egg, egg/peanut, milk/peanut), Mixed (milk/egg/peanut/cashew/almond/shrimp/walnut/wheat/salmon/hazelnut at low, medium, or high doses).

Table 3. Patient demographics.

Demographic Characteristics at Baseline	Control N = 45	Active Milk (N = 15)	Active Egg (N = 15)	Active Peanut (N = 15)	Active Peanut/ Milk (N = 15)	Active Milk/ Egg (N = 15)	Active Peanut/ Egg (N = 15)	Active Mixture Low (N = 15)	Active Mixture Medium (N = 15)	Active Mixture High (N = 15)
# Female	23	8	7	8	7	8	7	8	8	7
Age months (median and range)	6 (2–12)	5 (2–12)	5 (2–12)	6 (2–12)	5 (2–12)	5 (2–12)	6 (2–12)	6 (2–12)	6 (2–12)	5 (2–12)
Weight in kg (median and range)	7 (5–9)	7 (5–9)	6 (5–8)	7 (5–9)	6 (4–8)	6 (5–9)	7 (6–10)	7 (5–9)	8 (6–10)	7 (5–9)
# breast feeding until 6 mo	45	15	15	15	15	15	15	15	15	15
# no eczema (scored 0–9.9)	12	4	3	4	4	3	4	4	3	4
# Mild eczema (scored 10 to 28.9)	10	4	4	3	4	4	4	3	4	4
# Moderate eczema (scored 29.0 to 48.9)	15	4	4	4	4	4	4	4	4	3
# Severe eczema (scored 49.0 to 103)	8	3	4	4	3	4	3	4	4	4
# High risk * Family hx	23	7	8	8	7	8	7	8	7	8
Ethnicity										
Hispanic	4	2	2	1	1	1	2	1	1	1
Afro American	5	1	1	2	2	1	0	2	1	1
Caucasian	23	7	8	6	7	6	7	7	8	7
Pacific Islander	6	4	3	3	4	4	3	4	4	3
Asian	7	1	1	2	1	3	3	1	1	3

* High risk was defined as one first degree relative with FA/atopic dermatitis or two first degree relatives with atopic disease.

For safety parameters, across all active groups, there were no increases in allergic reactions reported in participants regardless of risk stratification and eczema comorbid condition. Reactions, including all mild skin rashes, were reported in both the control group, $n = 4$ (9%), and active groups, $n = 11$ (8%). None of those with the mild skin rashes had evidence of eczema or documented family history. Eczema (mild, moderate, and severe) decreased in both controls and in all active groups (Table 4) over time. There were no other adverse events such as vomiting, diarrhea, anaphylaxis, wheezing, cough, or epinephrine use within 2 h of consumption of the allergenic foods. The percentage of participants consuming real foods at the beginning and end of the study is shown in Table 5.

Table 4. Safety: Adverse reactions during study.

Characteristics	Control N = 45 at Baseline	Control Arm Reactions During Study	Active N = 135 at Baseline	Active Arm Reactions During Study
No eczema	8 (18%)	4 (all mild rash) (9%)	22 (16%)	11 (all mild rash) (8%)
Mild eczema	22 (49%)	1 (2%)	61 (45%)	2 (1%)
Moderate eczema	10 (22%)	none	35 (26%)	4 (3%)
Severe eczema	5 (11%)	1 (2%)	17 (13%)	none
High risk * Family hx	N = 23 (51%)	1 (2%)	N = 69 (51%)	3 (2%)
Other adverse events within 2 h of serving		Control arm reactions during study		Active arm reactions during study
Vomiting		0		0
Diarrhea		0		0
Anaphylaxis (more than two organ systems involved)		0		0
Wheezing		0		0
Cough		0		0
Epinephrine use		0		0

* High risk was defined as one first degree relative with FA/atopic dermatitis or two first degree relatives with atopic disease.

Table 5. Percentage of participants consuming real foods at beginning and end of study.

Food Item Consumed by Participant at Start of Study	Participants Consuming Food Item at Start of and during the Study		Participants Consuming All 10 Food Items as Table Foods at End of 1st Year	
	N	%	N	%
Milk	15	100	6	40
Egg	15	100	5	33
Peanut	15	100	6	40
Milk/egg	15	100	7	47
Egg/peanut	15	100	7	47
Milk/peanut	15	100	8	53
Milk/egg/peanut/cashew/almond/shrimp/walnut/wheat/fish/hazelnut (300 mg)	15	100	15	100
Milk/egg/peanut/cashew/almond/shrimp/walnut/wheat/fish/hazelnut (900 mg)	15	100	15	100
Milk/egg/peanut/cashew/almond/shrimp/walnut/wheat/fish/hazelnut (3000 mg)	15	100	15	100

Figure 2 indicates the results of oral food challenges (OFCs). The percent of participants able to consume 8 g of protein was significantly higher in all mixed protein groups compared to the controls (q < 0.05). There were 44, 14, and 14 participants who had available OFC outcomes in the control, peanut, and mixture high groups, respectively. Interestingly, results from questionnaires demonstrated that those on the mixture diet were more apt to diversify the diet of their infant compared to single, double, and control groups (Appendix A Table A1).

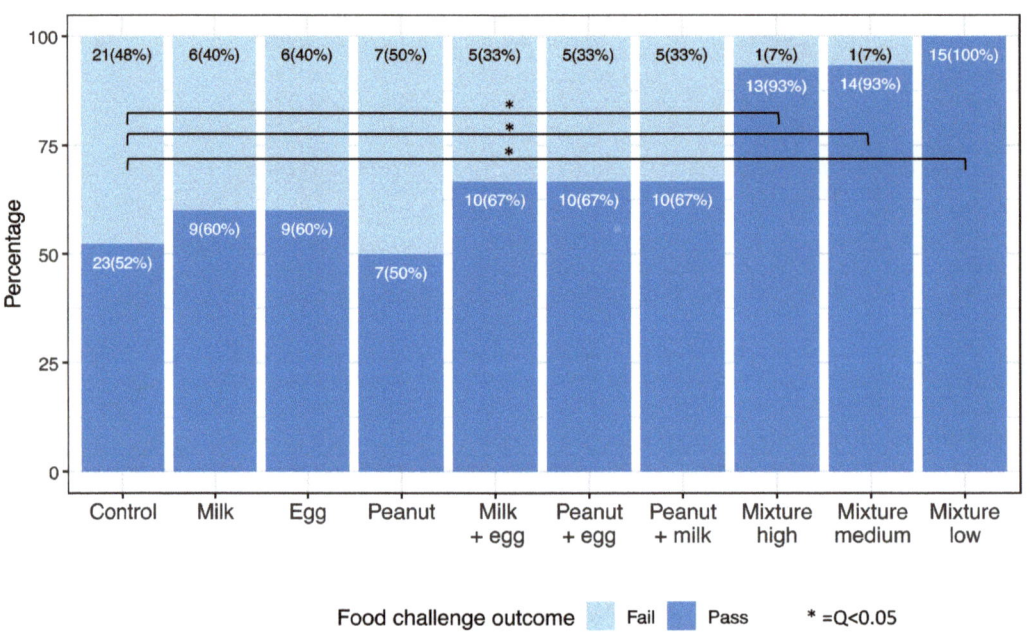

Figure 2. Oral Food Challenges: Food challenge outcome in active (singles, doubles, and mixtures) and control groups 2–4 years after start of study. Oral food challenges (up to 8 g of total protein from the 10-food allergen mixture) were conducted between 2–4 years after the start of the study in a facility with trained personnel with staged, monitored standard methods. Each food challenge consisted of several escalating doses of the food protein in flour or powder form concealed in an appropriate vehicle, such as applesauce or pudding, ingested by the participant every 15 min as tolerated. Typically challenges started with 2 mg and escalated upto a max of 8 g of total food protein as per our validated methods [26–28].

Specific IgG4, sIgE and IgG4/IgE ratios for all 10 allergens are shown in Figure 3a–j. The IgG4/IgE ratios for all mixed protein groups (low, medium, and high) were significantly higher at end of study compared to baseline (q < 0.1), even for peanut, egg, or milk compared to single early intervention active arms. The increase in the ratio can be mainly attributed to increases in IgG4 concentration rather than decreases in IgE. Peanut, milk, and egg biomarkers show improvement compared to control, however specificity was demonstrated only with peanut, milk, and egg containing food, respectively.

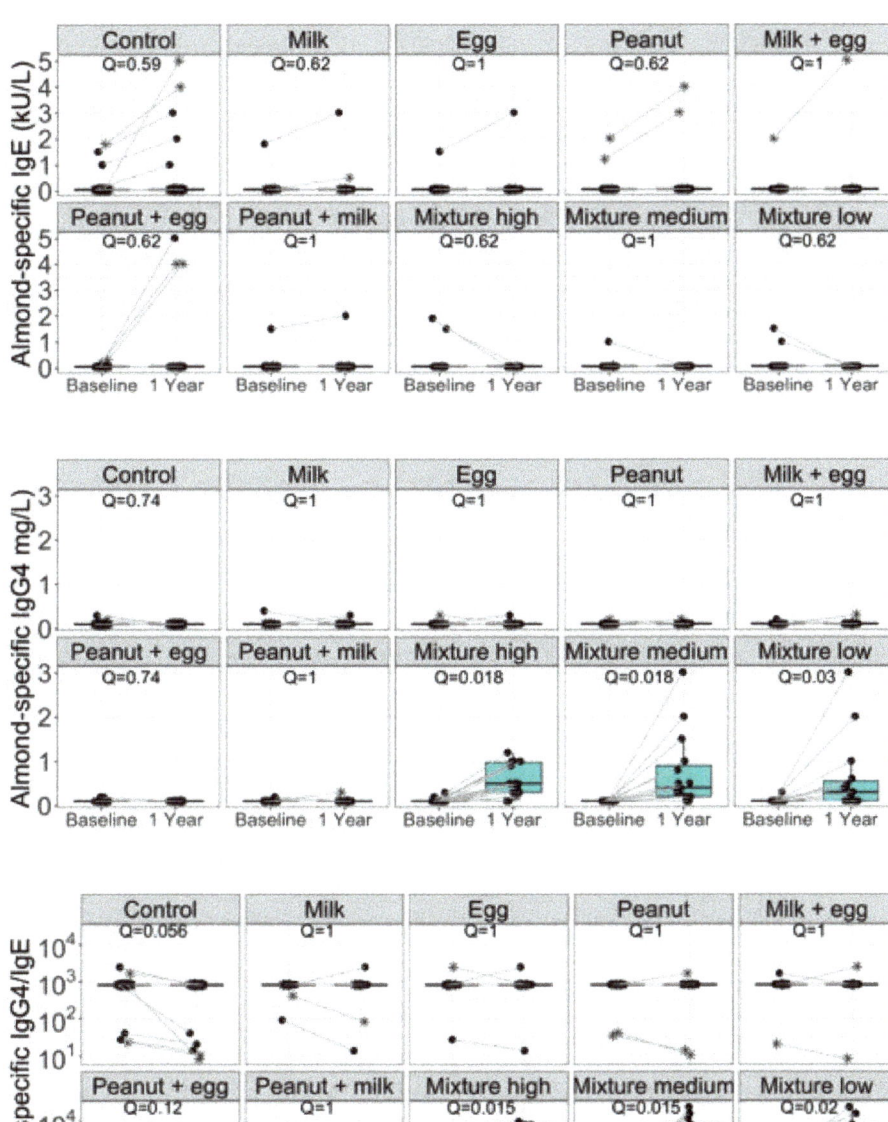

Figure 3. *Cont.*

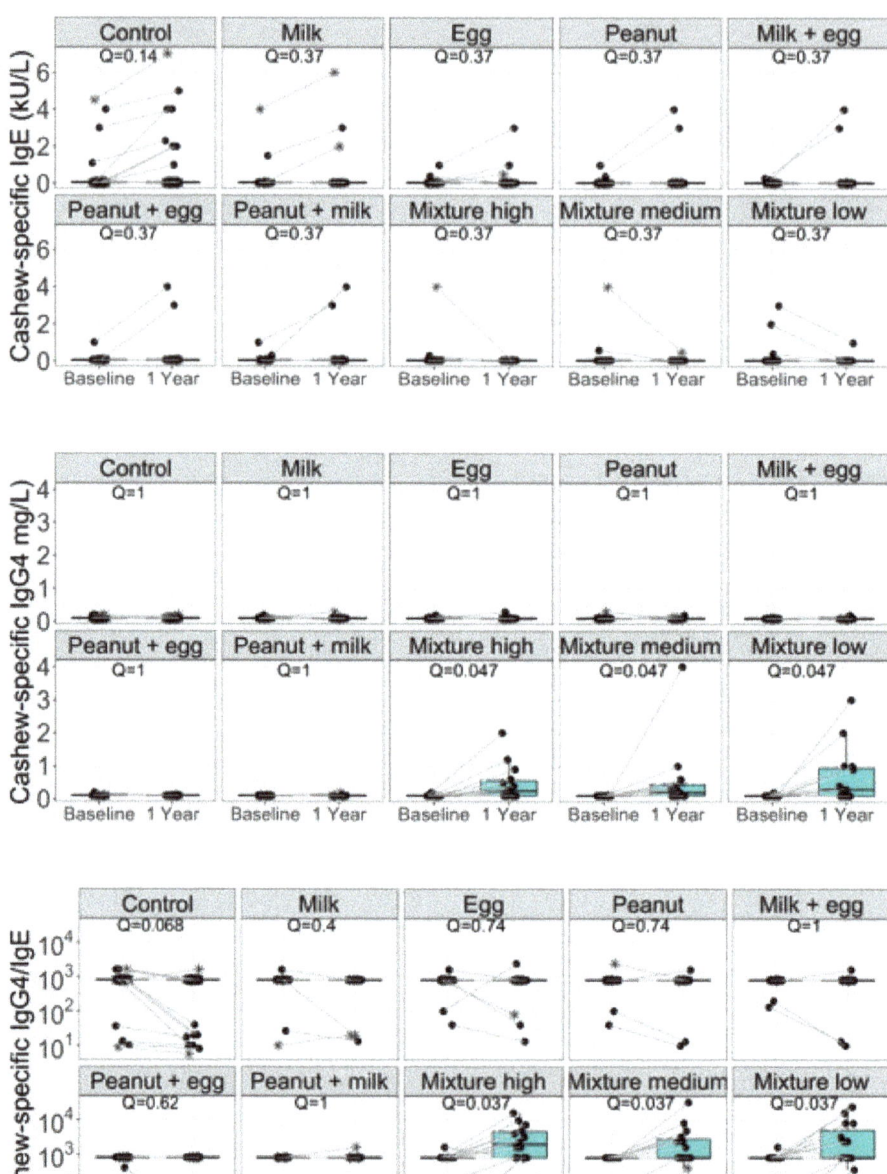

(b)

Figure 3. *Cont.*

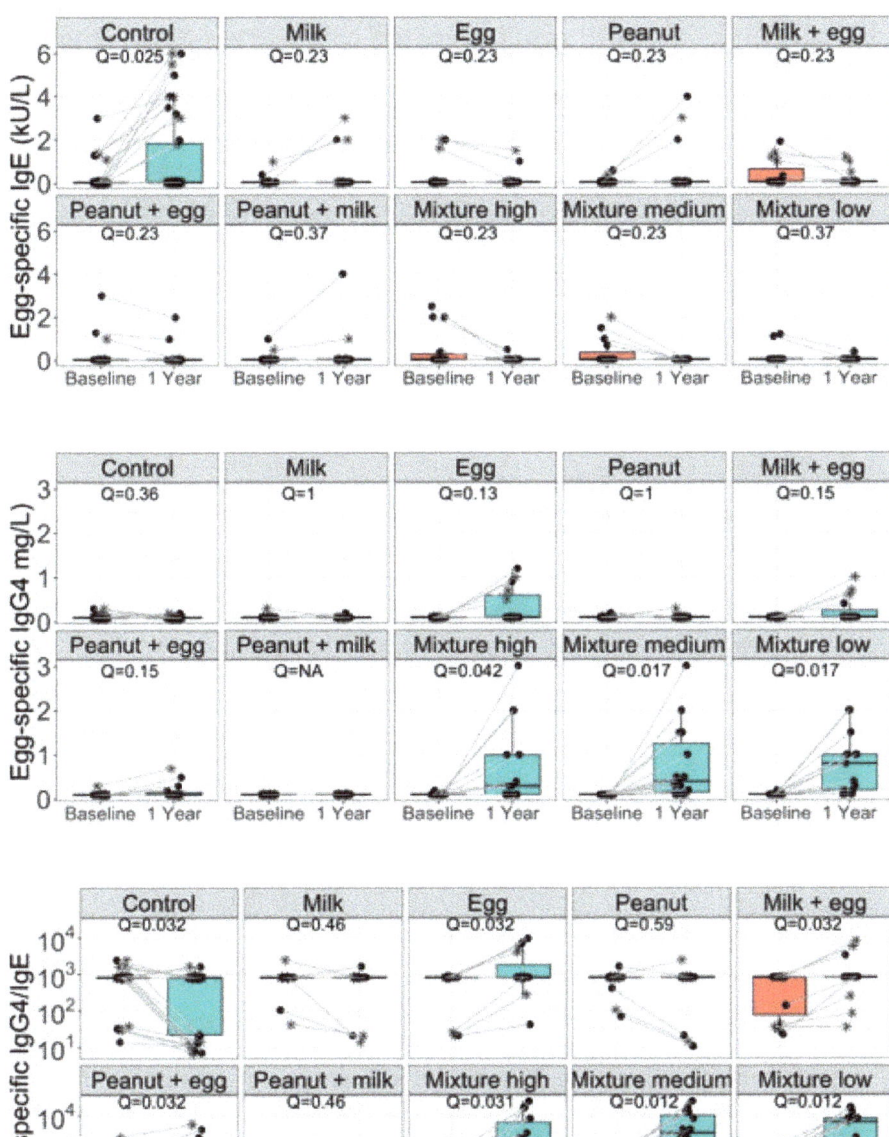

(c)

Figure 3. *Cont.*

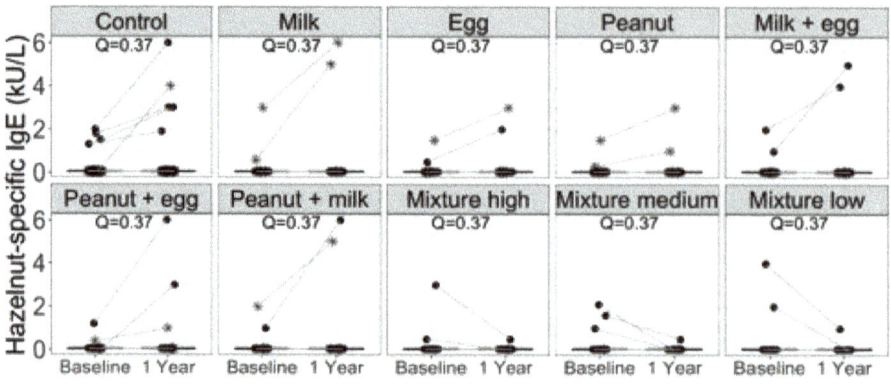
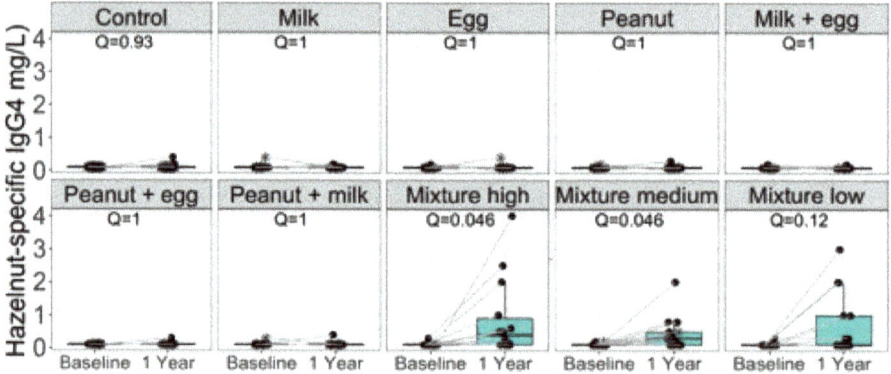
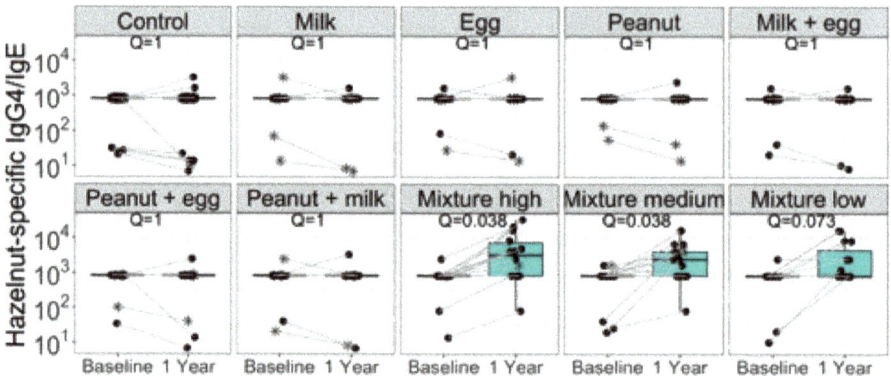

(d)

Figure 3. *Cont.*

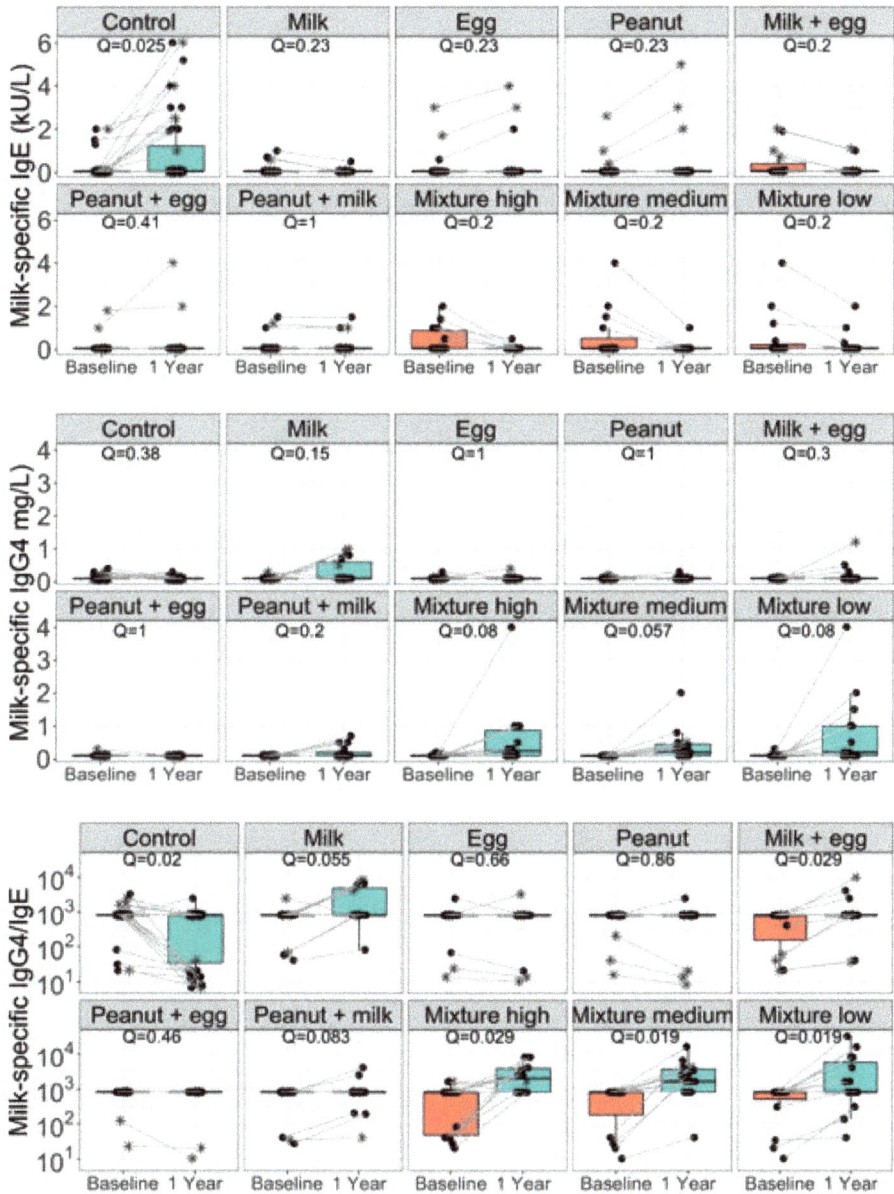

(e)

Figure 3. Cont.

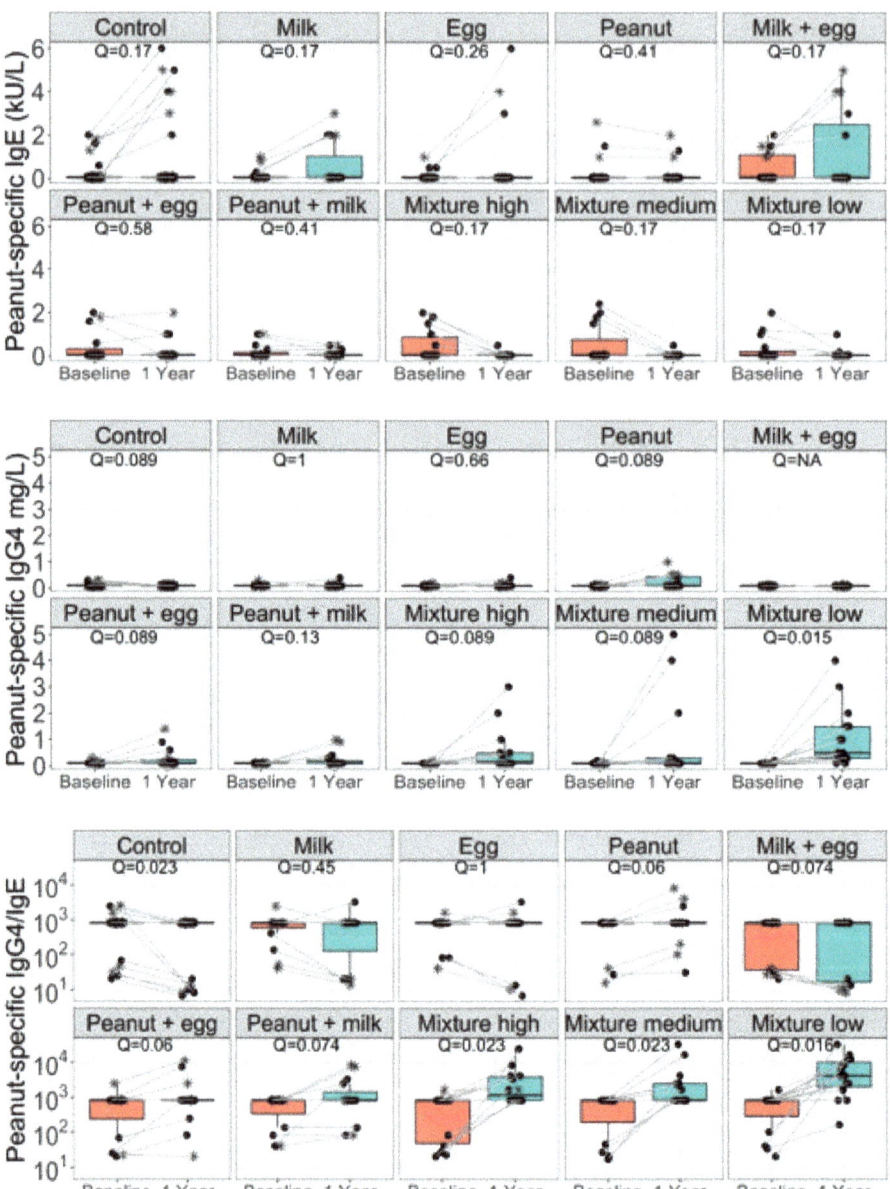

(f)

Figure 3. *Cont.*

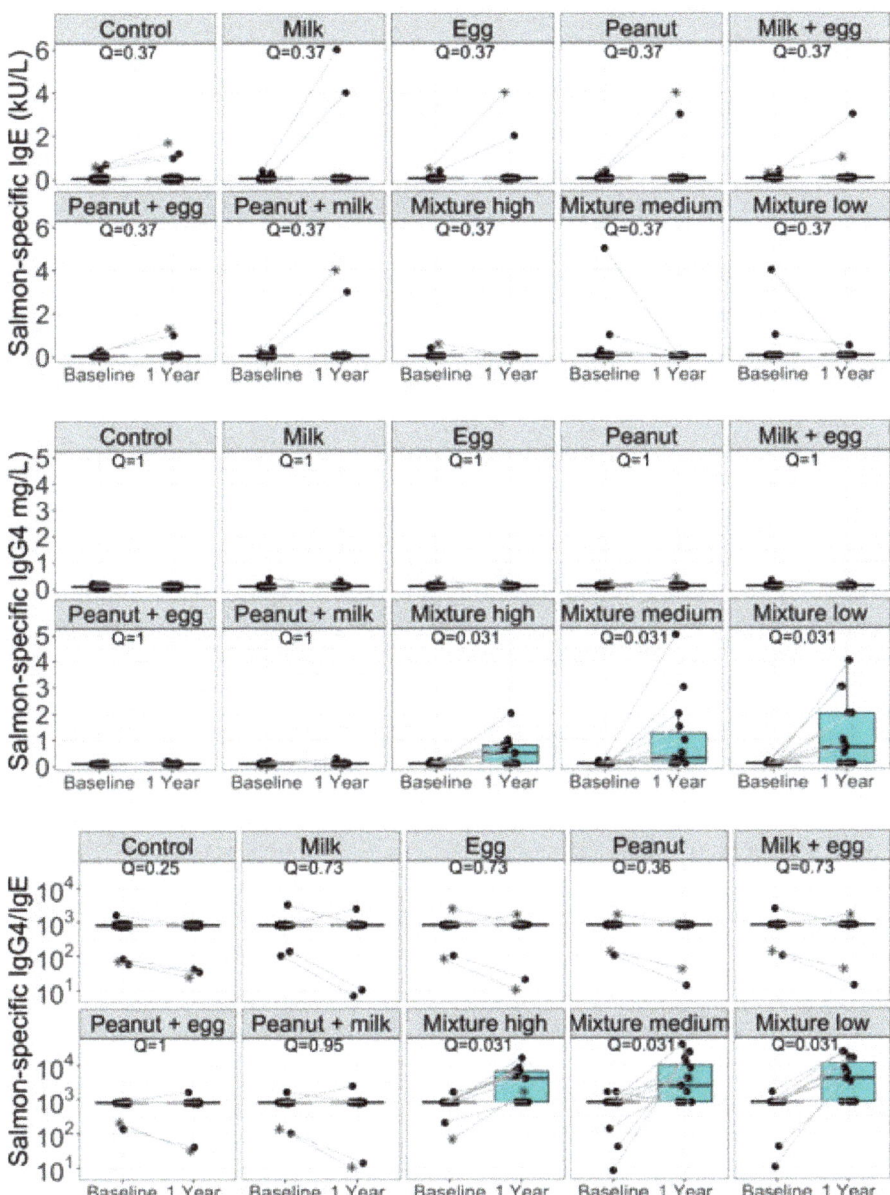

(g)

Figure 3. *Cont.*

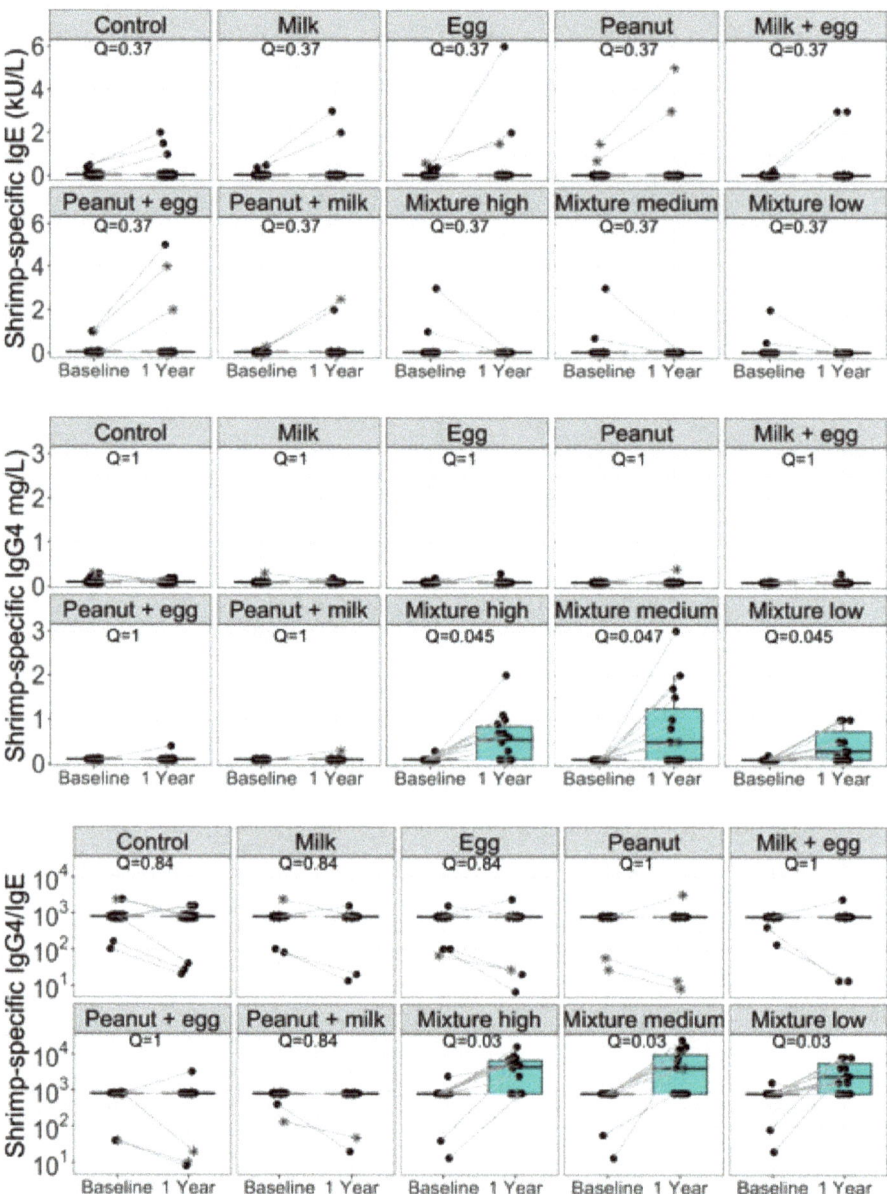

(h)

Figure 3. Cont.

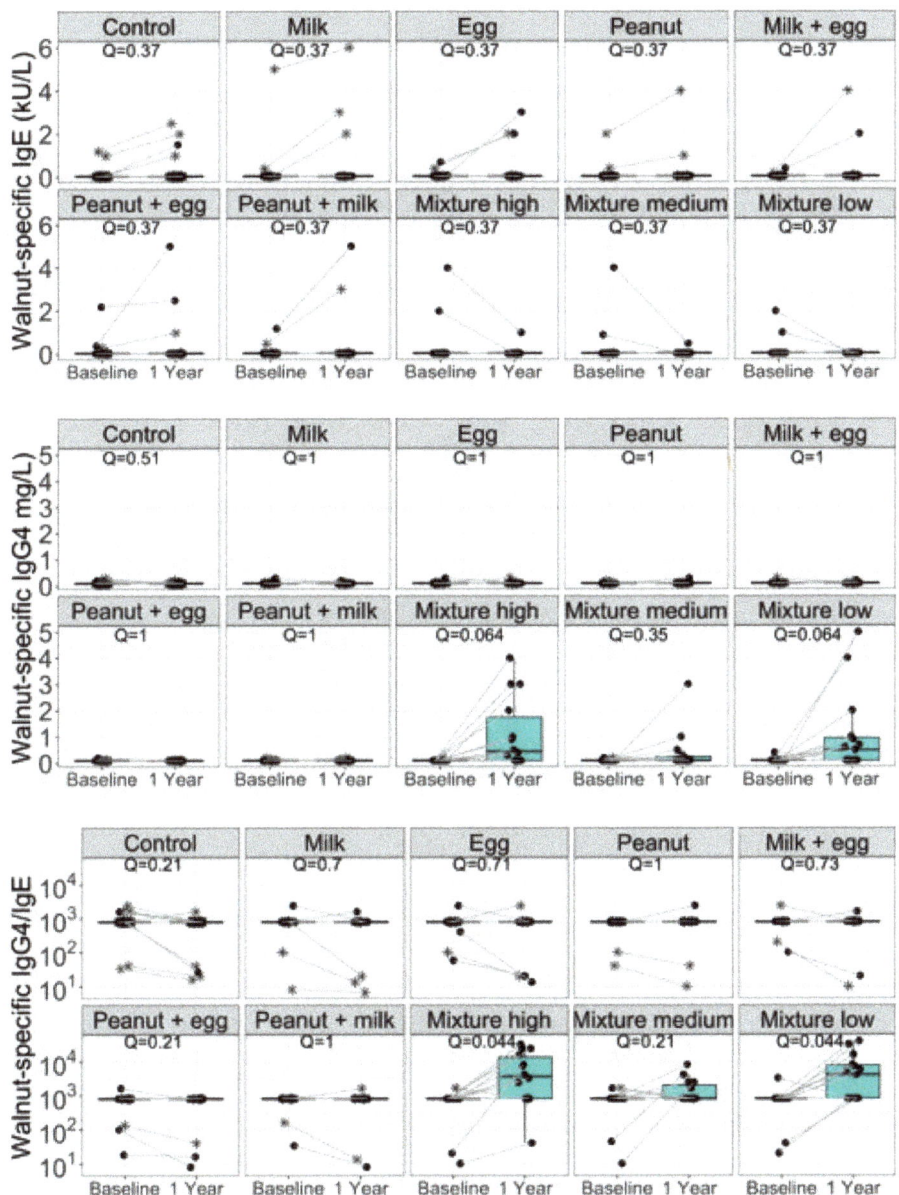

(i)

Figure 3. Cont.

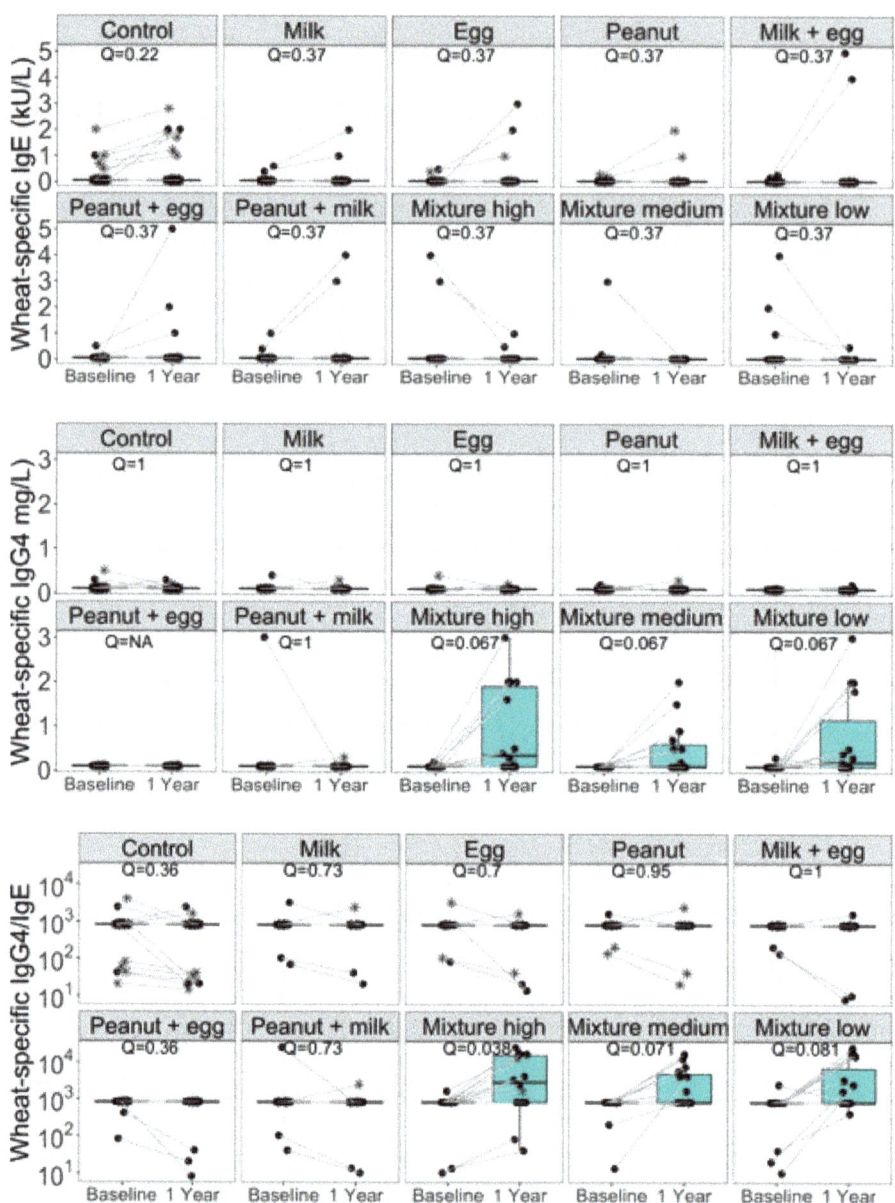

(j)

Figure 3. Allergen-specific IgG4, IgE and IgG4/IgE ratios for (**a**) Almond; (**b**) Cashew; (**c**) Egg; (**d**) Hazelnut; (**e**) Milk; (**f**) Peanut; (**g**) Salmon; (**h**) Shrimp; (**i**) Walnut and (**j**) Wheat are compared for controls, single, double, and multi-allergen groups (high, medium, and low) at baseline and after one year from the start of the study.

4. Discussion and Conclusions

While a number of studies have established the safety and efficacy of the early introduction of single allergens in infants for the prevention of FA, few studies have evaluated the dose, timing, and number of allergens that can be safely introduced in infants, particularly in those with eczema or those at high risk of atopy [29]. We therefore conducted a study to determine the safety and efficacy of the early introduction of single, double, and multiple allergens in infants for the prevention of FAs.

Our data from this pilot study suggest that consumption of single, double, and multiple allergens daily in infants is likely safe at up to 3000 mgs of protein. No increases in the incidence of eczema were observed in infants in the control or active groups, even in infants who had eczema at enrollment or those at high risk of atopy. The safety of multiple allergen introduction has been supported by a few other studies. The Holl study fed infants up to 16 allergens simultaneously with no adverse events. However, it should be noted that in the Holl study, the total protein amount in the allergen mix was only 480 mg, an amount much lower than the highest amount used in our study. Furthermore, the study only recruited healthy infants with no severe eczema. The EAT study, which also concluded that the early introduction of multiple allergens in infants was safe, differed from our study in that multiple allergens were introduced sequentially rather than simultaneously, and infants were recruited from the general population. The amount used in the EAT study (2000 mgs) was also lower than that used in our study (3000 mgs). The study by Cox et al. found infrequent reactions (0.1%) to early introduction of allergenic products similar or lower to what would be expected in a typical US infant population, indicating that early introduction with low doses is within safety parameters for typical feeding [30].

In our study, each food challenge consisted of several escalating doses of the food protein in flour or powder form concealed in an appropriate vehicle, such as applesauce or pudding, ingested by the participant every 15 min as tolerated. Typically, challenges started with 2 mg and escalated upto a max of 8 g of total food protein as per our validated methods [26–28]. Results from these food challenges as well as biomarker data from our study suggest that a daily dose of multiple allergens may be efficacious for the prevention of FA, even at low amounts (total 300 mg or 30 mg of each protein). This amount was found to be sufficient for decreasing positive food challenge responses and increasing specific food allergens IgG4/IgE. Our study found no difference in sIgE levels for all ten allergens between baseline and one year in the active groups. However, the sIgG4/sIgE ratio for all 10 allergens were significantly increased for mixtures (low, medium, and high) at the one-year time point compared to baseline. The change in the sIgG4/sIgE ratio was due to increases in IgG4 rather than decreases in sIgE. The results of this study are similar to other studies which have shown that sIgE and sIgG4 are indicative of allergy and tolerance, respectively. In the LEAP study, peanut-specific IgG4 increased in the peanut consumption group while a greater percentage of participants in the avoidance group had elevated titers of peanut-specific IgE [11]. A large randomized trial of egg introduction from 4 months of age in infants at risk for egg allergy found that levels of IgG4 to egg proteins and IgG4/IgE ratios were higher in those randomized to egg than in controls at 12 months; however, there was no significant difference in egg-specific sIgE levels at 12 months [31]. Numerous immunotherapy studies in children for FA have also found an increased ratio of sIgG4/sIgE to be indicative of tolerance [26,32–36]. Overall, the results from this pilot study demonstrate superior efficacy in food challenge outcomes in those individuals fed with the multiple mixture vs. single and vs. double as early introduction. A possible reason why the efficacy data shown in our study for multiple allergens is improved over single or double food early intervention could be due to a synchronous effect in inducing tolerance. It has been hypothesized that consumption of multiple allergens simultaneously increases polyclonal T cell memory subsets, increasing Th1 receptor diversity, leading to enhanced protection against potentially allergenic proteins compared to double or single food early intervention [37].

We believe regular daily dosing of small amounts of mixed food proteins was key to the success of this study. Participants reported that remembering to eat the powder mixture daily in small amounts was easier than if they were to dose 2–3 times a week with a larger serving of many foods. In comparison, in the EAT study [18], the mixture of allergens was prepared at patients' homes; individually prepared allergen mixes could be associated with dosing/serving size variations. Use of premixed allergens as used in this study would reduce this variability. Lastly, families who had taken the mixture of foods as an early intervention felt more comfortable having their children eat table foods.

The results of this pilot study suggest that the consumption of small convenient amounts of multiple allergens daily (even those with eczema or those at high risk of atopy) for the prevention of food allergies may be safe and efficacious. Larger, randomized controlled studies are needed to confirm these results. Although 3000 mg of allergenic protein was found to be safe, this high amount is impractical and can lead to noncompliance [19]. It would not impede optimal nutrient intake in the infant per USDA feeding guidelines for infants. The low mixture amount (300 mg protein) used in our study does not add significant calories and is not a substitute for foods, but instead the clinical data here shows that it can be easily used with breast feeding and/or table foods when the child is ready.

5. Patents

The following patent is associated with this work: "Special Oral Formula for Decreasing Food Allergy Risk and Treatment for Food Allergy".

Author Contributions: A.Z.Q., T.A.L. and V.S. wrote the article; R.D. and K.G.J. wrote article and drew figures; A.T. and M.W. manufactured the (allergenic) substance; R.S.C. and S.S. conducted the study, S.C. created the statistical analysis plan, performed the analysis, reviewed, and revised the manuscript, and K.C.N. conducted the study and wrote and reviewed the article. All authors have read and agreed to the published version of the manuscript.

Funding: Sean N. Parker Center for Allergy and Asthma Research at Stanford University.

Institutional Review Board Statement: This study was conducted according to the guidelines of the Declaration of Helsinki and approved by Stanford IRB study protocol (8629) approved June 2015.

Informed Consent Statement: Informed consent was obtained from all subjects involved in the study

Data Availability Statement: The data presented in this study are available on request from the corresponding author. The data are not publicly available as the patent is owned by a company and Stanford and permission is needed before release of data.

Conflicts of Interest: Sindher reports grants from NIH, Regeneron, DBV, AIMMUNE, Novartis, CoFAR, and FARE. She receives personal fees from Astra Zeneca, DBV, and honoraria from FARE. Chinthrajah reports grants from NIAID, CoFAR, Aimmune, DBV Technologies, Astellas, Regeneron, Stanford Maternal and Child Health Research Institute (MCHRI), and FARE. She is an Advisory Board Member at Alladapt Therapeutics, Novartis, Genentech, Sanofi, Allergenis, and Nutricia. Nadeau reports grants from National Institute of Allergy and Infectious Diseases (NIAID), National Heart, Lung, and Blood Institute (NHLBI), National Institute of Environmental Health Sciences (NIEHS), and Food Allergy Research & Education (FARE); stock options from IgGenix, Seed Health, ClostraBio, and ImmuneID; is Director of World Allergy Organization (WAO), Advisor at Cour Pharma, Consultant for Excellergy, Red tree ventures, Eli Lilly, and Phylaxis, Co-founder of Before Brands, Alladapt, Latitude, and IgGenix; and National Scientific Committee member at Immune Tolerance Network (ITN), and National Institutes of Health (NIH) clinical research centers, outside the submitted work; patents include, "Mixed allergen composition and methods for using the same", "Granulocyte-based methods for detecting and monitoring immune system disorders", "Methods and Assays for Detecting and Quantifying Pure Subpopulations of White Blood Cells in Immune System Disorders," and "Methods of isolating allergen-specific antibodies from humans and uses thereof." All other authors indicated no Conflict of Interest.

Appendix A

Table A1. Number of infants fed more than 10 foods as table foods by one year of age.

Allergen Group	N
Mixture (low dose)	15 (100%)
Mixture (medium dose)	14 (93%)
Mixture (high dose)	15 (100%)
Control	7 (15.5%)
Peanut	10 (66.7%)
Milk	8 (53.3%)
Egg	9 (60.0%)
Peanut/milk	11 (73.3%)
Milk/egg	10 (66.7%)
Egg/peanut	8 (53.3%)

References

1. Allen, K.J.; Koplin, J.J. The Epidemiology of IgE-Mediated Food Allergy and Anaphylaxis. *Immunol. Allergy Clin. N. Am.* **2012**, *32*, 35–50. [CrossRef] [PubMed]
2. Jackson, K.D.; Howie, L.D.; Akinbami, L.J. Trends in allergic conditions among children: United States, 1997–2011. *NCHS Data Brief* **2013**, *121*, 1–8.
3. Tang, M.L.K.; Mullins, R.J. Food allergy: Is prevalence increasing? *Intern. Med. J.* **2017**, *47*, 256–261. [CrossRef]
4. Gupta, R.S.; Warren, C.M.; Smith, B.M.; Blumenstock, J.A.; Jiang, J.; Davis, M.M.; Nadeau, K.C. The Public Health Impact of Parent-Reported Childhood Food Allergies in the United States. *Pediatrics* **2018**, *142*, e20181235. [CrossRef] [PubMed]
5. Gupta, R.S.; Warren, C.M.; Smith, B.M.; Jiang, J.; Blumenstock, J.A.; Davis, M.M.; Schleimer, R.P.; Nadeau, K.C. Prevalence and Severity of Food Allergies Among US Adults. *JAMA Netw. Open* **2019**, *2*, e185630. [CrossRef] [PubMed]
6. Greenhawt, M. Food allergy quality of life and living with food allergy. *Curr. Opin. Allergy Clin. Immunol.* **2016**, *16*, 284–290. [CrossRef]
7. Bergmann, M.M.; Caubet, J.-C.; Boguniewicz, M.; Eigenmann, P. Evaluation of Food Allergy in Patients with Atopic Dermatitis. *J. Allergy Clin. Immunol. Pract.* **2013**, *1*, 22–28. [CrossRef]
8. Cox, A.; Sicherer, S.H. Peanut and Tree Nut Allergy. *Monoclonal Antibody Therapy* **2015**, *101*, 131–144. [CrossRef]
9. Ebisawa, M.; Ito, K.; Fujisawa, T. Japanese guidelines for food allergy 2017. *Allergol. Int.* **2017**, *66*, 248–264. [CrossRef]
10. Zeiger, R.S. Food allergen avoidance in the prevention of food allergy in infants and children. *Pediatrics* **2003**, *111*, 1662–1671. [CrossRef]
11. Du Toit, G.; Roberts, G.; Sayre, P.H.; Bahnson, H.T.; Radulovic, S.; Santos, A.; Brough, H.; Phippard, D.; Basting, M.; Feeney, M.; et al. Randomized Trial of Peanut Consumption in Infants at Risk for Peanut Allergy. *N. Engl. J. Med.* **2015**, *372*, 803–813. [CrossRef] [PubMed]
12. Ierodiakonou, D.; Larsen, V.G.; Logan, A.; Groome, A.; Cunha, S.; Chivinge, J.; Robinson, Z.; Geoghegan, N.; Jarrold, K.; Reeves, T.; et al. Timing of Allergenic Food Introduction to the Infant Diet and Risk of Allergic or Autoimmune Disease. *JAMA J. Am. Med. Assoc.* **2016**, *316*, 1181–1192. [CrossRef]
13. Roduit, C.; Frei, R.; Depner, M.; Schaub, B.; Loss, G.; Genuneit, J.; Pfefferle, P.; Hyvärinen, A.; Karvonen, A.M.; Riedler, J.; et al. Increased food diversity in the first year of life is inversely associated with allergic diseases. *J. Allergy Clin. Immunol.* **2014**, *133*, 1056–1064. [CrossRef]
14. Venter, C.; Maslin, K.; Holloway, J.; Silveira, L.J.; Fleischer, D.M.; Dean, T.; Arshad, S.H. Different Measures of Diet Diversity During Infancy and the Association with Childhood Food Allergy in a UK Birth Cohort Study. *J. Allergy Clin. Immunol. Pract.* **2020**, *8*, 2017–2026. [CrossRef] [PubMed]
15. Venter, C.; Greenhawt, M.; Meyer, R.W.; Agostoni, C.; Reese, I.; du Toit, G.; Feeney, M.; Maslin, K.; Nwaru, B.I.; Roduit, C.; et al. EAACI position paper on diet diversity in pregnancy, infancy and childhood: Novel concepts and implications for studies in allergy and asthma. *Allergy* **2020**, *75*, 497–523. [CrossRef]
16. Koplin, J.J.; Allen, K.J.; Tang, M.L.K. Important risk factors for the development of food allergy and potential options for prevention. *Expert Rev. Clin. Immunol.* **2019**, *15*, 147–152. [CrossRef] [PubMed]
17. Du Toit, G.; Sayre, P.H.; Roberts, G.; Lawson, K.; Sever, M.L.; Bahnson, H.T.; Fisher, H.; Feeney, M.; Radulovic, S.; Basting, M.; et al. Allergen specificity of early peanut consumption and effect on development of allergic disease in the Learning Early About Peanut Allergy study cohort. *J. Allergy Clin. Immunol.* **2018**, *141*, 1343–1353. [CrossRef] [PubMed]
18. Perkin, M.; Logan, K.; Tseng, A.; Raji, B.; Ayis, S.; Peacock, J.; Brough, H.; Marrs, T.; Radulovic, S.; Craven, J.; et al. Randomized Trial of Introduction of Allergenic Foods in Breast-Fed Infants. *N. Engl. J. Med.* **2016**, *374*, 1733–1743. [CrossRef]
19. USDA. Infant Nutrition and Feeding. 2019. Available online: https://wicworks.fns.usda.gov/resources/infant-nutrition-and-feeding-guide (accessed on 12 January 2022).

20. Holl, J.L.; Bilaver, L.A.; Finn, D.J.; Savio, K. A randomized trial of the acceptability of a daily multi-allergen food supplement for infants. *Pediatr. Allergy Immunol.* **2020**, *31*, 418–420. [CrossRef]
21. Ashley, S.; Dang, T.; Koplin, J.; Martino, D.; Prescott, S. Food for thought. *Curr. Opin. Allergy Clin. Immunol.* **2015**, *15*, 237–242. [CrossRef]
22. Halken, S.; Muraro, A.; de Silva, D.; Khaleva, E.; Angier, E.; Arasi, S.; Arshad, H.; Bahnson, H.T.; Beyer, K.; Boyle, R.; et al. EAACI guideline: Preventing the development of food allergy in infants and young children (2020 update). *Pediatr. Allergy Immunol.* **2021**, *32*, 843–858. [CrossRef] [PubMed]
23. Fleischer, D.M.; Chan, E.S.; Venter, C.; Spergel, J.M.; Abrams, E.M.; Stukus, D.; Groetch, M.; Shaker, M.; Greenhawt, M. A Consensus Approach to the Primary Prevention of Food Allergy Through Nutrition: Guidance from the American Academy of Allergy, Asthma, and Immunology; American College of Allergy, Asthma, and Immunology; and the Canadian Society for Allergy and Clinical Immunology. *J. Allergy Clin. Immunol. Pract.* **2021**, *9*, 22–43. [CrossRef] [PubMed]
24. Greer, F.R.; Sicherer, S.H.; Burks, A.W.; Committee on Nutrition, Section on Allergy and Immunology. The Effects of Early Nutritional Interventions on the Development of Atopic Disease in Infants and Children: The Role of Maternal Dietary Restriction, Breastfeeding, Hydrolyzed Formulas, and Timing of Introduction of Allergenic Complementary Foods. *Pediatrics* **2019**, *143*, e20190281. [CrossRef] [PubMed]
25. Koplin, J.J.; Allen, K.J.; Gurrin, L.C.; Peters, R.L.; Lowe, A.J.; Tan, H.-T.T.; Dharmage, S.C. The Impact of Family History of Allergy on Risk of Food Allergy: A Population-Based Study of Infants. *Int. J. Environ. Res. Public Health* **2013**, *10*, 5364–5377. [CrossRef]
26. Chinthrajah, R.S.; Purington, N.; Andorf, S.; Long, A.; O'Laughlin, K.L.; Lyu, S.C.; Manohar, M.; Boyd, S.D.; Tibshirani, R.; Maecker, H.; et al. Sustained outcomes in oral immunotherapy for peanut allergy (POISED study): A large, randomised, double-blind, placebo-controlled, phase 2 study. *Lancet* **2019**, *394*, 1437–1449. [CrossRef]
27. Jones, S.M.; Kim, E.H.; Nadeau, K.C.; Nowak-Wegrzyn, A.; Wood, R.A.; Sampson, H.A.; Scurlock, A.M.; Chinthrajah, S.; Wang, J.; Pesek, R.D.; et al. Efficacy and safety of oral immunotherapy in children aged 1–3 years with peanut allergy (the Immune Tolerance Network IMPACT trial): A randomised placebo-controlled study. *Lancet* **2022**, *399*, 359–371. [CrossRef]
28. Purington, N.; Chinthrajah, R.S.; Long, A.; Sindher, S.; Andorf, S.; O'Laughlin, K.; Woch, M.A.; Scheiber, A.; Assa'ad, A.; Pongracic, J.; et al. Eliciting Dose and Safety Outcomes From a Large Dataset of Standardized Multiple Food Challenges. *Front. Immunol.* **2018**, *9*, 2057. [CrossRef]
29. Schroer, B.; Groetch, M.; Mack, D.P.; Venter, C. Practical Challenges and Considerations for Early Introduction of Potential Food Allergens for Prevention of Food Allergy. *J. Allergy Clin. Immunol. Pract.* **2021**, *9*, 44–56. [CrossRef]
30. Cox, A.L.; Shah, A.; Groetch, M.; Sicherer, S.H. Allergic reactions in infants using commercial early allergen introduction products. *J. Allergy Clin. Immunol. Pract.* **2021**, *9*, 3517–3520. [CrossRef]
31. Tan, J.W.-L.; Valerio, C.; Barnes, E.H.; Turner, P.J.; van Asperen, P.A.; Kakakios, A.M.; Campbell, D.E. A randomized trial of egg introduction from 4 months of age in infants at risk for egg allergy. *J. Allergy Clin. Immunol.* **2017**, *139*, 1621–1628. [CrossRef]
32. Kulis, M.; Yue, X.; Guo, R.; Zhang, H.; Orgel, K.; Ye, P.; Li, Q.; Liu, Y.; Kim, E.; Burks, A.W.; et al. High- and low-dose oral immunotherapy similarly suppress pro-allergic cytokines and basophil activation in young children. *Clin. Exp. Allergy* **2019**, *49*, 180–189. [CrossRef] [PubMed]
33. Santos, A.F.; Brough, H. Making the Most of In Vitro Tests to Diagnose Food Allergy. *J. Allergy Clin. Immunol. Pract.* **2017**, *5*, 237–248. [CrossRef] [PubMed]
34. Jones, S.M.; Pons, L.; Roberts, J.L.; Scurlock, A.M.; Perry, T.T.; Kulis, M.; Shreffler, W.G.; Steele, P.; Henry, K.A.; Adair, M.; et al. Clinical efficacy and immune regulation with peanut oral immunotherapy. *J. Allergy Clin. Immunol.* **2009**, *124*, 292–300. [CrossRef] [PubMed]
35. Vickery, B.P.; Lin, J.; Kulis, M.; Fu, Z.; Steele, P.H.; Jones, S.M.; Scurlock, A.M.; Gimenez, G.; Bardina, L.; Sampson, H.A.; et al. Peanut oral immunotherapy modifies IgE and IgG4 responses to major peanut allergens. *J. Allergy Clin. Immunol.* **2013**, *131*, 128–134. [CrossRef]
36. Varshney, P.; Jones, S.M.; Scurlock, A.M.; Perry, T.T.; Kemper, A.; Steele, P.; Hiegel, A.; Kamilaris, J.; Carlisle, S.; Yue, X.; et al. A randomized controlled study of peanut oral immunotherapy: Clinical desensitization and modulation of the allergic response. *J. Allergy Clin. Immunol.* **2011**, *127*, 654–660. [CrossRef]
37. Sampath, V.; Nadeau, K.C. Newly identified T cell subsets in mechanistic studies of food immunotherapy. *J. Clin. Investig.* **2019**, *129*, 1431–1440. [CrossRef]

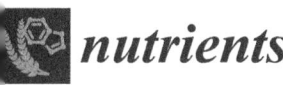

Review

Relevance of Early Introduction of Cow's Milk Proteins for Prevention of Cow's Milk Allergy

Laurien Ulfman [1], Angela Tsuang [2], Aline B. Sprikkelman [3,4], Anne Goh [5] and R. J. Joost van Neerven [1,6,*]

1. FrieslandCampina, 3818 LA Amersfoort, The Netherlands; laurien.ulfman@frieslandcampina.com
2. Division of Allergy & Immunology, Department of Pediatrics, Icahn School of Medicine at Mount Sinai, New York, NY 10029, USA; angela.tsuang@mountsinai.org
3. Department of Pediatric Pulmonology and Pediatric Allergology, University Medical Center Groningen, University of Groningen, 9713 GZ Groningen, The Netherlands; a.b.sprikkelman@umcg.nl
4. University Medical Center Groningen, GRIAC Research Institute, University of Groningen, 9713 RB Groningen, The Netherlands
5. Department of Paediatrics, KK Women's and Children's Hospital, Singapore 229899, Singapore; anne.goh.e.n@singhealth.com.sg
6. Cell Biology and Immunology, Wageningen University, 6700 AH Wageningen, The Netherlands
* Correspondence: joost.vanneerven@wur.nl

Abstract: Food allergy incidence has increased worldwide over the last 20 years. For prevention of food allergy, current guidelines do not recommend delaying the introduction of allergenic foods. Several groundbreaking studies, such as the Learning Early About Peanut Allergy study, showed that the relatively early introduction of this allergenic food between 4–6 months of age reduces the risk of peanut allergy. However, less is known about the introduction of cow's milk, as many children already receive cow's-milk-based formula much earlier in life. This can be regular cow's milk formula with intact milk proteins or hydrolyzed formulas. Several recent studies have investigated the effects of early introduction of cow's-milk-based formulas with intact milk proteins on the development of cow's milk allergy while breastfeeding. These studies suggest that depending on the time of introduction and the duration of administration of cow's milk, the risk of cow's milk allergy can be reduced (early introduction) or increased (very early introduction followed by discontinuation). The aim of this narrative review is to summarize these studies and to discuss the impact of early introduction of intact cow's milk protein—as well as hydrolyzed milk protein formulas—and the development of tolerance versus allergy towards cow's milk proteins.

Keywords: early introduction; food allergy; milk protein; prevention; cow's milk allergy (CMA)

1. Introduction

Food allergy is an immune reaction to the ingestion of food that is either IgE-mediated or non-IgE-mediated. The IgE-mediated allergic reaction is best understood and develops as a type 1 allergic reaction [1]. In food-allergen-sensitized individuals, the allergen induces an immediate response, typically within the first 2 h, leading to clinical symptoms that may involve the following systems: gastrointestinal, skin, respiratory, and cardiovascular [2]. Allergic reactions can occur to over 100 different foods, but egg, milk, and peanut allergens are the most common among children in Western countries, with egg and milk being particularly common under one year of age [3]. In analogy with the increased prevalence of asthma [4], the incidence in food allergies has increased considerably over the last few decades [5–8]. This is reflected by the atopic march theory that states that allergic diseases start in infancy with atopic dermatitis and food allergy and later progress to the development of allergic asthma and allergic rhinitis [9]. Allergic diseases are strongly associated with Westernized lifestyle and feeding practices, as prevalence in developing countries is also rising [10].

One of the key questions in relation to food allergy is when potentially allergenic foods should be introduced into the diet of infants to induce tolerance. As a result of several intervention trials on early introduction of food allergens, such as peanut and egg, there is increasing scientific consensus that earlier introduction of these foods can be recommended [11].

However, compared to other food allergens, the situation is quite different for the introduction of cow's milk, as infants may in practice—when not exclusively breastfed—be exposed to cow's milk proteins in cow's-milk-based formula (CMF) at any time before 4 months and sometimes already in the first days of their life. Moreover, infants can also be exposed to low amounts of milk and other food proteins through breastmilk [12–18]. A large proportion of exclusively breastfed infants will not be introduced to dairy until they are weaned from breastfeeding. The most common allergens in cow's milk are beta-lactoglobulin and caseins (beta, alpha s1 and s2, and kappa). The high prevalence of allergic patients with beta-lactoglobulin-specific IgE is explained by the absence of this protein in human milk. However, other whey proteins (bovine alpha-lactalbumin and bovine serum albumin (BSA)) have also been described as cow's milk allergens [19].

Recent insights have increased our knowledge about the relationship between the timing and dose of cow's milk exposure and the development of cow's milk allergy (CMA). Therefore, the aim of this review is to summarize what is known about the timing of introduction of cow's milk protein in early life and its influence on the development of tolerance versus allergy. We will discriminate between very early (first days of life) and early (first weeks to months of life) introduction and discuss the role of hydrolysates in the prevention of cow's milk allergy.

2. Early Introduction of Food Allergens

For many years, dietary guidelines to prevent food allergy recommended a delayed introduction of food allergens into the diet of infants. This has changed in recent years following the publication of several studies that indicated that early introduction of food allergens may actually help to induce tolerance and thus prevent the development of food allergy, specifically for peanut and egg [20–23]. In addition, several studies have shown that the diversity of the diet in the first year of life is also associated with a lower incidence of food allergies [24]. The first insights for a tolerance-inducing effect when exposed to allergens early in life came from observational studies. It was found that the prevalence of peanut allergy among Jewish children in the UK was much higher compared to Israel, and the main difference was that a much higher percentage of children had ingested peanut protein in their diets by the age of 9 months in Israel compared to the UK [25]. This observation led to the Learning Early About Peanut Allergy (LEAP) study, in which the development of peanut allergy was studied in high-risk infants with eczema with or without egg allergy. The infants were enrolled between 4 to 11 months of age and randomized to avoid or consume peanut at a dose of 6 g of peanut protein/week. This study clearly demonstrated that the risk of peanut allergy at 5 years of age was significantly lower in the group that consumed peanuts (3.4%) compared to the avoidance group (20.3%) (ITT, 95% CI; 3.4 to 20.3; $p < 0.001$) [20,26]. The subsequent Enquiring About Tolerance (EAT) Study evaluated the effects of early introduction of six foods (peanut, egg, cow's milk, sesame, whitefish, and wheat) in infants between 3 to 6 months of age alongside continued breastfeeding in comparison to exclusive breastfeeding until 6 months of age. The EAT study reported a significant decrease in the number of children from a general population developing peanut and egg allergy by 3 years of age in the per protocol analysis despite reported difficulties in adherence to the protocol [22]. However, the rates of other food allergies, including milk allergy, were not high enough to show significant effects. Nevertheless, the average relative risk of a positive skin-prick test at the age of 36 months to six food allergens was 79% lower in the early-introduction group compared to the standard food introduction group; These findings reached significance for peanut ($p = 0.007$), milk ($p = 0.02$), and sesame ($p = 0.04$). In addition to the EAT study, there are several randomized controlled trials that have investigated the effects of early egg introduction (STAR [27], HEALTHNUTS [28], STEP [29], HEAP [30], EAT [22], BEAT [31], PETIT [32]). A meta-analysis by Ierodiakonou [21] included five trials (1915 participants) and concluded that there was evidence with moderate certainty that introduction of egg at 4 to 6 months was associated with a lower egg allergy risk (risk ratio [RR], 0.56; 95% CI, 0.36–0.87; I^2 = 36%; p = 0.009). Although a recent pilot study suggested that the early introduction of mixtures of many allergenic foods may be safe and efficacious for preventing food allergy [33], the practicality and safety of this approach should be carefully evaluated in future studies with such products. To prevent food allergy, the dosage of allergens should be sufficient and has been reported to be too low in some other commercial preparations [34]. Furthermore, a disadvantage of providing a mixture of multiple allergens is that when an allergic reaction occurs, it requires additional investigations to ascertain which allergen was responsible for the reaction. It is not clear if such a reaction to one of the allergens would also affect responses to other allergens in the mix.

As a result of all these new insights, guidelines have been updated in many different countries. These guidelines have been reviewed in a systematic review by Vale et al [11]. These changes are also illustrated in the policy document of the American Academy of Pediatrics [35,36] that shifted from the statement that "there are insufficient data to document a protective effect of any dietary intervention beyond 4 to 6 months of age for the development of atopic disease" in 2008 [35] to "There is no evidence that delaying the introduction of allergenic foods, including peanuts, eggs, and fish, beyond 4 to 6 months prevents atopic disease. There is now evidence that early introduction of peanuts may prevent peanut allergy" in 2019 [36]. In line with this, Fleischer et al. [37] recently published a consensus document with guidance to prevent food allergy on behalf of the American Academy of Allergy, Asthma & Immunology (AAAAI), American College of Allergy, Asthma & Immunology (ACAAI), and the Canadian Society of Allergy and Clinical Immunology (CSACI). Here, it was stated "to prevent peanut and/or egg allergy, both peanut and egg should be introduced around 6 months of life, but not before 4 months" and "other allergens should be introduced around this time as well. "Also, in other parts of the world, guidelines have been renewed [38] with careful guidance on the early introduction of allergenic food (egg, peanut) in high-risk infants (British Society for Allergy and Clinical Immunology (BSACI) 2018 [39], European Society for Paediatric Gastroenterology Hepatology and Nutrition (ESPGHAN) 2017 [40], National Institute of Allergy and Infectious Diseases (NIAID) 2017 [41]. The most recent European Academy of Allergy and Clinical Immunology (EAACI) guideline [42] not only provides guidance on egg and peanut introduction but also cow's milk introduction (as discussed below).

3. Early Introduction of Cow's Milk and Development of Cow's Milk Allergy

Multiple studies have shown that introduction of cow's milk protein in the first hours to days after birth followed by inconsistent incorporation into the diet is associated with increased risk of developing CMA (Table 1). Early studies showed that brief exposure to cows' milk during the first three days of life in breast fed children was not associated with atopic disease or allergic symptoms up to age 5 [43,44]. However, cow's milk allergy was not determined in these studies. Indeed, very early introduction of cow's milk formula supplementation in the first 24 h of life increased the development of CMA in infants who were exclusively breastfed, as shown by a retrospective case–controlled study conducted in Ireland on 55 cow's-milk-allergic infants born between 2010–2011 [45].

Using logistic regression, the only risk factor for developing CMA was formula supplementation in the first 24 h of life in exclusively breastfed infants (OR 7.01; 95%CI 1.79–27.01, p < 0.001). There was no increased risk of CMA in infants who were exclusively breastfed (without need for formula supplementation) or exclusively formula fed from birth onwards [45]. In another prospective study [46], it was found that infants that had been exclusively breastfed from birth and subsequently developed CMA had been supplemented with cow's milk formula in the first 3 days of life. In another retrospective observational study in IgE-mediated CMA children, exposure to isolated doses of formula feeding in the hospital followed by exclusive breastfeeding was identified as a risk factor in the development of CMA [47].

Furthermore, a prospective study in more than 6000 infants [48] supported this finding by showing that infants who required supplementary feeding and received CMF while in the maternity hospital in the first 3 days of life had an increased risk for developing CMA (OR, 1.54; 95% CI, 1.04–2.30; p = 0.03) as compared to infants who received an extensively hydrolyzed whey formula (OR 0.61;95%CI, 0.38–1.00). Thus, preventing exposure to intact cow's milk proteins through supplementation with extensively hydrolyzed cow's milk devoid of allergenic proteins in the first 3 days of life may reduce the risk of developing CMA. Of interest is the observation that the infants that developed CMA in the breastfeeding group supplemented with CMF had a lower intake of formula in the first 8 weeks of life compared to the infants that did not develop CMA in that group [48]. The early exposure to cow's milk followed by a period of avoidance of the cow's-milk-based formula once breastfeeding is established likely leads to this increase in CMA. Based on these insights, EAACI recommended to "Avoid supplementing with cow's milk formula in breastfed infants in the first week of life to prevent cow's milk allergy in infants and young children" [42].

In contrast, observational studies have found that early introduction (after the first days of life but within the first weeks of life) of cow's milk and continuation in the diet is associated with a lower chance of developing CMA [49,51,52], see Table 1. Thus, besides timing, the duration and frequency of allergen introduction during breastfeeding is of importance. The case–control study by Onizawa et al. demonstrated that early introduction of formula based on cow's milk was associated with a decrease in the incidence of cow's milk allergy of 51 IgE-mediated-cow's-milk-allergic infants compared to 102 healthy controls [49]. There were significantly increased odds (aOR 23.4, 95%CI 5.39–104.52) of developing CMA when introduction was delayed (starting > 1 month after birth) or ingestion was irregular (less than once daily), further supporting the importance of duration and frequency. Likewise, using data from a large Japanese birth cohort involving over 100,000 mother–child pairs, analysis performed on 80,408 children showed that the regular consumption of cow's milk based formula within the first 3 months of life was associated with a lower risk of CMA at 6 and 12 months (aRR 0.42, 95%CI 0.30–0.57 and aRR 0.44, 95%CI 0.38–0.51, respectively). [50]. Furthermore, prospective cohort studies from Melbourne, Australia [51] and Israel [52] also found evidence for an association between early introduction of cow's milk before the third and first month of life and a reduced likelihood of developing CMA. In the Australian study, the early exposure to cow's milk (before 3 months of life) in a predominantly breastfed group (87%) was associated with a significant risk reduction of cow's milk allergy (aOR 0.31, 95% CI 0.10–0.91) at 12 months of age. In the Israeli cohort, the greatest risk of developing cow's milk allergy was apparent in the group that introduced cow's milk between 3.5 and 6.5 months of age after being exclusively breastfed. They observed that the risk of IgE-mediated CMA was lower in the infants of Arab women than Jewish women, and this difference was attributed to the decreased likelihood for Arab mothers to exclusively breastfeed their infants, instead providing cow's-milk-based formula while breastfeeding. This finding supports the hypothesis that early and regular exposure to cow's milk in the context of breastfeeding is important. In line with this, a retrospective study by Sakihara et al. [53] showed that continuous ingestion of cow's milk reduced the risk of cow's milk allergy in a population of infants with hen's egg allergy based on positive oral food challenge. The infants were categorized into 4 groups: exclusively breast-fed, discontinuation of cow's milk formula before the age of 3 months (temporary formula group), continuous but not daily ingestion of cow's milk formula up to 3 months of age (non-daily group) and continuous ingestion of cow's milk formula at least once daily (daily group). The non-daily group and daily group had significantly lower odds to develop CMA (OR 0.43, p = 0.02 and OR 0.11, p < 0.001, respectively) compared to the breastfeeding reference group, whereas the temporary group did not show a significant difference in CMA (OR 0.75, p = NS). However, a systematic review and meta-analysis by

Ierodiakonou [21] showed that early introduction of cow's milk did not significantly reduce the risk for development of CMA compared to late introduction (early n = 762 vs. late n = 788) and was based on two intervention studies [54,55]. A possible effect in the Lowe study [54] could have been missed due to the selection of infants (high risk) and/or the relative low number of infants that were exposed early to milk and/or avoided allergenic foods—including dairy—in the first year of life. In the study by Perkin et al. [55], the aim was to investigate the effect of early introduction of cow's milk. The standard introduction group in the EAT study was allowed to supplement with CMF between 3 to 6 months of life if less than 300 mL, which already may have been enough to induce tolerance [55].

The best study design thus far to support early introduction and regular consumption of cow's milk to prevent CMA is provided by the SPADE study (Strategy for prevention of milk allergy by daily ingestion of infant formula in early infancy) [57]. This prospective multicenter, open-label randomized controlled trial conducted in Okinawa, Japan included infants from the general population who were ingesting cow's milk daily (ingestion group) from 1 to 2 months of age compared to an avoidance group that were supplemented with soy formula. Continuation of breastfeeding up to 3 and 6 months was high (89.5 vs. 89.7% and 72.2 vs. 67.7%, respectively, for ingestion vs. avoidance group). The ingestion group showed a significant reduction in CMA as diagnosed by open oral cow's milk challenge at 6 months compared to the avoidance group (risk ratio = 0.12; 95% CI = 0.01–0.50; $p < 0.001$). Furthermore, infants in the avoidance group also showed higher sensitization to cow's milk manifested as a positive skin prick test. Infants in the intervention group had higher casein-specific IgG4, supporting the hypothesis that tolerance induction is due to skewing of the immune response. The authors [57] concluded that cow's milk formula should be started early, before the first month of life, and should be continued daily to reduce the risk of cow's milk allergy while maintaining breastfeeding. The relatively high number of cow's-milk-allergic-infants in the soy formula group may be the result of avoidance of cow's milk allergen in the first 2 months of life. This is in line with earlier observations that avoidance may be detrimental [47]. Furthermore, in a subsequent subgroup analysis, Sakihara [57] showed that infants who received cow's milk supplementation in the first 3 days of life who were subsequently randomized to the avoidance group also showed an increased risk of developing CMA. This is again in line with a difference in risk for CMA between very early introduction of cow's milk in the first days of life followed by long duration of avoidance compared to early but continuous supplementation of cow's milk from the first months of life. More observational and intervention studies are needed and are, according to clinicaltrials.gov, underway [58,59].

Table 1. Studies on very early introduction of cow's milk in first days of life [45–49] and early introduction of cow's milk [50–57].

Study	Design	Population	Infants/Children	Age Onset Introduction CM	CM Formula	Breastfeeding	CMA Diagnosis	Outcome
Kelly et al. [45] 2019	Retro- and prospective	Infants at risk	55 infants	Within 24 h after birth	Regular CMF	BF only vs. BF + CMF	Allergy-focused clinical history, SPT, SpIgE measurement, and open food challenge, if necessary	Increased risk when CMF supplementation in first 24 h (OR 7.01; 95CI 1.79 27.01, $p < 0.001$)
Host et al. [46] 1988	Prospective	General population	1749 infants	Within first 3 days after birth	Regular CMF	BF population +/− early introduction of CMF in nursery	IgE and non-IgE, elimination/challenge test	39/1539 infants that received supplementation with CMF in the first 3 days had confirmed CMA while none of 210 exclusively BF neonates developed CMA (0/210), $p < 0.05$
Gil et al [47] 2017	Retrospective	CMA + infants	211 infants/group	Diverse	Regular CMF	Study focused on duration of IgE	IgE + CMA cases by clinical examination, provocation tests, serology	Increased risk when CMF supplementation in hospital, BF duration < 1 mo and 4–6 mo associated with higher risk of CMA while no increased risk of BF duration of 1–3 mo
Saarinen [48] 1999	Prospective	General population	6209 infants	Within first 20 h of life, and average feeding time of 2 days after birth	Pasteurized breastmilk Regular CMF Ext.Hydrolyzed whey formula	BF population (exclusively or supplemented with CMF, Hydrolyzed or pasteurized breastmilk	Interview, elimination/challenge test, SPT	Feeding of CM at maternity hospitals increases the risk of CMA when compared with feeding of other supplements, but exclusive breast-feeding does not eliminate the risk

Table 1. *Cont.*

Study	Design	Population	Infants/Children	Age Onset Introduction CM	CM Formula	Breastfeeding	CMA Diagnosis	Outcome
Sakihara [49] 2022	Data from SPADE study. Randomized controlled trial	Participants who ingested CMF in the first 3 days of life	431 children	4 groups of breastfed infants who discontinued CMF ingestion before age 1 month ("DISC < 1-month group"), during age 1 to 2 months ("DISC 1-2-month group"), during age 3 to 5 months ("DISC 3-5-month group") not until age 6 months ("continuous group")	Mixed feeding groups (breastfeeding and cow's milk formula (CMF) who discontinued CMF at different ages)	Breastfeeding + CMF in first 3 days of life +/− continuous CMF supplementation	Oral food challenge was performed to assess CMA development	CMA incidence was significantly higher in the DISC < 1 month group ($n = 7$ of 17, 41.2%; RR, 65.7; 95% CI, 14.7–292.5; $p < 0.001$), DISC 1-2-month group ($n = 3$ of 26, 11.5%; RR, 18.4; 95% CI, 3.2–105.3; $p = 0.003$), and DISC 3-5-month group ($n = 7$ of 69, 10.1%; RR, 16.2; 95% CI, 3.4–76.2; $p < 0.001$) than in the continuous group ($n = 2$ of 319, 0.6%)
Tezuka [50] 2020	Prospective	General population	>80,000 children	CMF consumption was categorized in < 3 mo, 3–6 mo or 6–12 mo at introduction	Regular CMF	BF and mixed fed.	CMA was defined as an allergic reaction to a CM product in an individual not consuming CM products at the time of evaluation, combined with physician-diagnosed food allergy	Introducing regular consumption of formula within the first 3 months of age was associated with lower risk of CMA at 12 months. Regular consumption at 3–6 months was strongly associated with a reduction in 12-month CMA (adjusted relative risks [95% confidence intervals]: 0.22 [0.12–0.35]), whereas no association was observed at 0–3 months (1.07 [0.90–1.27]

Table 1. Cont.

Study	Design	Population	Infants/Children	Age Onset Introduction CM	CM Formula	Breastfeeding	CMA Diagnosis	Outcome
Peters [51] 2018	Longitudinal	General population	5276	Exposed to CMF 0–3 months or not	Regular CMF	Excl BF; mixed feeding, excl FF	Parental report of a reaction to cow's milk consistent with IgE-mediated symptoms and a positive cow's milk skin prick test	Early exposure to cow's milk protein was associated with a reduced risk of cow's milk sensitization (adjusted odds ratio [aOR] 0.44, 95% confidence interval [CI] 0.23–0.83), parent-reported reactions to cow's milk (aOR 0.44, 95% CI 0.29–0.67), and cow's milk allergy (aOR 0.31, 95% CI 0.10–0.91) at age 12 months
Katz [52] 2010	Prospective	General population	13019	Age at CMF exposure 0–14 days 15–104 days 105–194 days 195–374 days	Regular CMF	Excl BF; mixed feeding, excl FF feeding	Interview followed by SPT and open food challenge	The mean age of cow's milk protein (CMP) introduction was significantly different ($p < 0.001$) between the healthy infants (61.6 ± 92.5 days) and those with IgE-mediated CMA (116.1 ± 64.9 days). Only 0.05% of the infants who were started on regular CMP formula within the first 14 days versus 1.75% who were started on formula between the ages of 105 and 194 days had IgE-mediated CMA ($p < 0.001$). The odds ratio was 19.3 (95% CI, 6.0–62.1) for development of IgE-mediated CMA among infants with exposure to CMP at the age of 15 days or more ($p < 0.001$)

Table 1. Cont.

Study	Design	Population	Infants/Children	Age Onset Introduction CM	CM Formula	Breastfeeding	CMA Diagnosis	Outcome
Sakihara [53] 2016	Prospective	Hen's-egg-allergic patients	397, <6 years of age	Excl BF group, discont ingestion of CMF before 3 mo of age (temp group; continuous ingestion of CMF, but not daily, up to 3 months of age (nondaily group); continuous ingestion of CMF at least once daily (daily group)	Regular CMF	Excl BF and mixed feeding groups	(1) a positive OFC result or any convincing episode of immediate reaction within 2 h after the ingestion of a cow's milk product and [2] positive cow's milk-specific IgE (CM-sIgE, > 0.34 KUA/L)	The incidence of developing CMA between the breast-fed group and temporary group did not show any statistical difference. Nondaily group and daily group had significantly lower incidence of developing CMA in comparison to the breast-fed group (nondaily group odds ratio 0.43; $p = 0.02$, daily group odds ratio 0.11; $p < 0.001$).
Lowe [54] 2011	Single-blind (participant) randomized controlled trial	Children with a family history of allergic disease	620, 0–2 y old children. Follow up at 6–7 years	randomized to receive the allocated formula at cessation of breast-feeding	cow's milk formula, a pHWF, or a soy formula (after cessation of breastfeeding)	breast-feeding until cessation, followed by formula (cow's milk formula, a pHWF, or a soy formula)	Skin prick tests to 6 common allergens (milk, egg, peanut, dust mite, rye grass, and cat dander) were performed at 6, 12, and 24 months.	The primary outcome was any allergic manifestation (cumulative incidence) up to 2 years of age. There was no evidence that infants allocated to the pHWF (odds ratio, 1.21; 95% CI, 0.81–1.80) or the soy formula (odds ratio, 1.26; 95% CI, 0.84–1.88) were at a lower risk of allergic manifestations in infancy compared with conventional formula. There was also no evidence of reduced risk of skin prick test reactivity or childhood allergic disease.

Table 1. Cont.

Study	Design	Population	Infants/Children	Age Onset Introduction CM	CM Formula	Breastfeeding	CMA Diagnosis	Outcome
Perkin [55] 2016	Randomized controlled study	Exclusively breast-fed infants who were 3 months of age	1303 exclusively breast-fed infants randomized to (a) early introduction group of six allergenic foods (b) standard introduction group	As of 3 months of age for early introduction and as of 6 months for standard introduction group	peanut, cooked egg, cow's milk, sesame, whitefish, and wheat	In the standard-introduction group, there was no consumption of peanut, egg, sesame, fish, or wheat before 5 months of age and consumption of less than 300 mL per day of formula milk between 3 and 6 months of age	Double blind placebo controlled food challenges, skin prick testing	The primary outcome was challenge-proven food allergy to one or more of the six early-introduction foods between 1 year and 3 years of age. In the intention-to-treat analysis, no significant differences were found. In the per-protocol analysis, the prevalence of any food allergy was significantly lower in the early-introduction group than in the standard introduction group (2.4% vs. 7.3%, $p = 0.01$), as was the prevalence of peanut allergy (0% vs. 2.5%, $p = 0.003$) and egg allergy (1.4% vs. 5.5%, $p = 0.009$); there were no significant effects with respect to milk, sesame, fish, or wheat. The early introduction of all six foods was not easily achieved but was safe

Table 1. Cont.

Study	Design	Population	Infants/Children	Age Onset Introduction CM	CM Formula	Breastfeeding	CMA Diagnosis	Outcome
Sakihara [56] 2021	Randomized controlled trial (SPADE study)	Breastfed infants who (a) ingested at least 10 mL of CMF daily (b) avoided CMF but were given soy formula if needed	491 participants (242 in the ingestion group and 249 in the avoidance group)	Start CMF between 1 and 2 months of age	ingest at least 10 mL of CMF daily (ingestion group)	Breastfeeding +/− CMF or soy formula	Oral food challenge was performed to assess CMA development, skin prick test, serum titers specific IgE and IgG4	Primary outcome was CMA by oral food challenge. Secondary outcomes were proportion of infants with positive SPT and serum titers of specific IgE and IgG4. There were 2 CMA cases (0.8%) among the 242 members of the ingestion group and 17 CMA cases (6.8%) among the 249 participants in the avoidance group (risk ratio = 0.12; 95% CI = 0.01–0.50; $p < 0.001$). The risk difference was 6.0% (95% CI = 2.7–9.3). Approximately 70% of the participants in both groups were still being breast-fed at 6 months of age. Of the 227 ingestion group participants, 11 (4.8%) had a positive SPT response to cow's milk at 6 months of age, as did 38 (16.2%) of the 235 avoidance group participants (RR 0.26; 95% CI 0.12–0.55; $p < 0.001$). The median titer of casein-specific IgG4 was 2.61 mgA/L (range, 0.45–10.46 mgA/L) in the ingestion group and 0.12 mgA/L (range, 0.08–0.33 mgA/L) in the avoidance group (P 0.02). Specific IgE titers did not significantly differ between the groups.

Table 1. Cont.

Study	Design	Population	Infants/Children	Age Onset Introduction CM	CM Formula	Breastfeeding	CMA Diagnosis	Outcome
Onizawa [57] 2016	Retrospectively	CMA-allergic patients and non-allergic controls	51 IgE-CMA, 102 controls, 32 unmatched patients IgE egg. Over 1 year of age	Supplemented with CMF maternity clinic, excl BF, early regular CMF, delayed CMF, no early regular continuous CMF	Regular CMF	BF and mixed feeding population	Immediate allergic reactions, CM specific IgE ($\geq$0.7 kUA/L), doctors diagnose of allergy	In a multivariable logistic regression analysis, the adjusted odds ratio of delayed (started more than 1 month after birth) or no regular cow's milk formula (less than once daily) was 23.74 (95% CI, 5.39–104.52) comparing the CMA group with the Control group

4. Prevention of Cow's Milk Allergy: Hydrolysates

As discussed above, the very early introduction of cow's milk in the first days of life followed by a period of avoidance is associated with increased risk of developing CMA. Therefore, it is important to know which supplements can be provided to support breastfeeding early in life without increasing this risk. Saarinen et al. [48] compared the supplementation of healthy infants during their stay in the maternity hospital with an extensively hydrolyzed whey formula, regular CMF, or pasteurized human milk to an exclusively breastfed group as the control. These infants were followed for 18 to 34 months for the development of CMA. In the group of infants receiving the whey hydrolysate, 1.5% of the infants developed cow's milk allergy (OR 0.61; 95% CI, 0.38–1.00) compared to 2.4% in the group of infants receiving regular cow's milk formula. In the infants receiving pasteurized human milk, 1.7% developed CMA (0.70; 95% CI, 0.44–1.12). These trends, however, did not reach statistical significance. In addition to early exposure to cow's milk, parental history of allergy—defined as asthma, atopic dermatitis, allergic rhinitis, or conjunctivitis as determined by a questionnaire—also increased the risk of developing CMA in line with current knowledge on genetic risk. A randomized clinical trial [60] investigated the risk of sensitization towards cow's milk and the development of allergic disease by early supplementation (in the first 3 days of life, but without continuous exposure) of breastfed infants with cow's milk formula (CMF) or an amino-acid-based formula (AAF) in high-risk infants (defined as one immediate family member with atopic disease). Sensitization to cow's milk (IgE level $\geq$ 0.35 allergen units [UA]/mL) occurred in 16.8% in the AAF group compared to 32.3% in the CMF group. Prevalence of food allergy at the second birthday was also significantly lower in the AAF group (2.6%) compared to the CMF group (13.2%) (RR 0.2; 95% CI, 0.07–0.57). The differences were not only present for cow's-milk-induced allergic reactions but also egg- and wheat-related allergic reactions, which were increased in the CMF group. The mechanism for this is not clear. It may also be that those diagnosed with cow's milk allergy are more likely to delay introduction of other allergenic foods, thereby missing the window of tolerance acquisition. Furthermore, the risk of asthma and recurrent wheeze was reduced in those who avoided early CMF when followed up to their second birthday [61]. The EAACI guidelines therefore suggest hydrolyzed formula as one of the possible temporary supplementary options depending on clinical, cultural, and economic factors [42].

The effectiveness of hydrolysates, either extensive or partial, on the reduction of cow's milk allergy introduced later in life (beyond 14 days) is less clear. In fact, the conclusion of a recent EAACI guideline by Halken et al. [42] concluded that "There is no recommendation for or against using partially or extensively hydrolyzed formula to prevent CMA in infants. When exclusive breastfeeding is not possible many substitutes are available for families to choose from, including hydrolyzed formulas." Halken et al. based this recommendation on nine trials [54,62–69] that either tested partially or extensively hydrolyzed casein or whey formulas on the occurrence of cow's milk protein allergy. Cow's milk allergy was diagnosed by means of clinical examination with either an open oral cow's milk challenge which was followed by a double-blind challenge when the results were equivocal for the open challenge [65,68,69], single-blind challenge [66], double-blind challenge [62,63,67], clinical examination without an oral food challenge [64], or telephone interview [54]. In line with the EAACI statement, the recommendation from the AAAAI/ACAAI/CSACI Consensus Document [37] was "There is no protective benefit from the use of hydrolyzed formula in the first year of life against food allergy or food sensitization". Furthermore, an earlier systematic review concluded that the use of hydrolyzed formula to prevent allergic disease in high-risk infants should not be recommended [70]. Many of the studies investigating the effect of hydrolyzed formula on the prevention of CMA have limitations which may have contributed to the lack of robust outcomes, such as (i) small sample size, (ii) design of the study, (iii) diagnostic criteria used, and (iv) characterization of the hydrolysate. With respect to the latter, peptide distribution, source of protein (casein and/or whey), and processing steps are thought to impact efficacy of hydrolysates [71–73]. Indeed, the lack of information on the distribution of peptides in a hydrolyzed formula was the main reason why the European Food Safety Authority (EFSA) recently concluded that a cause–effect relationship could not be established between the consumption of hydrolyzed infant formula and the risk reduction of atopic dermatitis [74]. Careful documentation and publication of the specifications of the hydrolysates used in clinical intervention studies will therefore be needed to overcome this shortcoming.

Thus, based on current literature, there is a role for hydrolysates in the first days of life in infants whose mothers are planning to subsequently breastfeed exclusively but cannot do so yet in the first days after giving birth. This should help to reduce early sensitization to cow's milk protein. The role of continuous consumption of hydrolysates versus early cow's milk formula consumption in the prevention of CMA is not so clear.

5. Limitations

A limitation of this narrative review is that it did not discuss other risk factors that may also play a role in development of CMA. These factors include, but are not limited to, preterm birth, the mode of delivery, and microbiota composition. Another limitation is that the review does not discuss non-IgE manifestations of CMA, and neither did it discuss the effect of combined preventive strategies.

6. Conclusions

The studies on early introduction of cow's milk proteins into the infant diet via infant formulas have taught us that if mothers plan to exclusively breastfeed the infant, no cow's milk formula should be given in the first weeks of life while breastfeeding is being established. If (donor) breast milk is not or insufficiently available in this very early period, extensively hydrolyzed milk formula or amino acid formula may be considered as an alternative [42].

Breastfeeding from birth with early introduction of cow's milk supplementation within the first month of life and continued daily consumption of small amounts without hampering breastfeeding may reduce the risk of developing cow's milk allergy. Additionally, the introduction of cow's milk should not be followed by prolonged periods of avoidance, as this seems to increase the risk of developing cow's milk allergy. Finally, even though many studies have been performed to date, there is currently no strong evidence that supports the use of hydrolyzed formula after 2 weeks of life for the prevention of CMA, indicating the need for additional studies with specific attention to the number of infants in the study, better characterization of the hydrolysates and their properties, and robust study design.

Author Contributions: All authors contributed to the design and writing of this review. All authors have read and agreed to the published version of the manuscript.

Funding: This research received no external funding.

Institutional Review Board Statement: Not applicable.

Informed Consent Statement: Not applicable.

Conflicts of Interest: A.T., A.B.S. and A.G. declare no conflict of interest. L.U. and R.J.J.v.N. are employed by FrieslandCampina.

Abbreviations

AAF	Amino-acid-based formula
AAAAI	American Academy of Allergy, Asthma & Immunology
ACAAI	American College of Allergy, Asthma & Immunology
BSACI	British Society for Allergy and Clinical Immunology
CSACI	Canadian Society of Allergy and Clinical Immunology
CMA	Cow's milk allergy
CMF	Cow's-milk-based formula
EAACI	European Academy of Allergy and Clinical Immunology
EFSA	European Food Safety Authority
ESPGHAN	European Society for Paediatric Gastroenterology Hepatology and Nutrition
LEAP	Learning Early About Peanut
NIAID	National Institute of Allergy and Infectious Diseases

References

1. Justiz Vaillant, A.A.; Vashisht, R.; Zito, P.M. Immediate Hypersensitivity Reactions. *Statpearls*. 2022. Available online: https://pubmed.ncbi.nlm.nih.gov/30020687/ (accessed on 12 April 2022).
2. Sampson, H.A.; Muñoz-Furlong, A.; Campbell, R.L.; Adkinson, N.F.J.; Bock, S.A.; Branum, A.; Brown, S.G.A.; Camargo, C.A.; Cydulka, R.; Galli, S.J.; et al. Second symposium on the definition and management of anaphylaxis: Summary report—Second National Institute of Allergy and Infectious Disease/Food Allergy and Anaphylaxis Network symposium. *J. Allergy Clin. Immunol.* **2006**, *117*, 391–397. [CrossRef] [PubMed]
3. Nwaru, B.I.; Hickstein, L.; Panesar, S.S.; Muraro, A.; Werfel, T.; Cardona, V.; Dubois, A.E.J.; Halken, S.; Hoffmann-Sommergruber, K.; Poulsen, L.K.; et al. The epidemiology of food allergy in Europe: A systematic review and meta-analysis. *Allergy* **2014**, *69*, 62–75. [CrossRef] [PubMed]
4. Eder, W.; Ege, M.J.; von Mutius, E. The asthma epidemic. *N. Engl. J. Med.* **2006**, *355*, 2226–2235. [CrossRef] [PubMed]
5. Mullins, R.J.; Dear, K.B.G.; Tang, M.L.K. Characteristics of childhood peanut allergy in the Australian Capital Territory, 1995 to 2007. *J. Allergy Clin. Immunol.* **2009**, *123*, 689–693. [CrossRef] [PubMed]
6. McGowan, E.C.; Peng, R.D.; Salo, P.M.; Zeldin, D.C.; Keet, C.A. Changes in Food-Specific IgE Over Time in the National Health and Nutrition Examination Survey (NHANES). *J. Allergy Clin. Immunol. Pract.* **2016**, *4*, 713–720. [CrossRef] [PubMed]
7. Prescott, S.L. Early-life environmental determinants of allergic diseases and the wider pandemic of inflammatory noncommunicable diseases. *J. Allergy Clin. Immunol.* **2013**, *131*, 23–30. [CrossRef] [PubMed]
8. Motosue, M.S.; Bellolio, M.F.; Van Houten, H.K.; Shah, N.D.; Campbell, R.L. National trends in emergency department visits and hospitalizations for food-induced anaphylaxis in US children. *Pediatr. Allergy Immunol. Off. Publ. Eur. Soc. Pediatr. Allergy Immunol.* **2018**, *29*, 538–544. [CrossRef]
9. Tsuge, M.; Ikeda, M.; Matsumoto, N.; Yorifuji, T.; Tsukahara, H. Current Insights into Atopic March. *Child* **2021**, *8*, 1067. [CrossRef]
10. Leung, A.S.Y.; Wong, G.W.K.; Tang, M.L.K. Food allergy in the developing world. *J. Allergy Clin. Immunol.* **2018**, *141*, 76–78.e1. [CrossRef]
11. Vale, S.L.; Lobb, M.; Netting, M.J.; Murray, K.; Clifford, R.; Campbell, D.E.; Salter, S.M. A systematic review of infant feeding food allergy prevention guidelines—Can we AGREE? *World Allergy Organ. J.* **2021**, *14*, 100550. [CrossRef]
12. Metcalfe, J.R.; Marsh, J.A.; D'Vaz, N.; Geddes, D.T.; Lai, C.T.; Prescott, S.L.; Palmer, D.J. Effects of maternal dietary egg intake during early lactation on human milk ovalbumin concentration: A randomized controlled trial. *Clin. Exp. Allergy J. Br. Soc. Allergy Clin. Immunol.* **2016**, *46*, 1605–1613. [CrossRef]
13. Palmer, D.J.; Gold, M.S.; Makrides, M. Effect of cooked and raw egg consumption on ovalbumin content of human milk: A randomized, double-blind, cross-over trial. *Clin. Exp. Allergy. J. Br. Soc. Allergy Clin. Immunol.* **2005**, *35*, 173–178. [CrossRef]
14. Sorva, R.; Mäkinen-Kiljunen, S.; Juntunen-Backman, K. Beta-lactoglobulin secretion in human milk varies widely after cow's milk ingestion in mothers of infants with cow's milk allergy. *J. Allergy Clin. Immunol.* **1994**, *93*, 787–792. [CrossRef]
15. Chirdo, F.G.; Rumbo, M.; Añón, M.C.; Fossati, C.A. Presence of high levels of non-degraded gliadin in breast milk from healthy mothers. *Scand. J. Gastroenterol.* **1998**, *33*, 1186–1192.
16. Schocker, F.; Scharf, A.; Kull, S.; Jappe, U. Detection of the Peanut Allergens Ara h 2 and Ara h 6 in Human Breast Milk: Development of 2 Sensitive and Specific Sandwich ELISA Assays. *Int. Arch. Allergy Immunol.* **2017**, *174*, 17–25. [CrossRef]
17. Vadas, P.; Wai, Y.; Burks, W.; Perelman, B. Detection of peanut allergens in breast milk of lactating women. *JAMA* **2001**, *285*, 1746–1748. [CrossRef]
18. Schocker, F.; Baumert, J.; Kull, S.; Petersen, A.; Becker, W.-M.; Jappe, U. Prospective investigation on the transfer of Ara h 2, the most potent peanut allergen, in human breast milk. *Pediatr. Allergy Immunol. Off. Publ. Eur. Soc. Pediatr. Allergy Immunol.* **2016**, *27*, 348–355. [CrossRef]
19. Savilahti, E.; Kuitunen, M. Allergenicity of cow milk proteins. *J. Pediatr.* **1992**, *121*, S12–S20. [CrossRef]

20. Du Toit, G.; Roberts, G.; Sayre, P.H.H.; Bahnson, H.T.; Radulovic, S.; Santos, A.F.; Brough, H.A.; Phippard, D.; Basting, M.; Feeney, M.; et al. Randomized Trial of Peanut Consumption in Infants at Risk for Peanut Allergy. *N. Engl. J. Med.* **2015**, *372*, 803–813. [CrossRef]
21. Ierodiakonou, D.; Garcia-Larsen, V.; Logan, A.; Groome, A.; Cunha, S.; Chivinge, J.; Zoe, R.; Natalie, G.; Katharine, J.; Tim, R.; et al. Timing of Allergenic Food Introduction to the Infant Diet and Risk of Allergic or Autoimmune Disease: A Systematic Review and Meta-analysis. *JAMA* **2016**, *316*, 1181–1192. [CrossRef]
22. Perkin, M.R.; Logan, K.; Marrs, T.; Radulovic, S.; Craven, J.; Flohr, C.; Lack, G.; Young, L.; Offord, V.; DeSousa, M.; et al. Enquiring About Tolerance (EAT) study: Feasibility of an early allergenic food introduction regimen. *J. Allergy Clin. Immunol.* **2016**, *137*, 1477–1486.e8. [CrossRef] [PubMed]
23. Koplin, J.J.; Allen, K.J. Optimal timing for solids introduction—Why are the guidelines always changing? *Clin. Exp. Allergy J. Br. Soc. Allergy Clin. Immunol.* **2013**, *43*, 826–834. [CrossRef] [PubMed]
24. Roduit, C.; Frei, R.; Depner, M.; Schaub, B.; Loss, G.; Genuneit, J.; Pfefferle, P.; Hyvärinen, A.; Karvonen, A.M.; Riedler, J.; et al. Increased food diversity in the first year of life is inversely associated with allergic diseases. *J. Allergy Clin. Immunol.* **2014**, *133*, 1056–1064. [CrossRef]
25. Du Toit, G.; Katz, Y.; Sasieni, P.; Mesher, D.; Maleki, S.J.; Fisher, H.R.; Fox, A.T.; Turcanu, V.; Amir, T.; Zadik-Mnuhin, G.; et al. Early consumption of peanuts in infancy is associated with a low prevalence of peanut allergy. *J. Allergy Clin. Immunol.* **2008**, *122*, 984–991. [CrossRef] [PubMed]
26. Toit, G.; Tsakok, T.; Lack, S.; Lack, G. Prevention of food allergy. *J. Allergy Clin. Immunol.* **2016**, *137*, 998–1010. [CrossRef] [PubMed]
27. Palmer, D.J.; Metcalfe, J.; Makrides, M.; Gold, M.S.; Quinn, P.; West, C.E.; Loh, R.; Prescott, S.L. Early regular egg exposure in infants with eczema: A randomized controlled trial. *J. Allergy Clin. Immunol.* **2013**, *132*, 387–392.e1. [CrossRef]
28. Koplin, J.; Osborne, N.; Wake, M.; Martin, P.E.; Gurrin, L.; Robinson, M.N.; Tey, D.; Slaa, M.; Thiele, L.; Miles, L. Can early introduction of egg prevent egg allergy in infants? A population-based study. *J. Allergy Clin. Immunol.* **2010**, *126*, 807–813. [CrossRef] [PubMed]
29. Palmer, D.J.; Sullivan, T.R.; Gold, M.S.; Prescott, S.L.; Makrides, M. Randomized controlled trial of early regular egg intake to prevent egg allergy. *J. Allergy Clin. Immunol.* **2017**, *139*, 1600–1607.e2. [CrossRef]
30. Bellach, J.; Schwarz, V.; Ahrens, B.; Trendelenburg, V.; Aksünger, Ö.; Kalb, B.; Niggemann, B.; Keil, T.; Beyer, K. Randomized placebo-controlled trial of hen's egg consumption for primary prevention in infants. *J. Allergy Clin. Immunol.* **2017**, *139*, 1591–1599.e2. [CrossRef]
31. Tan, J.W.L.; Valerio, C.; Barnes, E.H.; Turner, P.J.; Van Asperen, P.A.; Kakakios, A.M.; Campbell, D.E.; Beating Egg Allergy Trial BEAT Study Group. A randomized trial of egg introduction from 4 months of age in infants at risk for egg allergy. *J. Allergy Clin. Immunol.* **2017**, *139*, 1621–1628.e8.
32. Natsume, O.; Kabashima, S.; Nakazato, J.; Yamamoto-Hanada, K.; Narita, M.; Kondo, M.; Saito, M.; Kishino, A.; Takimoto, T.; Inoue, E.; et al. Two-step egg introduction for prevention of egg allergy in high-risk infants with eczema (PETIT): A randomised, double-blind, placebo-controlled trial. *Lancet* **2017**, *389*, 276–286. [CrossRef]
33. Quake, A.Z.; Liu, T.A.; D'Souza, R.; Jackson, K.G.; Woch, M.; Tetteh, A.; Sampath, V.; Nadeau, K.C.; Sindher, S.; Chinthrajah, R.S.; et al. Early Introduction of Multi-Allergen Mixture for Prevention of Food Allergy: Pilot Study. *Nutrients* **2022**, *14*, 737. [CrossRef]
34. Cox, A.L.; Shah, A.; Groetch, M.; Sicherer, S.H. Allergic reactions in infants using commercial early allergen introduction products. *J. Allergy Clin. Immunol. Pract.* **2021**, *9*, 3517–3520.e1. [CrossRef]
35. Greer, F.R.; Sicherer, S.H.; Burks, A.W. Effects of early nutritional interventions on the development of atopic disease in infants and children: The role of maternal dietary restriction, breastfeeding, timing of introduction of complementary foods, and hydrolyzed formulas. *Pediatrics* **2008**, *121*, 183–191. [CrossRef]
36. Greer, F.R.; Sicherer, S.H.; Burks, A.W. The Effects of Early Nutritional Interventions on the Development of Atopic Disease in Infants and Children: The Role of Maternal Dietary Restriction, Breastfeeding, Hydrolyzed Formulas, and Timing of Introduction of Allergenic Complementary Foods. *Pediatrics* **2019**, *143*, e20190281. [CrossRef]
37. Fleischer, D.M.; Chan, E.S.; Venter, C.; Spergel, J.M.; Abrams, E.M.; Stukus, D.; Groetch, M.; Shaker, M.; Greenhawt, M. A Consensus Approach to the Primary Prevention of Food Allergy Through Nutrition: Guidance from the American Academy of Allergy, Asthma, and Immunology; American College of Allergy, Asthma, and Immunology; and the Canadian Society for Allergy and Clinical. *J. Allergy Clin. Immunol. Pract.* **2021**, *9*, 22–43.e4. [CrossRef]
38. Chan, A.W.; Chan, J.K.; Lee, T.; Leung, T.; Tam, A.Y. Guidelines for Allergy Prevention in Hong Kong on Behalf of the Hong Kong Institute of Allergy. September 2015. Available online: https://www.allergy.org.hk/publications/Guidelines%20for%20Allergy%20Prevention%20in%20Hong%20Kong%20(Published%20version%20on%20HKMJ).pdf (accessed on 12 April 2022).
39. Turner, P.J.; Feeney, M.; Meyer, R.; Perkin, M.R.; Fox, A.T. Implementing primary prevention of food allergy in infants: New BSACI guidance published. Vol. 48, Clinical and experimental allergy. *J. Br. Soc. Allergy Clin. Immunol.* **2018**, *48*, 912–915. [CrossRef]
40. Fewtrell, M.; Bronsky, J.; Campoy, C.; Domellöf, M.; Embleton, N.; Fidler Mis, N.; Hojsak, I.; Hulst, J.M.; Indrio, F.; Lapillonne, A.; et al. Complementary Feeding: A Position Paper by the European Society for Paediatric Gastroenterology, Hepatology, and Nutrition (ESPGHAN) Committee on Nutrition. *J. Pediatr. Gastroenterol. Nutr.* **2017**, *64*, 119–132. [CrossRef]

1. Togias, A.; Cooper, S.F.; Acebal, M.L.; Assa'ad, A.; Baker, J.R.J.; Beck, L.A.; Block, J.; Byrd-Bredbenner, C.; Chan, E.S.; Eichenfield, L.F.; et al. Addendum guidelines for the prevention of peanut allergy in the United States: Report of the National Institute of Allergy and Infectious Diseases-sponsored expert panel. *J. Allergy Clin. Immunol.* **2017**, *139*, 29–44. [CrossRef]
2. Halken, S.; Muraro, A.; de Silva, D.; Khaleva, E.; Angier, E.; Arasi, S.; Arshad, H.; Bahnson, H.T.; Beyer, K.; Boyle, R.; et al. EAACI guideline: Preventing the development of food allergy in infants and young children (2020 update). *Pediatr. Allergy Immunol.* **2021**, *32*, 843–858. [CrossRef]
3. de Jong, M.H.; Scharp-Van Der Linden, V.T.; Aalberse, R.C.; Oosting, J.; Tijssen, J.G.; de Groot, C.J. Randomised con-trolled trial of brief neonatal exposure to cows' milk on the development of atopy. *Arch. Dis. Child.* **1998**, *79*, 126–130. [CrossRef]
4. de Jong, M.H.; Scharp-Van Der Linden, V.T.M.; Aalberse, R.; Heymans, H.S.A.; Brunekreef, B. The effect of brief neo-natal exposure to cows' milk on atopic symptoms up to age 5. *Arch. Dis. Child.* **2002**, *86*, 365–369. [CrossRef]
5. Kelly, E.; DunnGalvin, G.; Murphy, B.P.; Hourihane, J.O.; Hourihane, J.O. Formula supplementation remains a risk for cow's milk allergy in breast-fed infants. *Pediatr. Allergy Immunol.* **2019**, *30*, 810–816. [CrossRef] [PubMed]
6. Høst, A.; Husby, S.; Osterballe, O. A prospective study of cow's milk allergy in exclusively breast-fed infants. Incidence, pathogenetic role of early inadvertent exposure to cow's milk formula, and characterization of bovine milk protein in human milk. *Acta Paediatr. Scand.* **1988**, *77*, 663–670. [CrossRef] [PubMed]
7. Gil, F.; Amezqueta, A.; Martinez, D.; Aznal, E.; Etayo, V.; Durá, T.; Sánchez-Valverde, F. Association between Caesarean Delivery and Isolated Doses of Formula Feeding in Cow Milk Allergy. *Int. Arch. Allergy Immunol.* **2017**, *173*, 147–152. [CrossRef] [PubMed]
8. Saarinen, K.M.; Juntunen-Backman, K.; Järvenpää, A.L.; Kuitunen, P.; Lope, L.; Renlund, M.; Siivola, M.; Savilahti, E. Supplementary feeding in maternity hospitals and the risk of cow's milk allergy: A prospective study of 6209 infants. *J. Allergy Clin. Immunol.* **1999**, *104*, 457–461. [CrossRef]
9. Sakihara, T.; Otsuji, K.; Arakaki, Y.; Hamada, K.; Sugiura, S.; Ito, K. Early Discontinuation of Cow's Milk Protein Ingestion Is Associated with the Development of Cow's Milk Allergy. *J. Allergy Clin. Immunol. Pract.* **2022**, *10*, 172–179. [CrossRef]
10. Tezuka, J.; Sanefuji, M.; Ninomiya, T.; Kawahara, T.; Matsuzaki, H.; Sonoda, Y.; Ogawa, M.; Shimono, M.; Suga, R.; Honjo, S.; et al. Possible association between early formula and reduced risk of cow's milk allergy: The Japan Environment and Children's Study. *Clin. Exp. Allergy J. Br. Soc. Allergy Clin. Immunol.* **2021**, *51*, 99–107. [CrossRef]
11. Peters, R.L.; Koplin, J.J.; Dharmage, S.C.; Tang, M.L.K.; McWilliam, V.L.; Gurrin, L.C.; Neeland, M.R.; Lowe, A.J.; Ponsonby, A.L.; Allen, K.J. Early Exposure to Cow's Milk Protein Is Associated with a Reduced Risk of Cow's Milk Allergic Outcomes. *J. Allergy Clin. Immunol. Pract.* **2019**, *7*, 462–470.e1. [CrossRef]
12. Katz, Y.; Rajuan, N.; Goldberg, M.R.; Eisenberg, E.; Heyman, E.; Cohen, A.; Leshno, M. Early exposure to cow's milk protein is protective against IgE-mediated cow's milk protein allergy. *J. Allergy Clin. Immunol.* **2010**, *126*, 77–82.e1. [CrossRef]
13. Sakihara, T.; Sugiura, S.; Ito, K. The ingestion of cow's milk formula in the first 3 months of life prevents the development of cow's milk allergy. *Asia Pac. Allergy* **2016**, *6*, 207–212. [CrossRef]
14. Lowe, A.J.; Hosking, C.S.; Bennett, C.M.; Allen, K.J.; Axelrad, C.; Carlin, J.B.; Abramson, M.J.; Dharmage, S.C.; Hill, D.J. Effect of a partially hydrolyzed whey infant formula at weaning on risk of allergic disease in high-risk children: A randomized controlled trial. *J. Allergy Clin. Immunol.* **2011**, *128*, 360–365.e4. [CrossRef]
15. Perkin, M.R.; Logan, K.; Tseng, A.; Raji, B.; Ayis, S.; Peacock, J.; Brough, H.; Marrs, T.; Radulovic, S.; Craven, J.; et al. Randomized Trial of Introduction of Allergenic Foods in Breast-Fed Infants. *N. Engl. J. Med.* **2016**, *374*, 1733–1743. [CrossRef]
16. Sakihara, T.; Otsuji, K.; Arakaki, Y.; Hamada, K.; Sugiura, S.; Ito, K. Randomized trial of early infant formula introduction to prevent cow's milk allergy. *J. Allergy Clin. Immunol.* **2021**, *147*, 224–232.e8. [CrossRef]
17. Onizawa, Y.; Noguchi, E.; Okada, M.; Sumazaki, R.; Hayashi, D. The Association of the Delayed Introduction of Cow's Milk with IgE-Mediated Cow's Milk Allergies. *J. Allergy Clin. Immunol. Pract.* **2016**, *4*, 481–488.e2. [CrossRef]
18. Preventing Atopic Dermatitis and ALLergies in Children (PreventADALL). ClinicalTrials.gov Identifier: NCT02449850. Available online: https://clinicaltrials.gov/ct2/show/NCT02449850 (accessed on 12 April 2022).
19. The Influence of Early and Continuous Exposure of Infants to Cow's Milk Formula on the Prevention of Milk Allergy. ClinicalTrials.gov Identifier: NCT02785679. Available online: https://clinicaltrials.gov/ct2/show/NCT02785679 (accessed on 12 April 2022).
20. Urashima, M.; Mezawa, H.; Okuyama, M.; Urashima, T.; Hirano, D.; Gocho, N.; Tachimoto, H. Primary Prevention of Cow's Milk Sensitization and Food Allergy by Avoiding Supplementation with Cow's Milk Formula at Birth: A Randomized Clinical Trial. *JAMA Pediatr.* **2019**, *173*, 1137–1145. [CrossRef]
21. Tachimoto, H.; Imanari, E.; Mezawa, H.; Okuyama, M.; Urashima, T.; Hirano, D.; Gocho, N.; Urashima, M. Effect of Avoiding Cow's Milk Formula at Birth on Prevention of Asthma or Recurrent Wheeze Among Young Children: Extended Follow-up From the ABC Randomized Clinical Trial. *JAMA Netw. Open* **2020**, *3*, e2018534. [CrossRef]
22. Vandenplas, Y. Atopy at 3 years in high-risk infants fed whey hydrolysate or conventional formula. *Lancet* **1992**, *339*, 1118. [CrossRef]
23. Zeiger, R.S.; Heller, S.; Mellon, M.H.; Forsythe, A.B.; O'Connor, R.D.; Hamburger, R.N.; Schatz, M. Effect of combined maternal and infant food-allergen avoidance on development of atopy in early infancy: A randomized study. *J. Allergy Clin. Immunol.* **1989**, *84*, 72–89. [CrossRef]
24. Mallet, E.; Henocq, A. Long-term prevention of allergic diseases by using protein hydrolysate formula in at-risk infants. *J. Pediatr.* **1992**, *121*, S95–S100. [CrossRef]

65. Halken, S.; Høst, A.; Hansen, L.G.; Osterballe, O. Preventive effect of feeding high-risk infants a casein hydrolysate formula or an ultrafiltrated whey hydrolysate formula. A prospective, randomized, comparative clinical study. *Pediatr. Allergy Immunol. Off. Publ. Eur. Soc. Pediatr. Allergy Immunol.* **1993**, *4*, 173–181. [CrossRef]
66. Odelram, H.; Vanto, T.; Jacobsen, L.; Kjellman, N.I. Whey hydrolysate compared with cow's milk-based formula for weaning at about 6 months of age in high allergy-risk infants: Effects on atopic disease and sensitization. *Allergy* **1996**, *51*, 192–195. [CrossRef] [PubMed]
67. Oldaeus, G.; Anjou, K.; Björkstén, B.; Moran, J.R.; Kjellman, N.I. Extensively and partially hydrolysed infant formulas for allergy prophylaxis. *Arch. Dis. Child.* **1997**, *77*, 4–10. [CrossRef] [PubMed]
68. Halken, S.; Hansen, K.S.; Jacobsen, H.P.; Estmann, A.; Faelling, A.E.; Hansen, L.G.; Kier, S.R.; Lassen, K.; Lintrup, M.; Mortensen, S.; et al. Comparison of a partially hydrolyzed infant formula with two extensively hydrolyzed formulas for allergy prevention: A prospective, randomized study. *Pediatr. Allergy Immunol.* **2000**, *11*, 149–161. [CrossRef] [PubMed]
69. von Berg, A.; Koletzko, S.; Grübl, A.; Filipiak-Pittroff, B.; Wichmann, H.-E.; Bauer, C.P.; Reinhardt, D.; Berdel, D. The effect of hydrolyzed cow's milk formula for allergy prevention in the first year of life: The German Infant Nutritional Intervention Study, a randomized double-blind trial. *J. Allergy Clin. Immunol.* **2003**, *111*, 533–540. [CrossRef]
70. Boyle, R.J.; Ierodiakonou, D.; Khan, T.; Chivinge, J.; Robinson, Z.; Geoghegan, N.; Jarrold, K.; Afxentiou, T.; Reeves, T.; Cunha, S.; et al. Hydrolysed formula and risk of allergic or autoimmune disease: Systematic review and meta-analysis. *Br. Med. J.* **2016**, *352*, i974. [CrossRef]
71. Nutten, S.; Maynard, F.; Järvi, A.; Rytz, A.; Simons, P.J.; Heine, R.G.; Kuslys, M. Peptide size profile and residual immunogenic milk protein or peptide content in extensively hydrolyzed infant formulas. *Allergy Eur. J. Allergy Clin. Immunol.* **2020**, *75*, 1446–1449. [CrossRef]
72. Knol, E.F.; de Jong, N.W.; Ulfman, L.H.; Tiemessen, M.M. Management of cow's milk allergy from an immunological perspective: What are the options? *Nutrients* **2019**, *11*, 81–90. [CrossRef]
73. Lambers, T.T.; Gloerich, J.; van Hoffen, E.; Alkema, W.; Hondmann, D.H.; van Tol, E.A. Clustering analyses in peptidomics revealed that peptide profiles of infant formulae are descriptive. *Food Sci. Nutr.* **2015**, *3*, 81–90. [CrossRef]
74. EFSA Panel on Nutrition NF and FA (NDA); Castenmiller, J.; Hirsch-Ernst, K.-I.; Kearney, J.; Knutsen, H.K.; Maciuk, A.; Mangelsdorf, I.; McArdle, H.J.; Naska, A.; Pelaez, C.; et al. Efficacy of an infant formula manufactured from a specific protein hydrolysate derived from whey protein isolate and concentrate produced by Société des Produits Nestlé, S.A. in reducing the risk of developing atopic dermatitis. *EFSA J.* **2021**, *19*, e06603.

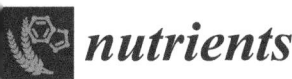

Article

Proportions of Polyunsaturated Fatty Acids in Umbilical Cord Blood at Birth Are Related to Atopic Eczema Development in the First Year of Life

Malin Barman [1,2,*], Mia Stråvik [1], Karin Broberg [2,3], Anna Sandin [4], Agnes E. Wold [5] and Ann-Sofie Sandberg [1]

1. Food and Nutrition Science, Department of Biology and Biological Engineering, Chalmers University of Technology, 41296 Gothenburg, Sweden; mia.stravik@chalmers.se (M.S.); ann-sofie.sandberg@chalmers.se (A.-S.S.)
2. Institute of Environmental Medicine, Karolinska Institutet, 17177 Stockholm, Sweden; karin.broberg@ki.se
3. Occupational and Environmental Medicine, Department of Laboratory Medicine, Lund University, 22363 Lund, Sweden
4. Pediatrics, Department of Clinical Sciences, Umeå University, 90187 Umeå, Sweden; anna.sandin@umu.se
5. Department of Infectious Diseases, Institute of Biomedicine, The Sahlgrenska Academy, University of Gothenburg, 40530 Gothenburg, Sweden; agnes.wold@microbio.gu.se
* Correspondence: malin.barman@chalmers.se; Tel.: +46-31-772-1000

Abstract: Atopic eczema, the most common atopic disease in infants, may pave the way for sensitization and allergy later in childhood. Fatty acids have immune-regulating properties and may regulate skin permeability. Here we examine whether the proportions of fatty acids among the infant and maternal plasma phospholipids at birth were associated with maternal dietary intake during pregnancy and development of atopic eczema during the first year of age in the Nutritional impact on Immunological maturation during Childhood in relation to the Environment (NICE) birth cohort. Dietary data were collected with a semi-quantitative food frequency questionnaire, fatty acids were measured with GC-MS and atopic eczema was diagnosed by a pediatric allergologist at 12 months of age. We found that higher proportions of n-6 PUFAs (including arachidonic acid) but lower proportions of n-3 PUFAs (including DPA) in the infant's phospholipids at birth were associated with an increased risk of atopic eczema at 12 months of age. The n-6 and n-3 PUFAs were related to maternal intake of meat and fish, respectively. Our results suggest that prenatal exposure to unsaturated fatty acids is associated with eczema development in the infant. Maternal diet during pregnancy may partly explain the fatty acid profiles *in utero*.

Keywords: diet; pregnancy; cord blood; fatty acids; n-3 PUFAs; n-6 PUFAs; arachidonic acid; phospholipids; atopic eczema; NICE birth cohort

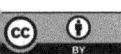

1. Introduction

Atopic eczema is the most common skin disease in children, affecting up to 20% of all children and up to 3% of adults [1]. Atopic eczema is a multifaceted, chronic, inflammatory skin condition with age-specific distribution patterns [1]. The first manifestations of atopic eczema usually appear early in life and often precede other allergic manifestations such as allergic rhinitis and asthma [2]. The etiology of atopic eczema is not completely understood but depends on complex interactions between genetic and different environmental and lifestyle factors. Filaggrin is a protein essential for healthy skin barrier function. Loss-of-function mutations in the filaggrin (*FLG*) gene have been associated with higher total IgE levels, sensitization to more allergens, and increased risk of atopic diseases [3]. This suggests that skin barrier function is one important factor in atopic eczema development.

One environmental factor that has been implicated in allergic diseases is diet [4]. Since atopic eczema often appears during the first year of life, maternal diet during pregnancy has been suggested to be of importance for the development of this disease in the infant [5,6]. Food contains certain nutrients that have immunomodulatory properties, such as different types of fatty acids. Fatty acids may be saturated, monounsaturated (MUFA), or polyunsaturated (PUFA). The PUFAs belong to either the n-6 or n-3 series. Different n-6 PUFAs may be endogenously synthesized by elongation of the precursor linoleic acid (LA, 18:2 n-6), which is a fatty acid that is abundant in vegetable oils and margarine. The n-3 PUFAs, on the other hand, may be synthesized from the n-3 precursor α-linolenic acid (ALA, 18:3 n-3), which is found in, for example, rapeseed oil. This elongation process is more effective in pregnant women, possibly due to the increased need for long-chain n-3 PUFAs during infancy [7,8]. In addition to the fatty acid elongation process that occurs in the human body, long-chain n-3 PUFAs are derived from intake of fish and other seafood.

Both n-6 and n-3 PUFAs have well-known immunomodulatory effects [5,6,9,10]. For example, PUFAs bind to fatty acid receptors (such as the ligand-activated transcription factor peroxisome proliferator-activated receptors, PPARs) [11,12] on the membranes of immune cells [13,14]. PUFAs also act as precursors for different lipid mediators, such as the eicosanoids. While eicosanoids produced from the n-6 PUFA arachidonic acid promote allergic sensitization and allergic inflammation, it has been suggested that the n-3 PUFAs act to oppose these actions [6]. Based on the molecular and cellular mechanisms of the eicosanoids produced from arachidonic acid, Black and Sharp, in 1997, already suggested a causal linkage between increased n-6 PUFA intake and increased prevalence of allergic diseases [4]. In a review published in 2017, Miles and Calder further discussed the association between early n-3 PUFA exposure and allergic disease risk and suggested that eating oily fish or fish oil supplements during pregnancy could be a strategy to prevent infant and childhood allergic diseases [6]. This hypothesis is supported by results from observational studies that have reported protective effects of maternal fish intake during pregnancy on atopic eczema development in infants [15,16].

Here, the aims were to: (1) examine the associations between the fatty acid profiles of maternal and infant cord plasma at delivery and the incidence of atopic eczema during the first year of life in a large Swedish birth cohort; and (2) examine the correlations between maternal and infant plasma phospholipid fatty acid proportions, as well as the association between these proportions and maternal dietary intake during pregnancy.

2. Materials and Methods

2.1. Study Population

The current study is based on the Nutritional impact on Immunological maturation during Childhood in relation to the Environment (NICE) birth cohort study conducted in Luleå, northern Sweden [17]. Pregnant women who were able to communicate in Swedish and planned on giving birth at Sunderby Hospital were informed about the birth cohort during their first visit to the local maternity clinic in GW 10–12. Recruitment was conducted between February 2015 and March 2018, at the hospital in connection with a routine ultrasound at GW 18. In total, 655 pregnant women were included in the NICE birth cohort. Three women gave birth to twins, five fetuses died before birth, one woman had a late miscarriage after inclusion in the birth cohort, and one woman withdrew her participation. Thus, 645 singleton liveborn infants were included in the birth cohort. Of these, 16 families participated in the birth cohort with two subsequent pregnancies and were, thus, excluded from the current study. Plasma samples from the infants' umbilical cords were available for fatty acid analyses for 290 of the 629 families eligible for inclusion in the current study, and 249 of these attended the 12-month follow-up and could be classified either as having atopic eczema or being non-allergic. Infants who did not have atopic eczema but had other allergic manifestations (such as food allergy or asthma) or were sensitized (N = 43) were excluded from the statistical analyses because they could not be classified as non-allergic. This resulted in a total of 206 infants being included in the statistical calculations in the current study, of which 14 were diagnosed with atopic eczema (see Figure 1 for flow chart). Plasma samples from the mothers were available for

193 of the mother and infant pairs, i.e., 13 in the allergic group and 180 in the non-allergic control group.

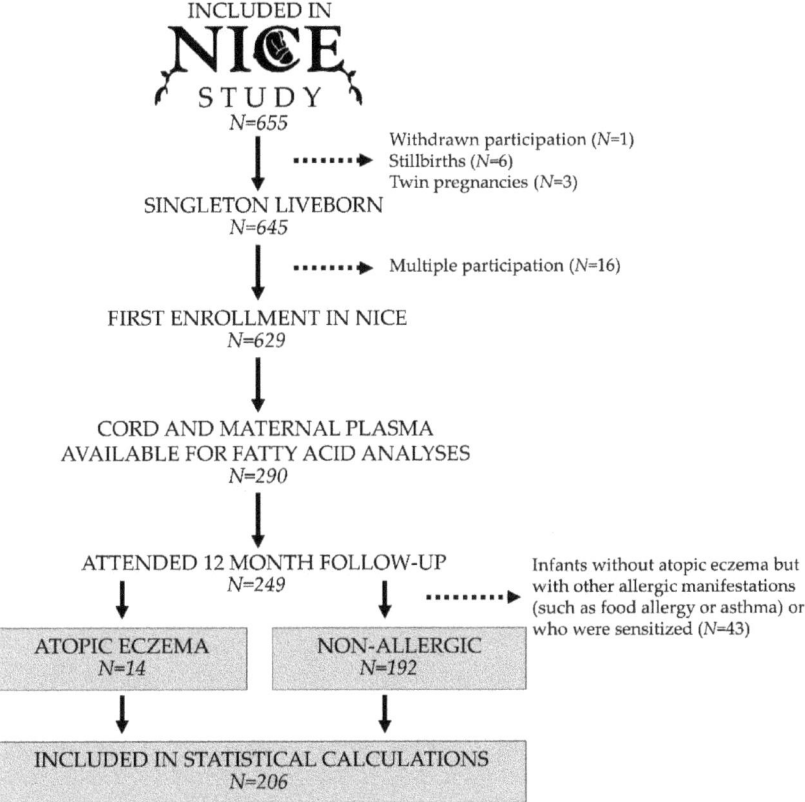

Figure 1. Flow chart of the study population.

2.2. Collection of Maternal and Infant Blood

Infant cord blood was collected from the umbilical cord directly after delivery. The cord was clamped and severed before cord blood was squeezed out into 6 mL EDTA tubes (Becton Dickinson, Franklin Lakes, NJ, USA). Peripheral venous blood samples from the mothers were collected in 10 mL EDTA vacutainer tubes (Becton Dickinson) in connection with the delivery (usually when arriving at the delivery ward). Blood samples were stored refrigerated (4 °C) at the delivery ward until transported to the research laboratory, where they were centrifuged and the plasma was decanted, aliquoted, and stored at −80 °C. The research laboratory was only staffed on weekdays, which meant that samples acquired during deliveries that occurred during weekends could be stored at 4 °C for up to 3 days before centrifugation and subsequent freezing.

2.3. Analysis of Fatty Acid Proportions in Plasma Phospholipids

Plasma samples (200 µL) were thawed slowly in cold water, vortexed, and mixed with 50 µL of internal standard (fatty acid 17:0, 1 mg/mL). Fatty acids were extracted by adding 4 mL of chloroform:methanol 1:1 (v/v) and 2 mL of 0.5% NaCl. After vortexing and centrifugation, 1 mL of the chloroform phase was collected and evaporated at 40 °C under nitrogen gas. The remaining precipitate was dissolved in 200 µL chloroform and run through solid-phase extraction (SPE) columns (Supelco, Bellefonte, PA, USA, NH$_2$, 500 mg/3 mL), preconditioned with 2 × 2 mL hexane. The columns were rinsed with 2 × 2 mL chloroform:isopropanol 2:1 (v/v) and 2 × 2 mL of 2% acetic acid in diethyl ether. Thereafter, the adsorbed phospholipids were eluted with 2 × 2 mL of methanol. Methylation of fatty acids was carried out as follows: the methanol was evaporated and the precipitate was dissolved in 2 mL of toluene and 2 mL of 10% acetyl chloride in methanol and vortexed for 1 min. The mixture was incubated at 70 °C for 2 h with vortexing every 30 min. Thereafter, 1 mL of Milli-Q water and 2 mL of petroleum ether were added to the samples. After vortexing and centrifugation, 3 mL of the organic phase was collected and evaporated at 40 °C under nitrogen gas.

2.4. Analysis of Fatty Acids by GC-MS

The fatty acids were separated by gas chromatography-mass spectrometry (GC-MS) using the 7890A GC-system, 5975C inert XL EI/CI MSD with Triple-Axis Detector, and 7693 Autosampler, together with a VF-WAXms GC column (30 m × 0.25 mm × 0.25 µm; P/N 7FD-G033-05) (all from Agilent Technologies Inc., Santa Clara, CA, USA). The liner used was the Ultra Inert Inlet Liner, Low PSI drop, wool (P/N 5190-3165; Agilent Technologies). The Non-Stick Bleed/Temperature-Optimized Non-Stick 11-mm Septa was used (Agilent Technologies).

Samples were dissolved in 100 µL iso-octane for the GC analysis. Three quality control samples were analyzed in parallel in each run. The standard GLC-463 mixed fatty acid methyl esters (Nu-Chek Prep, Elysian, MN, USA) were dissolved in toluene and used as an external standard for peak evaluation. The GC oven program consisted of: initial temperature of 100 °C, ramping at 4 °C/min to 205 °C and then at 1 °C/min to 230 °C with a 5-min hold. The instrumental settings were: helium as the carrier gas; inlet heater at 275 °C; pressure, 10.523 psi; total flow, 14 mL/min, septum purge flow, 3 mL/min; split flow, 10 mL/min; and split ratio, 10. The injection volume was 1 µL per sample, with an oven run time of 56 min.

The fatty acids in the phospholipids were identified by comparing the retention times of the external standard with the retention times of the samples, as well as a mass spectrum analysis of each peak and comparison with a library of the mass spectra of known fatty acids, which is maintained in the laboratory.

The following fatty acids were identified and quantified in the phospholipid fraction of the plasma: 14:0, 20:0, 18:1 n-9, 18:1 n-7, 18:2 n-6 (LA), 18:3 n-3 (ALA), 20:3 n-6 (DGLA), 20:4 n-6 (AA), 20:5 n-3 (EPA), 22:0, 22:4 n-6, 22:5 n-6, 22:5 n-3 (DPA) and 22:6 n-3 (DHA). The concentration of each fatty acid was calculated using the concentration of the internal standard 17:0. The proportions of specific fatty acids were expressed as the concentration of the particular fatty acid relative to the concentration of all 14 fatty acids. Fatty acids 16:0 and 18:0 were not quantified due to contamination from the SPE columns and, therefore, are not included in the total sum of fatty acids.

2.5. Dietary Assessments

Maternal daily intake of food and nutrients during pregnancy was assessed using a web-based, semi-quantitative, food frequency questionnaire (Meal-Q), as previously described in detail [18,19]. The questionnaire, which was distributed to the subjects when they were around GW 34, sought information regarding food intake during the previous month, measured on a frequency scale that ranged from no intake/intake less than once per month to ≥5 times/day. The intake of food in grams per day was calculated using either reported intake quantities or, if no quantities were specified, standard portions from the Swedish Food Composition Database [20].

2.6. Clinical Examination

Atopic eczema during the first year of life was diagnosed by an experienced pediatric allergologist (author AS) at a clinical visit that was scheduled at 12 months of age. Diagnosis followed the criteria proposed by Williams and coworkers [21–23]. The major criterion was an itchy condition or parental report of scratching/rubbing by the child. This resulted in a diagnosis when present in combination with three or more of the following criteria:

(1) history of infant eczema that was spreading generally or found in typical areas and creases, such as the cheeks, folds of the elbows, rear of knees, front of ankles or around the neck; (2) history of asthma or other atopic disease or a history of atopic disease in a first-degree relative; (3) history of generally dry skin in the previous year; and (4) visible infant eczema that was generally spreading or located in typical areas and creases, such as the cheeks, folds of the elbows, behind the knees, front of ankles or around the neck.

2.7. Assessment of Filaggrin Gene (FLG) Mutations

DNA extraction was performed on infant EDTA-treated blood or blood cells using the Omega E.Z.N.A. Blood DNA Mini Kit (Omega Bio-tek Inc., Norcross, GA, USA). The 260/280 nm and the 260/230 nm absorbance ratios were measured with the Nanodrop 1000 Spectrophotometer (Thermo Fisher Scientific, Waltham, MA, USA).

The *FLG* null mutations R501X, R2477X, S3247X, and 2282del4 (the most common mutations in Europe) were analyzed [24]. For R501X, R2477X, and S3247X the qPCR was carried out in a total reaction volume of 5 μL, containing: 0.125 μL of 40× custom-made SNP genotyping assay (Thermo Fisher Scientific), 2.5 μL of 2× TaqMan Master Mix (Thermo Fisher Scientific), and 2 μL of DNA (5 ng/μL). The PCR program was as follows: 10 min at 95 °C, followed by 45 cycles of 15 s at 92 °C, and a final step of 1 min and 30 s at 60 °C.

For 2282del4, 0.125 μL of the SNP assay, 2.5 μL of TaqMan MasterMix, 0.25 μL of a 10-μM stock of second primer (for increased specificity of the reaction), and 2 μL of DNA (5 ng/μL) were added to the reaction mixture. The PCR program was as above, except that the final step was for 1 min at 60 °C. The programs were run on the ABI 7900 instrument. The primer pairs for the different assays are listed in Supplementary Table S1. As a positive control, a synthesized DNA construct that included the R501X, R2447X, S3247X, and 2282del4 rare alleles and surrounding sequences was included in each qPCR run in duplicate (GeneArt; Thermo Fisher Scientific).

2.8. Data Variables

Data on maternal and birth characteristics were extracted from electronic hospital records. All data were anonymized before processing. Allergic heredity and pet ownership were assessed as part of a structured interview conducted during the study visit at 12 months of age. Data on the number of siblings in the house and residential area were extracted from questionnaires filled in by both parents around GW 20–25.

2.9. Statistical Methods

All statistical analyses were performed using the IBM SPSS Statistics ver. 27.0 (IBM, New York, NY, USA), the R ver. 3.6.2 software (R Foundation for Statistical Computing, Vienna, Austria), and Umetrics SIMCA ver. 16.0.1 (Sartorius Stedim Data Analytics AB, Umeå, Sweden). Participants' characteristics were analyzed using the χ^2 test or Fisher's exact test for categorical variables and the Mann–Whitney U-test for continuous variables. Differences in the levels of plasma fatty acids were analyzed using the Mann–Whitney U-test. Correlations were calculated by Spearman's rho. Logistic regression models were used to analyze associations between proportions of fatty acids and atopic eczema. One unadjusted model was performed and two adjusted models, one with adjustment for any allergy within the family (parent or sibling) and one with adjustment for *FLG* loss-of-function mutation. The logistic regression models were performed on standardized fatty acid levels (per interquartile range, IQR). Therefore, the results refer to a change in an interquartile range for each fatty acid proportion. Partial least square (PLS) was used to investigate which of the food variables were most strongly related to the infant and maternal plasma proportions of n-3 and n-6 PUFAs. Orthogonal partial least square with discriminant analysis (OPLS-DA) was used to investigate which of the variables were most strongly related (positively or negatively) to atopic eczema.

3. Results

Cord blood and maternal peripheral venous blood were obtained at delivery from 206 infants and 196 mothers, respectively, and the fractions of different fatty acids in the plasma phospholipids were determined (expressed as the proportions of all measured fatty acids). Figure 2 and Supplementary Table S2 show the proportions of various PUFAs in the infant and maternal plasma phospholipids.

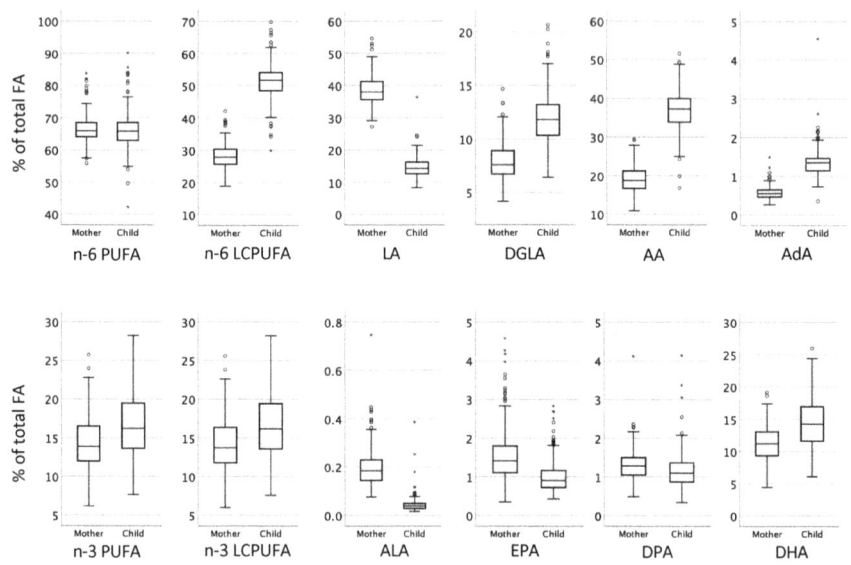

Figure 2. Proportions of fatty acids in the maternal and infant plasma samples at delivery. Abbreviations: PUFA, polyunsaturated fatty acids; LCPUFA, long-chain PUFA; LA, linolenic acid (18:2 n-6); DGLA, dihomo-gamma-linoleic acid (20:3 n-6); AA, arachidonic acid (20:4 n-6); AdA, Adrenic acid (22:4 n-6); ALA, α-linolenic acid (18:3 n-3); EPA, eicosapentaenoic acid (20:5 n-3); DPA, docosapentaenoic acid (22:5 n-3); DHA, docosahexaenoic acid (22:6 n-3).

As shown in Figure 2, compared to the maternal plasma phospholipids, the infant plasma phospholipids were enriched for the n-6 PUFAs arachidonic acid (AA, 20:4 n-6), dihomo-gamma-linoleic acid (DGLA, 20:3 n-6) and adrenic acid (22:4 n-6), as well as the n-3 PUFA docosahexaenoic acid (DHA, 22:6 n-3). In contrast, the maternal plasma phospholipids contained higher proportions of linoleic acid (LA, 18:2 n-6), α-linolenic acid (ALA, 18:3 n-3), eicosapentaenoic acid (EPA, 20:5 n-3), and docosapentaenoic acid (DPA, 22:5 n-3) (Figure 2, Supplementary Table S2).

Even though the proportions of many of the fatty acids differed substantially between the mothers and their infants (Figure 2), all the fatty acids, with the exception of α-linolenic acid, were strongly positively correlated ($p < 0.001$) between infants and mothers (Supplementary Table S2).

3.1. Prevalence of Eczema and Relationships between Eczema and Background Factors

The infants were clinically examined by a pediatric allergology specialist at 12 months of age. In total, 14 infants were diagnosed with atopic eczema, and 192 infants were classified as non-allergic and non-sensitized. Sensitized children without any allergy diagnosis and children with allergies other than eczema were excluded from the control group (N = 43). Children who had eczema and other allergic manifestations, such as food allergy (N = 5) or asthma (N = 3), were included in the eczema group. Thus, 8 of the 14 infants with eczema also had an additional atopic manifestation.

Table 1 lists the characteristics of the study participants, showing the differences between the allergic and non-allergic children. The vast majority of the infants were born by vaginal delivery and most were breastfed for at least 6 months. Children with eczema were more likely to have an allergic family member (p = 0.033). More specifically, allergy in a sibling was highly predictive of eczema development during the first year of life (p = 0.007). *FLG* loss of function mutation was not associated with the prevalence of atopic eczema. No other significant differences were found between the allergic and non-allergic children (Table 1).

Table 1. Characteristics of infants with atopic eczema and non-allergic infants.

	Non-Allergic (N = 192)		Atopic Eczema (N = 14)		p-Value
	N	(%)	N	(%)	
Male sex	82	(43)	5	(36)	0.609
Birth order					0.505
First-born	92	(48)	8	(57)	
Mother with ≥1 previous pregnancy	100	(52)	6	(43)	
Birthweight in grams					0.068
<2500	1	(<1)	1	(7)	
2500–4500	178	(93)	13	(93)	
>4500	13	(7)	0	(0)	
FLG null					1.000
Heterozygous (*FLG* null)	11	(6)	0	(0)	
Homozygous Wild-Type (WT)	159	(94)	11	(100)	
Breastfed					0.467
Never	6	(3)	0	(0)	
<4 months	13	(7)	2	(14)	
4–5 months	31	(17)	4	(29)	
≥6 months	130	(72)	8	(57)	
Missing	12		-		
Pet ownership (first year of life)					
Dog	62	(32)	4	(29)	1.000
Cat	47	(25)	3	(21)	1.000
Other	11	(6)	0	(0)	1.000
Allergic heredity					
Maternal	74	(39)	9	(64)	0.058
Paternal	80	(42)	9	(64)	0.099
Sibling	28	(15)	5	(71)	0.007
Any	125	(65)	13	(93)	0.033
Maternal age at delivery (years)					0.815
<25	19	(10)	2	(14)	
26–30	89	(46)	5	(36)	
31–35	56	(29)	6	(43)	
>35	28	(15)	1	(7)	
Mother's highest education level					0.138
Elementary school (9 years)	3	(2)	0	(0)	
Senior high school (12 years)	51	(27)	7	(50)	
University/other education (>12 years)	138	(72)	7	(50)	
Early pregnancy BMI, kg/m^2					0.910
Underweight (<18.5)	0	(0)	0	(0)	
Normal weight (18.5–24.9)	82	(56)	7	(54)	
Overweight (25–29.9)	46	(29)	4	(31)	
Obese (≥30)	28	(15)	2	(15)	
Missing	6		1		

Table 1. Cont.

	Non-Allergic (N = 192)		Atopic Eczema (N = 14)		p-Value
	N	(%)	N	(%)	
Residential address					
Town (central part)	82	(43)	5	(36)	0.696
Town (suburb)	46	(24)	4	(29)	
Countryside	64	(33)	5	(36)	
Maternal smoking before pregnancy					
Yes	11	(6)	0	(0)	1.000
No	180	(94)	14	(100)	
Missing	1		-		
Gestational length					
Preterm	4	(2)	1	(7)	0.365
Term	167	(87)	12	(86)	
Post-term	21	(11)	1	(7)	
Birth mode					
Vaginal delivery	180	(94)	12	(86)	0.244
Cesarean section	12	(6)	2	(14)	

Differences between allergic and non-allergic children were analyzed with the chi-square test. For dichotomized variables, Fisher's exact test or Pearson's chi-square test was used depending on the number of expected cases in each group. For analysis of trends in categorical data, Linear-by-linear associations were used. Birth order was categorized as 'no previous children' (nulliparous) and 'one or more previous children' (multiparous). The child was defined as having allergic heredity if the mother, father, or any sibling had any diagnosis of atopic eczema, food allergy, allergic rhinoconjunctivitis, and/or asthma with treatment. Smoking was categorized as 'yes' or 'no' regardless of the number of smoked cigarettes. Gestational age (presented as days of gestation from ultrasound or, if missing, from last menstrual period) was categorized as: preterm (GW < 36+6), term (GW 37+0–41+6), and post-term (GW $\geq$ 42+0).

3.2. Proportions of Fatty Acids in Plasma Phospholipids at Birth in Relation to Presence of Atopic Eczema during the First Year of Life

The fatty acid compositions of the plasma phospholipids in maternal venous plasma and infant cord plasma samples obtained at delivery were related to the diagnosis of atopic eczema at 12 months of age using OPLS. In the model, eczema was set as the outcome (Y) variable, and the proportions of individual fatty acids were set as explanatory (X) variables. Figure 3 shows a model that only includes those fatty acids with a variable of importance (VIP) value > 0.8; a model incorporating all fatty acids is shown in Supplementary Figure S1. The variables that showed the strongest associations with atopic eczema were further investigated using univariate analysis. As shown in Figure 3, the sum of the n-6 PUFA proportions in the infant's phospholipids was significantly positively associated with the risk of having atopic eczema at 12 months of age ($p = 0.002$). The same was true for the sum of the long-chain n-6 fatty acids (n-6 LCPUFA; $p = 0.001$), as well as in the case of arachidonic acid ($p = 0.002$). In contrast, higher proportions of the long-chain n-3 PUFA DPA in the infant's cord serum correlated negatively with atopic eczema ($p = 0.03$). Other n-3 PUFAs also appeared at the opposite side of eczema in the plot, although they were not significantly associated with the non-allergic state. In general, maternal and infant fatty acids appeared on the same side of the plot, although the maternal fatty acid composition was more weakly associated with allergy in the infant than was the infant's own fatty acid pattern (Figure 3). In addition, the presence of α-linolenic acid in the infant's cord blood was significantly associated with a decreased risk of developing eczema ($p = 0.02$) (Supplementary Figure S1), although this association was excluded by the VIP analysis due to a too-weak contribution to the model, such that it is not visible in Figure 3.

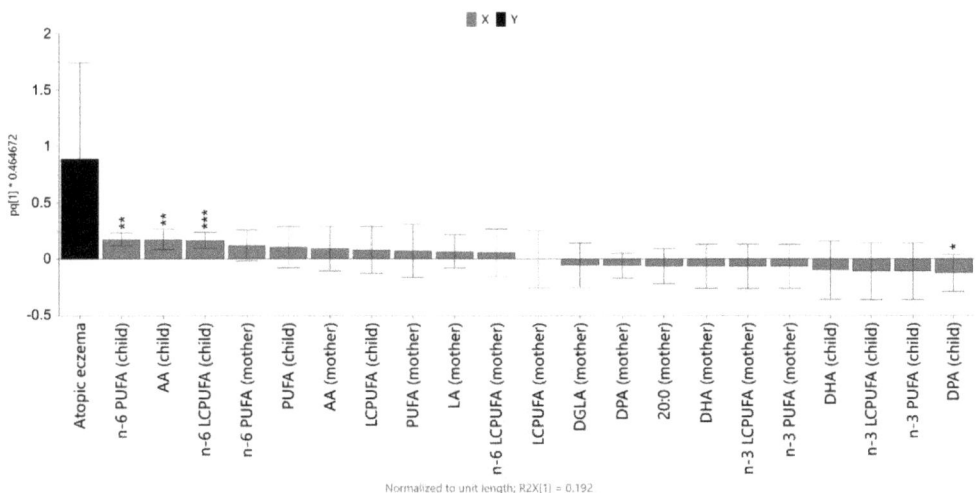

Figure 3. Orthogonal partial least squares (OPLS) loading column plot showing the associations between atopic eczema at 12 months of age and the proportion of selected fatty acids in maternal and infant cord plasma phospholipids. Fatty acids with a variable of importance (VIP) value >0.8 in the model that included all fatty acids (shown in Supplementary Figure S1) are included here. Associations that were significant in the univariate analyses (Mann–Whitney U-test) are indicated with an asterisk: * $p < 0.05$, ** $p < 0.01$, *** $p < 0.001$. Abbreviations: AA, arachidonic acid (20:4 n-6); DGLA, dihomo-gamma-linoleic acid (20:3 n-6); DHA, docosahexaenoic acid (22:6 n-3); DPA, docosapentaenoic acid (22:5 n-3); LCPUFA, long-chain PUFA; PUFA, polyunsaturated fatty acids.

The proportions of fatty acids in the cord blood of infants who subsequently developed eczema or remained non-allergic are listed in Supplementary Table S2, while the corresponding values for the maternal plasma are shown in Supplementary Table S3. Neither monounsaturated fatty acids (MUFA) nor saturated fatty acids in the infant's or mother's blood at delivery were related to the risk of developing eczema during the first year of life (Supplementary Tables S2 and S3).

3.3. Magnitude of the Association between Infant Cord Blood Fatty Acids and Atopic Eczema

The magnitude of the associations between the proportions of n-3 and n-6 fatty acids in the phospholipids present in infant cord serum at birth and atopic eczema were further explored with logistic regression models, without adjustment and with adjustment for either any allergic disease within the family (sibling or parent) or being a carrier of *FLG* loss-of-function mutation (Table 2). Primarily, arachidonic acid was found to account for the positive association between the infant's proportions of n-6 PUFAs and long-chain n-6 PUFAs and eczema at 12 months of age. An increase of one IQR in the proportion of arachidonic acid in the infant cord plasma phospholipids corresponded to a 2.8-fold increase in the odds of having atopic eczema during the first year of life in the unadjusted model. After adjustment for allergy within the family or for *FLG* mutation, the odds were similar (OR = 2.6 in both models). Arachidonic acid was the dominant n-6 fatty acid in the infant cord blood phospholipids, representing 71% of the long-chain n-6 PUFAs and 56% of the n-6 PUFAs. Thus, an increase of one IQR in the proportion of long-chain n-6 PUFAs or total n-6 PUFAs resulted in 2.1-fold or 1.8-fold higher odds of developing atopic eczema, respectively in the unadjusted models with slightly reduced but similar results in the adjusted models.

Table 2. Associations between one unit increase in IQR for the proportions of different polyunsaturated fatty acids (PUFAs) in cord serum phospholipids and atopic eczema during the first year of life.

		Association with Atopic Eczema During 1st Year of Life					
		Unadjusted Model		Adjusted Model [1]		Adjusted Model [2]	
Fatty Acid	% in Cord Blood Phospholipids Median (IQR)	OR [3] (95% CI)	p-Value	OR [3] (95% CI)	p-Value	OR [3] (95% CI)	p-Value
n-6 fatty acids							
Linoleic acid, 18:2 n-6	14 (3.7)	1.08 (0.66–1.79)	0.754	1.01 (0.61–1.68)	0.956	0.80 (0.36–1.76)	0.578
Arachidonic acid, 20:4 n-6	37 (6.1)	2.75 (1.38–5.47)	**0.004**	2.58 (1.32–5.04)	**0.005**	2.61 (1.21–5.64)	**0.014**
n-6 LCPUFAs	52 (5.7)	2.11 (1.23–3.63)	**0.007**	1.99 (1.17–3.39)	**0.012**	1.91 (1.05–3.48)	**0.035**
n-6 PUFAs	66 (5.6)	1.79 (1.18–2.70)	**0.006**	1.67 (1.11–2.51)	**0.015**	1.52 (0.94–2.46)	0.086
n-3 fatty acids							
α-linolenic acid, 18:3 n-3	0.039 (0.021)	0.33 (0.12–0.93)	**0.036**	0.34 (0.12–0.94)	**0.038**	0.39 (0.13–1.19)	0.099
EPA, 20:5 n-3	0.92 (0.48)	0.80 (0.41–1.53)	0.494	0.74 (0.38–1.44)	0.371	0.81 (0.39–1.70)	0.583
DPA, 22:5 n-3	1.1 (0.52)	0.41 (0.17–1.01)	0.052	0.40 (0.16–1.00)	**0.049**	0.56 (0.22–1.40)	0.215
DHA, 22:6 n-3	14 (5.5)	0.53 (0.22–1.29)	0.160	0.53 (0.22–1.30)	0.165	0.83 (0.32–2.16)	0.699
n-3 LCPUFAs	16 (5.9)	0.49 (0.20–1.19)	0.114	0.48 (0.20–1.18)	0.109	0.76 (0.30–1.95)	0.571
n-3 PUFAs	16 (5.9)	0.49 (0.20–1.18)	0.111	0.48 (0.20–1.17)	0.107	0.76 (0.29–1.95)	0.563

Atopic eczema was diagnosed at 12 months of age through clinical examination by an experienced pediatric allergologist. The proportions of various PUFAs were measured in the phospholipid fractions of cord plasma samples collected at delivery and related by multiple logistic regression to the occurrence of infant atopic eczema during the first year of life. [1] Adjusted for any allergic disease within the family (sibling or parent). [2] Adjusted for *FLG* loss-of-function mutations. [3] OR per interquartile range (IQR) of fatty acid proportions. Both the unadjusted and the model adjusted for allergy within the family included 14 infants with eczema and 192 non-allergic infants, the model adjusted for *FLG* mutations included 11 infants with atopic eczema and 170 non-allergic individuals. Significant p-values are indicated in bold. Abbreviations: CI, confidence interval; OR, odds ratio; PUFA, polyunsaturated fatty acids; LCPUFA, long-chain PUFA; EPA, eicosapentaenoic acid; DPA, docosapentaenoic acid; DHA, docosahexaenoic acid.

Conversely, an increase of one IQR in the proportion of ALA in the cord blood plasma phospholipids was associated with a 3.0-fold lower odds of having a diagnosis of atopic eczema at 12 months of age (2.9-fold after adjustment for allergic heredity while not significant after adjusting for *FLG*). An increase of one IQR in the proportion of DPA resulted in 2.6-fold lower odds, after adjusting for any allergy within the family, while not significant in the unadjusted model or in the model adjusted for *FLG* (Table 2).

3.4. Associations between Fatty Acids in Maternal and Infant Cord Plasma and Maternal Food Intake

The proportion of fatty acids in plasma phospholipids is partially determined by the diet. For example, a diet that is high in fish gives a higher proportion of the long-chain fatty acids EPA, DHA, and DPA. Partial least squares (PLS) analysis was used to examine whether maternal intake of different fat-containing foods was associated with the proportions of PUFAs in the plasma phospholipids of the infants and mothers. The proportions of n-3 PUFAs or n-6 PUFAs were set as the outcome (Y) variables, while the mother's reported intake of different fatty acid-rich foods was set as explanatory (X) variables (Figure 4). As is evident in Figure 4, the infant's and mother's proportions of n-6 PUFAs in their plasma phospholipids were positively associated with the maternal intake of different sorts of meat and chocolate. The total n-3 PUFAs in both the infant and maternal plasma were instead related to maternal intake of seafood, total fish, and fatty fish, which are known sources of n-3 PUFAs, as well as the intake levels of game meat, egg, cheese, and milk. Univariate statistical analysis using Spearman's correlation showed the only significant correlations between maternal dietary food intake and infant proportions of fatty acids were a negative correlation between the infant proportions of n-6 PUFAs and maternal intake of fatty fish (Rho = −0.17, p = 0.02) and total fish (Rho = −0.16, p = 0.03). For maternal fatty acid proportions more correlations were significant in univariate statistics: the maternal proportions of n-3 PUFAs correlated positively with their intake levels of fatty fish (Rho = 0.22, p = 0.003), total fish (Rho = 0.21, p = 0.005), egg (Rho = 0.17, p = 0.02), and nuts and seeds (Rho = 0.19, p = 0.01), whereas they correlated negatively with the intake of chocolate (Rho = −0.17, p = 0.02). The maternal proportions of n-6 PUFAs, on the other hand, correlated negatively with their intake levels of fatty fish (Rho = −0.15, p = 0.04), total fish (Rho = −0.15, p = 0.04), and cow's milk (Rho = −0.17, p = 0.02).

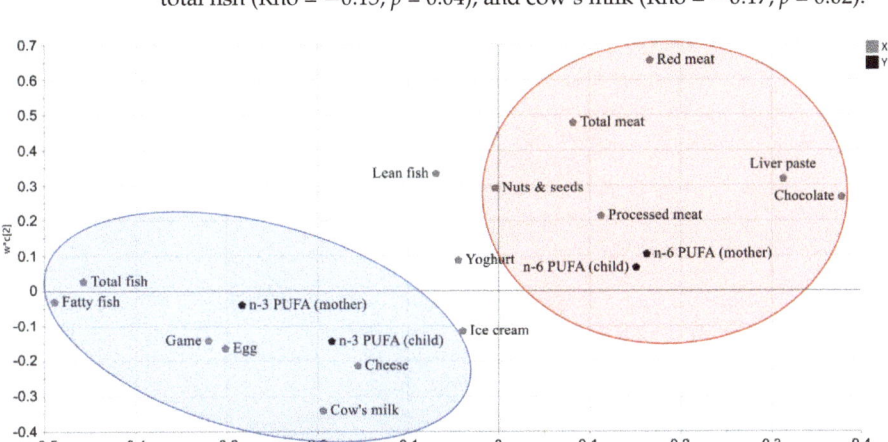

Figure 4. Partial least squares (PLS) loading plot showing the associations between maternal food intake during pregnancy and proportions of n-3 and n-6 polyunsaturated fatty acids (PUFAs) in the infant's and mother's plasma phospholipids at birth (N = 196 mothers and N = 196 children).

4. Discussion

In the present study, we show that the fatty acid profiles of phospholipids in the cord blood samples obtained from infants at birth are linked to a modified risk of developing atopic eczema during the first year of life. More specifically, higher proportions of n-6 LCP-UFAs in the infant's phospholipids at birth were associated with an increased risk of atopic eczema at 12 months of age, whereas higher proportions of n-3 PUFAs were associated with a decreased risk. The strongest association were found for the n-6 PUFA arachidonic acid where one IQR (interquartile range) increase in the proportion of arachidonic acid in infant cord plasma was associated with an over two-fold higher risk of eczema during the first year of life, after adjustment for allergic heredity as well as after adjustment for *FLG* loss of function mutations.

Since we examined the proportions of fatty acids among plasma phospholipids, a high proportion of one type of fatty acid inevitably yields lower proportions of the other types of fatty acids. Therefore, the apparent protective effects of α-linoleic acid and DPA with regards to atopic eczema may be due to a relatively lower percentage of arachidonic acid and vice versa. When α-linolenic acid and DPA were added to a logistic regression model together with arachidonic acid these fatty acids were no longer associated with lower odds of developing atopic eczema. Furthermore, as shown in Supplementary Figure S1, arachidonic acid was found to be more important than any of the n-3 fatty acids in terms of distinguishing infants with and without eczema. This indicates that arachidonic acid plays a negative role in eczema development in itself, and not only as a result of relatively lower n-3 PUFA proportions.

Fatty acids may play an important role both in atopic eczema development and disease. One association between fatty acids and atopic eczema is connected to the skin barrier function. The primary role of the skin is to prevent water loss and protect from UV light, entry of harmful compounds and organisms from the environment. The skin consists among other things of different lipids which contribute to skin barrier function, membrane structure, and cell function [25] The lipids in the extracellular lipid membranes of the outer layer of the skin, the stratum corneum, mediate the permeability barrier function [26]. Impaired skin barrier function is one important factor in atopic disease development [27]. It may, for example, increase the risk for sensitization to food allergens, according to "the dual exposure hypothesis", which suggests that tolerance to food antigens occurs in early life through high-dose oral exposure while a low dose cutaneous exposure of food allergens through a disrupted skin barrier increases allergic sensitization [28]. *FLG* loss-of-function mutations reduce the skin barrier function and these mutations have been identified as a risk factor for different allergic diseases such as atopic eczema [29,30]. No associations were found in this study between *FLG* and atopic eczema. Further, adjusting the logistic regression models for *FLG* (or allergy within the family which reflects heredity) did not influence the association between arachidonic acid and atopic eczema, suggesting that the association between arachidonic acid and increased risk of atopic eczema is not confounded by genetic variation in skin barrier function. However, the small sample size limits our conclusions.

Except for the effect on skin permeability, fatty acids have other characteristics of importance for allergy development and disease. The association between arachidonic acid and atopic eczema development found in this study may, for example, be attributed to lipid mediators (i.e., eicosanoids), which are produced from long-chain PUFAs such as arachidonic acid [6]. For instance, prostaglandin E2 (PGE2) play important roles in several mechanisms linked to allergic sensitization and allergic inflammation. It supports the activation of dendritic cells, and suppresses the functions of macrophages, neutrophils, and the Th1-, CTL-, and NK cell-mediated type 1 immunity. In addition, it promotes vascular permeability, as well as Th2, Th17, and regulatory T-cell responses [31], while it inhibits the production of Th1-type cytokines. PGE2 is also involved in the priming of naïve T cells, resulting in the production of interleukin (IL)-4 and IL-5, as well as the promotion of immunoglobulin (Ig) class switching in naive B cells towards the production of IgE [31]. Results from previous observational studies on the effects of fatty acids in infant cord plasma on allergy development are inconsistent [32–36]. In accordance with our results, we have previously reported that in the FARMFLORA birth cohort, that the proportions of n-3 LCPUFAs in infant cord serum, which correlated positively with maternal fish intake during pregnancy, were negatively associated with infant allergies at both 3 and 8 years of age [32]. In addition, a Spanish cohort [33] that included 211 mother-child pairs found that both DHA and the sum of total n-3 PUFAs correlated negatively with parental-reported atopic eczema at 14 months of age. They also reported a non-significant correlation between higher levels of arachidonic acid and lower prevalence of atopic eczema. Furthermore, in a nested case-control study of 70 children, the children with allergic sensitization and atopic dermatitis before the age of 3 years were shown to have lower levels of both EPA and α-linoleic acid in their cord blood plasma [36]. In a larger cohort study that comprised 1238 infants from the ALPSAC study, no associations were found for specific fatty acids, except for the ratio of arachidonic acid to EPA in infant's red blood cells at birth, which was positively associated with parental-reported eczema at 30 months of age [34]. In another European birth cohort, the Munich LISAplus cohort, no associations were found in 436 children between the concentrations of any n-3 or n-6 fatty acids in the infant cord serum and allergy (including eczema) at 6 and 10 years of age [35]. Hence, the results from previous epidemiological studies are inconsistent, although the majority suggests a protective effect of n-3. PUFA and further evaluation is needed.

During pregnancy, fatty acids are transported from the maternal circulation to the fetal circulation across the placenta, and for long-chain PUFAs, this is achieved through active transport mediated by transport proteins [37]. This active transport is evident when comparing the proportions of fatty acids in infant and maternal plasma, in that we found that the infant plasma contained lower proportions of linoleic acid, α-linolenic acid, EPA, and DPA but higher proportions of DGLA, arachidonic acid, adrenic acid, and DHA. These results are in accordance with our previous findings in the FARMFLORA study [38]. In the present study, we show that even though the proportions of many of the fatty acids differed between mothers and infants, all the fatty acids, with the exception of α-linolenic acid, were strongly positively correlated between infants and mothers. Therefore, the fatty acid composition of the fetus' blood is related to the fatty acid composition of the mother's blood, which in turn is related to the maternal intake of fat-rich food items and maternal fatty acid metabolism. Long-chain PUFAs of both the n-3 and n-6 series may be endogenously produced from short-chain fatty acid precursors, linoleic acid and α-linolenic acid, and the capacity for this conversion seems to be higher in women during pregnancy [7,8]. Fetal endogenous production of long-chain fatty acids has also been suggested, although it is not as well-studied and may be lower than maternal production [39]. When we used PLS to study how the proportions of n-3 and n-6 PUFAs in infant cord plasma and maternal plasma were related to maternal food intake, we found a positive association between n-3 PUFAs in both the infant and maternal plasma and maternal intake levels of seafood, total fish, and fatty fish, which are known sources of n-3 LCPUFAs. Moreover, a positive association between n-6 LCPUFAs and maternal intake of meat was detected.

In the present study, atopic eczema was associated with lower proportions of n-3 PUFAs and higher proportions of n-6 PUFAs, which in turn were associated with lower maternal intake of fish and higher intake of meat. These findings may suggest that maternal intake of fish during pregnancy is associated with a reduced risk of atopic eczema, and that maternal intake of meat during pregnancy is associated with an increased risk of atopic eczema during the first year of life. We have previously published data on the associations between the intake of food items and nutrients during pregnancy (and lactation) and infant allergy risk during the first year of life, among all the infants in the NICE cohort with data available for maternal food intake and allergy outcomes (N = 508). In the current study, a subset of the cohort was included based on the availability of cord plasma samples from the infants at birth and allergy outcomes (N = 206). In the previous study [19], as well as in the current study, no significant direct associations were identified between maternal fish intake and atopic eczema. This may reflect the difficulties associated with accurately measuring food intake using food frequency questionnaires [40–42]. Since n-3 LCPUFAs, especially EPA and DHA, are recognized biomarkers of fish intake [43,44], they may be well-suited to serve as a proxy for maternal fish intake. Thus, the inverse association observed between n-3 PUFAs and allergy in the current study may either arise from a protective effect of n-3 PUFAs *per se*. Alternatively, it could be a marker of higher maternal intake of fish, which may offer protection by means other than its content of n-3 PUFAs. The association seen between higher proportions of n-6 PUFAs and increased risk of atopic eczema is not as easily explained by maternal food intake, since arachidonic acid is found in many different food items in addition to meat. However, we found a correlation between meat intake and higher plasma arachidonic acid proportions, and this association has also been reported in previous studies [45,46]. Furthermore, the hypothesis that maternal fish intake during pregnancy protects against childhood atopic eczema is supported by several other observational studies [15,16,47,48], while the negative effects on infant allergy of maternal intake of meat are less widely reported. Still, a study on 1140 mother-infant pairs from the French EDEN cohort found that a higher maternal intake of meat during pregnancy was associated with increased risks of wheezing, allergic rhinitis, and atopic eczema in children at 3 years of age [49]. Several review articles have discussed the effects of maternal dietary intake during pregnancy on allergic outcomes in children, reaching different conclusions [6,50–52]. A systematic review by Kremmyda and colleagues in 2011 [53] reported on a protective association between maternal fish intake during pregnancy and allergic outcomes in the offspring based on five observational studies, while a systematic review by Netting and coworkers in 2014 [52] did not find any consistent linkages between mothers' dietary intake and atopic outcomes in their children. In 2017, another review was published by Venter et al. [50], who concluded that current evidence regarding the effects of maternal diet in pregnancy and lactation on allergic disease outcomes in the offspring is limited [50]. Our own conclusion is that there seems to be some beneficial association between maternal fish intake during pregnancy and allergy development in offspring, and this is supported by the results of the current study, but whether or not these effects are due to a protective effect of the n-3 fatty acids *per se* or due to other components of the fish remains to be elucidated.

Strengths and Limitations

The major strength of the present study is that atopic eczema was physician-diagnosed based on strict criteria and that all the children met with the same pediatrician specialized in allergy. A limitation of the current study is that the phospholipid fatty acids 16:0 and 18:0 could not be quantified due to contamination from the SPE columns. Therefore, as these are not included in the sum of the total phospholipids, the proportions of the different fatty acids that we show here are therefore not comparable with the levels or proportions of fatty acids reported in other studies. Furthermore, due to the observational design of our study, there is always a risk of residual confounding, and we cannot investigate causality.

5. Conclusions

Our results suggest that higher proportions of n-3 PUFAs and lower proportions of n-6 PUFAs in infant cord serum at birth may be associated with a reduced risk of developing atopic eczema during the first year of life. The proportions of n-3 PUFAs increase with a higher intake of fish, while the n-6 PUFAs are associated with meat consumption. Therefore, our findings imply that it might be beneficial, at least partly, to choose fish over meat during pregnancy, so as to prevent eczema in the offspring. However, it remains to be discovered whether this is due to a protective effect of the n-3 fatty acids *per se* or due to other components of the fish or if it is due to an allergy-promoting effect of arachidonic acid or meat intake.

Supplementary Materials: The following are available online at https://www.mdpi.com/article/10.3390/nu13113779/s1, Figure S1: Orthogonal partial least square (OPLS) model of the associations between atopic eczema at 12 months of age and fatty acids in maternal and cord plasma phospholipids, Table S1: Primer pairs for detecting variations in the filaggrin gene, Table S2: Median (25th–75th percentile) fatty acid proportions of phospholipids in maternal and infant plasma at birth, Table S3: Relative proportions of phospholipids in cord serum at birth in children with atopic eczema compared to non-allergic children, Table S4: Relative proportions of phospholipids in maternal serum at birth in mothers to children with atopic eczema compared to mothers to non-allergic children.

Author Contributions: Conceptualization, M.B., A.S., A.E.W. and A.-S.S.; data curation, M.B., M.S., K.B. and A.S.; formal analysis, M.B. and M.S.; funding acquisition, M.B., K.B., A.E.W. and A.-S.S.; investigation, M.B. and M.S.; methodology, M.B., M.S. and K.B.; project administration, A.S., A.E.W. and A.-S.S.; resources, A.S.; supervision, A.-S.S.; validation, M.B.; visualization, M.B. and M.S.; writing—original draft, M.B.; writing—review and editing, M.S., K.B., A.S., A.E.W. and A.-S.S. All authors have read and agreed to the published version of the manuscript.

Funding: This research was funded by the Swedish Research Council (VR) [521-2013-3154 and 2019-01317] to A.-S.S.; Swedish Research Council for Health, Working Life and Welfare (FORTE) [2014-0923, 2016-00700, 2018-00485] to A.E.W.; Västra Götaland Region (RUN) [612-0618-15] to A.-S.S.; Research and Innovation Unit at Region Norrbotten to A.S.; Magnus Bergvalls stiftelse [2017-02297] to M.B.; Wilhelm och Martina Lundgrens stiftelse [2018-2250 and 2019-3141] to M.B.; Dr Per Håkanssons stiftelse to M.B. (2019 and 2020); Stiftelsen Sigurd och Elsa Goljes Minne [LA2019-0105] to M.B.; The Royal Society of Arts and Sciences in Gothenburg to M.B.; and Jane och Dan Olssons stiftelse [2020-23] to A.-S.S.

Institutional Review Board Statement: The study was conducted according to the guidelines of the Declaration of Helsinki and approved by the Regional Ethical Review Board in Umeå, Sweden (2013/18-31M, 2015-71-32).

Informed Consent Statement: Informed consent was obtained from all subjects involved in the study. To be able to participate, all women and their partners had to sign a written consent form both for themselves and for their child. All participants were informed about the right to withdraw from the birth cohort at any point and to have their data removed.

Data Availability Statement: The food frequency questionnaires are not publicly available due to proprietary rights. The raw data used in this study are not publicly available because they relate to information that could compromise research participant privacy or consent. Explicit consent to deposit raw data was not obtained from the participants. Therefore, the data can only be made public if a new consent is filled in by the participants together with a new ethical permit being obtained.

Acknowledgments: We give our warmest thanks to all the participating families within the NICE cohort. We thank study coordinator Fiona Murray, study nurses Marjut Larsson and Ulrika Börlin, study midwives Lisa Sundén and Louise Lindgren and study assistant Elvira Sandin for excellent management of the cohort, including recruitment, sending out questionnaires, collecting and preparing samples, and meeting all the participating families at the different follow-up time points. We also thank statistician Robert Lundqvist at Region Norrbotten, Linda Englund-Ögge and Bo Jacobsson for collecting and managing data on pregnancy and birth outcomes from medical charts. We further thank Katarina Bälter for processing the Meal-Q questionnaires, master student Elin Johansson for performing all the fatty acid analysis, and Helena Korres de Paula for performing the DNA extractions and the filaggrin genotyping.

Conflicts of Interest: The authors declare no conflict of interest. The funders had no role in the design of the study; in the collection, analyses, or interpretation of data; in the writing of the manuscript, or in the decision to publish the results.

References

1. Nutten, S. Atopic dermatitis: Global epidemiology and risk factors. *Ann. Nutr. Metab.* **2015**, *66*, 8–16. [CrossRef]
2. Hill, D.A.; Spergel, J.M. The atopic march: Critical evidence and clinical relevance. *Ann. Allergy Asthma Immunol.* **2018**, *120*, 131–137. [CrossRef]
3. Werfel, T.; Allam, J.P.; Biedermann, T.; Eyerich, K.; Gilles, S.; Guttman-Yassky, E.; Hoetzenecker, W.; Knol, E.; Simon, H.U.; Wollenberg, A.; et al. Cellular and molecular immunologic mechanisms in patients with atopic dermatitis. *J. Allergy Clin. Immunol.* **2016**, *138*, 336–349. [CrossRef]
4. Black, P.N.; Sharpe, S. Dietary fat and asthma: Is there a connection? *Eur. Respir. J.* **1997**, *10*, 6–12. [CrossRef]
5. Sala-Vila, A.; Miles, E.A.; Calder, P.C. Fatty acid composition abnormalities in atopic disease: Evidence explored and role in the disease process examined. *Clin. Exp. Allergy* **2008**, *38*, 1432–1450. [CrossRef]
6. Miles, E.A.; Calder, P.C. Can early omega-3 fatty acid exposure reduce risk of childhood allergic disease? LID-784. *Nutrients* **2017**, *9*, 784. [CrossRef]
7. Burdge, G.C.; Calder, P.C. Conversion of alpha-linolenic acid to longer-chain polyunsaturated fatty acids in human adults. *Reprod. Nutr. Dev.* **2005**, *45*, 581–597. [CrossRef]
8. Burdge, G.C.; Wootton, S.A. Conversion of alpha-linolenic acid to eicosapentaenoic, docosapentaenoic and docosahexaenoic acids in young women. *Br. J. Nutr.* **2002**, *88*, 411–420. [CrossRef]
9. Calder, P.C. Dietary fatty acids and the immune system. *Nutr. Rev.* **1998**, *56*, S70–S83. [CrossRef]
10. Calder, P.C. Immunomodulation by omega-3 fatty acids. *Prostaglandins Leukot. Essent. Fat. Acids* **2007**, *77*, 327–335. [CrossRef]
11. Kliewer, S.A.; Sundseth, S.S.; Jones, S.A.; Brown, P.J.; Wisely, G.B.; Koble, C.S.; Devchand, P.; Wahli, W.; Willson, T.M.; Lenhard, J.M.; et al. Fatty acids and eicosanoids regulate gene expression through direct interactions with peroxisome proliferator-activated receptors alpha and gamma. *Proc. Natl. Acad. Sci. USA* **1997**, *94*, 4318–4323. [CrossRef]
12. Delerive, P.; Furman, C.; Teissier, E.; Fruchart, J.; Duriez, P.; Staels, B. Oxidized phospholipids activate PPARalpha in a phospholipase A2-dependent manner. *FEBS Lett.* **2000**, *471*, 34–38. [CrossRef]
13. Hirasawa, A.; Tsumaya, K.; Awaji, T.; Katsuma, S.; Adachi, T.; Yamada, M.; Sugimoto, Y.; Miyazaki, S.; Tsujimoto, G. Free fatty acids regulate gut incretin glucagon-like peptide-1 secretion through GPR120. *Nat. Med.* **2005**, *11*, 90–94. [CrossRef]
14. Oh, D.Y.; Talukdar, S.; Bae, E.J.; Imamura, T.; Morinaga, H.; Fan, W.; Li, P.; Lu, W.J.; Watkins, S.M.; Olefsky, J.M. GPR120 is an omega-3 fatty acid receptor mediating potent anti-inflammatory and insulin-sensitizing effects. *Cell* **2010**, *142*, 687–698. [CrossRef]
15. Romieu, I.; Torrent, M.; Garcia-Esteban, R.; Ferrer, C.; Ribas-Fito, N.; Anto, J.M.; Sunyer, J. Maternal fish intake during pregnancy and atopy and asthma in infancy. *Clin. Exp. Allergy* **2007**, *37*, 518–525. [CrossRef]
16. Sausenthaler, S.; Koletzko, S.; Schaaf, B.; Lehmann, I.; Borte, M.; Herbarth, O.; von Berg, A.; Wichmann, H.E.; Heinrich, J.; Group, L.S. Maternal diet during pregnancy in relation to eczema and allergic sensitization in the offspring at 2 y of age. *Am. J. Clin. Nutr.* **2007**, *85*, 530–537. [CrossRef]
17. Barman, M.; Murray, F.; Bernardi, A.I.; Broberg, K.; Bolte, S.; Hesselmar, B.; Jacobsson, B.; Jonsson, K.; Kippler, M.; Rabe, H.; et al. Nutritional impact on Immunological maturation during Childhood in relation to the Environment (NICE): A prospective birth cohort in northern Sweden. *BMJ Open* **2018**, *8*, e022013. [CrossRef]
18. Stravik, M.; Jonsson, K.; Hartvigsson, O.; Sandin, A.; Wold, A.E.; Sandberg, A.S.; Barman, M. Food and nutrient intake during pregnancy in relation to maternal characteristics: Results from the NICE Birth Cohort in Northern Sweden. *Nutrients* **2019**, *11*, 1680. [CrossRef]
19. Stravik, M.; Barman, M.; Hesselmar, B.; Sandin, A.; Wold, A.E.; Sandberg, A.S. Maternal intake of cow's milk during lactation is associated with lower prevalence of food allergy in offspring. *Nutrients* **2020**, *12*, 3680. [CrossRef]
20. Swedish Food Agency. The Food Database. Available online: https://www.livsmedelsverket.se/en/food-and-content/naringsamnen/livsmedelsdatabasen (accessed on 22 September 2021).

21. Williams, H.C.; Burney, P.G.; Hay, R.J.; Archer, C.B.; Shipley, M.J.; Hunter, J.J.; Bingham, E.A.; Finlay, A.Y.; Pembroke, A.C.; Graham-Brown, R.A.; et al. The U.K. Working Party's Diagnostic Criteria for Atopic Dermatitis. I. Derivation of a minimum set of discriminators for atopic dermatitis. *Br. J. Derm.* **1994**, *131*, 383–396. [CrossRef]
22. Williams, H.C.; Burney, P.G.; Pembroke, A.C.; Hay, R.J. The U.K. Working Party's Diagnostic Criteria for Atopic Dermatitis. III. Independent hospital validation. *Br. J. Derm.* **1994**, *131*, 406–416. [CrossRef]
23. Williams, H.C.; Burney, P.G.; Strachan, D.; Hay, R.J. The U.K. Working Party's Diagnostic Criteria for Atopic Dermatitis. II. Observer variation of clinical diagnosis and signs of atopic dermatitis. *Br. J. Derm.* **1994**, *131*, 397–405. [CrossRef]
24. Wahlberg, K.; Liljedahl, E.R.; Alhamdow, A.; Lindh, C.; Lidén, C.; Albin, M.; Tinnerberg, H.; Broberg, K. Filaggrin variations are associated with PAH metabolites in urine and DNA alterations in blood. *Envion. Res.* **2019**, *177*, 108600. [CrossRef]
25. Feingold, K.R.; Elias, P.M. Role of lipids in the formation and maintenance of the cutaneous permeability barrier. *Biochim. Biophys. Acta* **2014**, *1841*, 280–294. [CrossRef]
26. Khnykin, D.; Miner, J.H.; Jahnsen, F. Role of fatty acid transporters in epidermis: Implications for health and disease. *Dermatoendocrinology* **2011**, *3*, 53–61. [CrossRef]
27. Weidinger, S.; Illig, T.; Baurecht, H.; Irvine, A.D.; Rodriguez, E.; Diaz-Lacava, A.; Klopp, N.; Wagenpfeil, S.; Zhao, Y.; Liao, H.; et al. Loss-of-function variations within the filaggrin gene predispose for atopic dermatitis with allergic sensitizations. *J. Allergy Clin. Immunol.* **2006**, *118*, 214–219. [CrossRef]
28. Lack, G. Update on risk factors for food allergy. *J. Allergy Clin. Immunol.* **2012**, *129*, 1187–1197. [CrossRef]
29. Weidinger, S.; O'Sullivan, M.; Illig, T.; Baurecht, H.; Depner, M.; Rodriguez, E.; Ruether, A.; Klopp, N.; Vogelberg, C.; Weiland, S.K.; et al. Filaggrin mutations, atopic eczema, hay fever, and asthma in children. *J. Allergy Clin. Immunol.* **2008**, *121*, 1203–1209.e1201. [CrossRef]
30. Palmer, C.N.A.; Irvine, A.D.; Terron-Kwiatkowski, A.; Zhao, Y.; Liao, H.; Lee, S.P.; Goudie, D.R.; Sandilands, A.; Campbell, L.E.; Smith, F.J.D.; et al. Common loss-of-function variants of the epidermal barrier protein filaggrin are a major predisposing factor for atopic dermatitis. *Nat. Genet.* **2006**, *38*, 441–446. [CrossRef]
31. Kalinski, P. Regulation of immune responses by prostaglandin E2. *J. Immunol.* **2012**, *188*, 21–28. [CrossRef]
32. Barman, M.; Rabe, H.; Hesselmar, B.; Johansen, S.; Sandberg, A.S.; Wold, A.E. Cord blood levels of EPA, a marker of fish intake, correlate with infants' T- and B-lymphocyte phenotypes and risk for allergic disease. *Nutrients* **2020**, *12*, 3000. [CrossRef]
33. Montes, R.; Chisaguano, A.M.; Castellote, A.I.; Morales, E.; Sunyer, J.; Lopez-Sabater, M.C. Fatty-acid composition of maternal and umbilical cord plasma and early childhood atopic eczema in a Spanish cohort. *Eur. J. Clin. Nutr.* **2013**, *67*, 658–663. [CrossRef]
34. Newson, R.B.; Shaheen, S.O.; Henderson, A.J.; Emmett, P.M.; Sherriff, A.; Calder, P.C. Umbilical cord and maternal blood red cell fatty acids and early childhood wheezing and eczema. *J. Allergy Clin. Immunol.* **2004**, *114*, 531–537. [CrossRef] [PubMed]
35. Standl, M.; Demmelmair, H.; Koletzko, B.; Heinrich, J. Cord blood LC-PUFA composition and allergic diseases during the first 10 yr. Results from the LISAplus study. *Pediatr. Allergy Immunol.* **2014**, *25*, 344–350. [CrossRef]
36. Byberg, K.; Oymar, K.; Aksnes, L. Fatty acids in cord blood plasma, the relation to soluble CD23 and subsequent atopy. *Prostaglandins Leukot. Essent. Fat. Acids* **2008**, *78*, 61–65. [CrossRef] [PubMed]
37. Cunningham, P.; McDermott, L. Long chain PUFA transport in human term placenta. *J. Nutr.* **2009**, *139*, 636–639. [CrossRef]
38. Barman, M.; Jonsson, K.; Wold, A.E.; Sandberg, A.S. Exposure to a farm environment during pregnancy increases the proportion of arachidonic acid in the cord sera of offspring. *Nutrients* **2019**, *11*, 238. [CrossRef]
39. Carnielli, V.P.; Wattimena, D.J.; Luijendijk, I.H.; Boerlage, A.; Degenhart, H.J.; Sauer, P.J. The very low birth weight premature infant is capable of synthesizing arachidonic and docosahexaenoic acids from linoleic and linolenic acids. *Pediatr. Res.* **1996**, *40*, 169–174. [CrossRef] [PubMed]
40. Gemming, L.; Ni Mhurchu, C. Dietary under-reporting: What foods and which meals are typically under-reported? *Eur. J. Clin. Nutr.* **2016**, *70*, 640–641. [CrossRef]
41. Freedman, L.S.; Commins, J.M.; Moler, J.E.; Arab, L.; Baer, D.J.; Kipnis, V.; Midthune, D.; Moshfegh, A.J.; Neuhouser, M.L.; Prentice, R.L.; et al. Pooled results from 5 validation studies of dietary self-report instruments using recovery biomarkers for energy and protein intake. *Am. J. Epidemiol.* **2014**, *180*, 172–188. [CrossRef] [PubMed]
42. Kipnis, V.; Midthune, D.; Freedman, L.; Bingham, S.; Day, N.E.; Riboli, E.; Ferrari, P.; Carroll, R.J. Bias in dietary-report instruments and its implications for nutritional epidemiology. *Public Health Nutr.* **2002**, *5*, 915–923. [CrossRef]
43. Hjartaker, A.; Lund, E.; Bjerve, K.S. Serum phospholipid fatty acid composition and habitual intake of marine foods registered by a semi-quantitative food frequency questionnaire. *Eur. J. Clin. Nutr.* **1997**, *51*, 736–742. [CrossRef]
44. Lindberg, M.; Midthjell, K.; Bjerve, K.S. Long-term tracking of plasma phospholipid fatty acid concentrations and their correlation with the dietary intake of marine foods in newly diagnosed diabetic patients: Results from a follow-up of the HUNT Study, Norway. *Br. J. Nutr.* **2013**, *109*, 1123–1134. [CrossRef]
45. Seah, J.Y.; Gay, G.M.; Su, J.; Tai, E.S.; Yuan, J.M.; Koh, W.P.; Ong, C.N.; van Dam, R.M. consumption of red meat, but not cooking oils high in polyunsaturated fat, is associated with higher arachidonic acid status in singapore chinese adults. *Nutrients* **2017**, *9*, 101. [CrossRef] [PubMed]
46. Sinclair, A.J.; Johnson, L.; O'Dea, K.; Holman, R.T. Diets rich in lean beef increase arachidonic acid and long-chain omega 3 polyunsaturated fatty acid levels in plasma phospholipids. *Lipids* **1994**, *29*, 337–343. [CrossRef] [PubMed]

47. Willers, S.M.; Devereux, G.; Craig, L.C.; McNeill, G.; Wijga, A.H.; Abou El-Magd, W.; Turner, S.W.; Helms, P.J.; Seaton, A. Maternal food consumption during pregnancy and asthma, respiratory and atopic symptoms in 5-year-old children. *Thorax* **2007**, *62*, 773–779. [CrossRef]
48. Jedrychowski, W.; Perera, F.; Maugeri, U.; Mrozek-Budzyn, D.; Miller, R.L.; Flak, E.; Mroz, E.; Jacek, R.; Spengler, J.D. Effects of prenatal and perinatal exposure to fine air pollutants and maternal fish consumption on the occurrence of infantile eczema. *Int. Arch. Allergy Immunol.* **2011**, *155*, 275–281. [CrossRef]
49. Baiz, N.; Just, J.; Chastang, J.; Forhan, A.; de Lauzon-Guillain, B.; Magnier, A.M.; Annesi-Maesano, I.; The EDEN Mother-Child Cohort Study Group. Maternal diet before and during pregnancy and risk of asthma and allergic rhinitis in children. *Allergy Asthma Clin. Immunol.* **2019**, *15*, 40. [CrossRef]
50. Venter, C.; Brown, K.R.; Maslin, K.; Palmer, D.J. Maternal dietary intake in pregnancy and lactation and allergic disease outcomes in offspring. *Pediatr. Allergy Immunol.* **2017**, *28*, 135–143. [CrossRef] [PubMed]
51. Garcia-Larsen, V.; Ierodiakonou, D.; Jarrold, K.; Cunha, S.; Chivinge, J.; Robinson, Z.; Geoghegan, N.; Ruparelia, A.; Devani, P.; Trivella, M.; et al. Diet during pregnancy and infancy and risk of allergic or autoimmune disease: A systematic review and meta-analysis. *PLoS Med.* **2018**, *15*, e1002507. [CrossRef] [PubMed]
52. Netting, M.J.; Middleton, P.F.; Makrides, M. Does maternal diet during pregnancy and lactation affect outcomes in offspring? A systematic review of food-based approaches. *Nutrition* **2014**, *30*, 1225–1241. [CrossRef]
53. Kremmyda, L.S.; Vlachava, M.; Noakes, P.S.; Diaper, N.D.; Miles, E.A.; Calder, P.C. Atopy risk in infants and children in relation to early exposure to fish, oily fish, or long-chain omega-3 fatty acids: A systematic review. *Clin. Rev. Allergy Immunol.* **2011**, *41*, 36–66. [CrossRef] [PubMed]

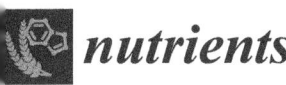

Opinion

Partial Hydrolyzed Protein as a Protein Source for Infant Feeding: Do or Don't?

Yvan Vandenplas [1,*], Janusz Książyk [2], Manuel Sanchez Luna [3], Natalia Migacheva [4], Jean-Charles Picaud [5,6], Luca A. Ramenghi [7], Atul Singhal [8] and Martin Wabitsch [9]

1. KidZ Health Castle, Vrije Universiteit Brussel (VUB), 1090 Brussel, Belgium
2. Department of Pediatrics, Nutrition, and Metabolic Diseases, The Children's Memorial Health Institute, 04-730 Warsaw, Poland; j.ksiazyk@ipczd.pl
3. Neonatology Division and NICU, Hospital General Universitario "Gregorio Marañón", Complutense University of Madrid, 28009 Madrid, Spain; msluna@salud.madrid.org
4. Department of Pediatrics, Samara State Medical University, 443084 Samara, Russia; nbmigacheva@gmail.com
5. Department of Neonatology, Hôpital de la Croix-Rousse, Hospices Civils de Lyon, F69677 Lyon, France; jean-charles.picaud@chu-lyon.fr
6. CarMen Laboratory, INSERM, INRA, Claude Bernard University Lyon1, F69310 Pierre-Benite, France
7. Department of Neuroscience, Ophthalmology, Genetics, Maternal and Child Health (DINOGMI), University of Genoa, 16147 Genoa, Italy; lucaramenghi@gaslini.org
8. Childhood Nutrition Research Centre, PPP Department, UCL GOS Institute of Child Health, London WC1N 1EH, UK; a.singhal@ucl.ac.uk
9. Division of Pediatric Endocrinology and Diabetes, Department of Pediatrics and Adolescent Medicine, University of Ulm, 89075 Ulm, Germany; martin.wabitsch@uniklinik-ulm.de
* Correspondence: yvan.vandenplas@uzbrussel.be; Tel.: +32-475748794

Citation: Vandenplas, Y.; Książyk, J.; Luna, M.S.; Migacheva, N.; Picaud, J.-C.; Ramenghi, L.A.; Singhal, A.; Wabitsch, M. Partial Hydrolyzed Protein as a Protein Source for Infant Feeding: Do or Don't? *Nutrients* 2022, 14, 1720. https://doi.org/10.3390/nu14091720

Academic Editors: RJ Joost Van Neerven, Janneke Ruinemans-Koerts and Alessio Fasano

Received: 6 March 2022
Accepted: 18 April 2022
Published: 21 April 2022

Publisher's Note: MDPI stays neutral with regard to jurisdictional claims in published maps and institutional affiliations.

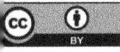

Copyright: © 2022 by the authors. Licensee MDPI, Basel, Switzerland. This article is an open access article distributed under the terms and conditions of the Creative Commons Attribution (CC BY) license (https://creativecommons.org/licenses/by/4.0/).

Abstract: Exclusive breastfeeding until the age of six months is the recommended feeding method for all infants. However, this is not possible for every infant. Therefore, a second choice of feeding, as close as possible to the gold standard, is needed. For historical reasons, this has been cow's-milk-based feeding. This paper discusses if this second-choice feeding method should contain intact protein or partially hydrolyzed proteins. The limited data available indicates that mother's milk is relatively rich in bioactive peptides. Whether partially hydrolyzed protein might be a protein source closer to human milk protein content than intact cow's milk needs further research. However, more research on protein and bioactive peptides in mother's milk should be a priority for future scientific development in this field. Results of such research will also provide an answer to the question of which option would be the best second choice for infant feeding if sufficient breast milk is not available.

Keywords: breastfeeding; functional gastrointestinal disorder; partial hydrolysate; peptide; prevention; protein

1. Introduction

Hydrolyzed formulas for infants who are not breastfed can be of two types: partially or extensively hydrolyzed cow's-milk-protein based. Protein hydrolysis means that proteins are broken down into smaller components or peptides. The size of the peptides determines the classification of a formula as partially hydrolyzed (most peptides with molecular weight of 3–10 kDa) or extensively hydrolyzed (peptides with molecular weight of <3 kDa) [1]. This definition is based on consensus rather than scientific evidence. Hydrolyzation results in a range or continuum of peptide sizes. However, different methods of protein hydrolysis (e.g., heat treatment, enzymatic hydrolysis) are applied by various manufacturers of infant formula. As a result, the end-products of each company differ. The peptide size of some formulas has been reported to be production dependent [2]. There is no evidence to indicate whether differences in peptide size result in different clinical outcomes, although some studies suggest that up to half of all children with a proven cow's milk allergy (CMA) have incomplete resolution of symptoms upon treatment with an extensive whey hydrolysate [3]. Similar differences are reported for partial hydrolysates, i.e., differences in peptide size, allergenicity, and induction of tolerance [4]. Peptide size was not necessarily associated with a reduction in allergenicity in vitro, nor with oral tolerance induction in vivo, as measured by a specific IgE level [4].

In summary, hypo-allergenicity and the induction of oral tolerance are hydrolysate specific. Therefore, it is not recommended to pool data obtained from clinical trials involving different hydrolysates.

2. Breastfeeding

Exclusive breastfeeding up to the age of 6 months is the preferred feeding method for all infants. However, there is no evidence that breastfeeding has a preventative effect on the risk of developing allergies [5]. A crucial factor in deciding the optimal second choice of protein source for infant formula is the knowledge of the protein structure in mother's milk. Unfortunately, this has been poorly studied. There is no evidence to suggest that intact cow's milk protein is the protein source closest to the protein found in human milk, and there is even some data suggesting that the protein in goat's milk, rather than cow's milk, might be closer to that in human milk. In any case, the total protein content in human milk is much lower than in animal milk, and the casein/whey ratios differ substantially. However, these differences relate to the intact protein structure, not the size of the peptides. According to the limited data available, human milk is relatively rich in peptides because of human milk proteases [6]. Human milk contains more than 1100 unique peptides derived from the 42 milk protein hydrolysates within the mammary gland, including 306 potential bioactive peptides [7]. Milk proteases actively cleave milk proteins within the mammary gland, initiating the release of functional peptides. This means that the breastfed infant receives pre-digested proteins and numerous bioactive peptides [7]. Consequently, the protein structure in a partially hydrolyzed cow's-milk-based whey protein infant formula may be closer to the protein structure in human milk than that in intact whey protein formulas. However, proteolysis in the milk is controlled by a balance of protease inhibitors and protease activators, so not all milk proteins are digested within the mammary gland. This seems to be important, as many bioactive milk proteins (e.g., lactoferrin, immunoglobulin) need to remain intact to function [5]. More research is needed on the protein structure in mother's milk to improve protein similarity between first- and second-choice infant feeding.

3. Partial Hydrolysates

The possibility of preventing CMA and other allergies in infants is not unequivocally accepted [8–10]. Partial hydrolysates have been available in many countries for more than 30 years. They have been marketed in Europe as "hypo-allergenic formulae". This terminology caused a lot of confusion, as the term "hypo-allergenic formula" is used in the US to describe a formula that is effective in the management of CMA in more than 90% of all infants, with a confidence interval of 95% [11]. In Europe, the use of "hypo-allergenic" ("HA") was intended to indicate "reduced allergenicity", as it was hypothesized that hydrolyzed cow's milk protein would reduce its allergenicity. The use of the term "HA" refers to the fact that hydrolyzed protein has a reduced allergenicity in in vitro models [4] and does not focus on the clinical impact. The use of "partial" and "extensively" hydrolyzed protein removes the confusion induced by the term "hypo-allergenic".

Qualitative changes of the peptides as a result of the method of hydrolysis may influence the potential risk of allergic disease. Consequently, the degree of hydrolysis does not always correlate with the clinical effects in trials. Since different techniques are used to hydrolyze protein, the residual allergenicity of each formula is likely to differ. Peptide size is not necessarily associated with the in vitro reduction of allergenicity, nor is it associated with oral tolerance induction in vivo, as measured by specific IgE level [2]. Infant formulas differ regarding their ability to induce T-cell proliferation and proinflammatory cytokine secretion, which could also explain the different outcomes obtained in clinical studies using infant formulas [12]. However, it should also be recognized that differences demonstrated in peptide length and structure do not necessarily imply a difference in clinical outcome.

Data from in vitro and animal studies suggest that partially hydrolyzed protein has a reduced allergenicity and increases oral tolerance [13–15]. Animal studies suggest that a specific partial hydrolysate decreases the risk of atopic dermatitis by improving the skin barrier [15]. However, the etiology of allergic disease, including CMA, is multifactorial, with the genetic background, environmental factors, and contact with the offending allergen all contributing to the risk of allergy. The fact that many, if not all, confounding variables can be controlled in in vitro conditions or animal studies, which is not the case in real-life clinical settings, may explain the contradictory data.

Feeding infants hydrolyzed formulas has not convincingly been shown to reduce the prevalence of allergic disease and, specifically, CMA. According to a systematic review and meta-analysis (in which all studies are grouped together independent of formula or study design), there is no evidence that partial or extensive hydrolysates reduce the risk of allergic or immune-mediated disease [9]. However, some individual studies show a different outcome.

The German Infant Nutritional Intervention (GINI) study was one of the first to report evidence for a role of a specific partially hydrolyzed whey protein in the short- and long-term prevention of allergic manifestations, mainly atopic eczema, in infants with a positive family history of atopic disease [16]. The most recent follow-up data of the GINI study also suggest a reduced risk of asthma after puberty (reduced period prevalence between 16 and 20 years) [17]. Furthermore, the outcome of the GINI study illustrates the specificity of hydrolysates, as an extensive casein hydrolysate and a partially hydrolyzed whey protein showed a significant and clinically relevant reduction in eczema risk in at-risk infants, but the extensively hydrolyzed whey protein formula did not [16,17].

Current guidelines and recommendations, which are based on defined search criteria, remain neutral and do not make recommendations for or against the use of partial hydrolysates in the prevention of allergies. For example, the European Academy of Allergy and Clinical Immunology (EAACI) issued no recommendations for or against using partially or extensively hydrolyzed formula to prevent IgE mediated food allergies in infants and young children [10]. The EAACI also recommended against feeding infants intact cow's milk protein during the first week of life [10]. Another analysis of studies on different protein hydrolysates has led to the conclusion that their role in preventing allergies is small. However, this analysis also pooled the results from different protein hydrolysates and, therefore, does not allow an evaluation of the individual hydrolysates [18]. A meta-analysis that focuses exclusively on only one type of hydrolysate showed that this specific hydrolysate reduced the risk of eczema among children at high risk for allergies, albeit not at all time points [19]. Therefore, the recommendation of the updated guidelines on Allergy Prevention DGKJ/GPA 20/21 for at-risk infants is to consider whether an infant formula with efficacy demonstrated in allergy prevention studies is available until complementary feeding is introduced [20]. Recent guidelines do no longer recommend considering a family history of atopic disease as a risk factor [21,22].

Currently, only one observational study has suggested a possible negative outcome regarding allergenicity with a partial hydrolysate [23]. This study analyzed data from a French longitudinal birth cohort study. All children who received a HA formula based on a partially hydrolyzed protein at 2 months were consolidated into one single HA group (N = 251) and compared with children who received a cow's milk formula at 2 months (N = 7149). Apart from the extreme imbalance of the groups, the study does not allow for any conclusions concerning the effect of a specific HA formula, as partially hydrolyzed protein HA formulas from different manufactures were used. As previously mentioned, the properties of a hydrolysate are not only determined by the degree of hydrolysis or protein source, but, crucially, are dependent on the hydrolysis process itself, which varies between manufacturers [14]. Therefore, combining data from studies using different hydrolysates is likely to be scientifically inappropriate [24].

Unfortunately, trials comparing different partial hydrolysates have not been performed.

All reviews suggest that partially hydrolyzed formulas are safe, well-tolerated, and lead to appropriate infant growth. Since formulas containing hydrolyzed proteins may be produced from any suitable protein source and by different enzymatic or chemical means, the EFSA emphasizes that the safety and suitability of each specific formula containing protein hydrolysates must be established by clinical studies [25].

Partial hydrolysates are more easily digested than intact proteins [26]. An accelerated transit time in preterm infants fed partially hydrolyzed formulas, compared to intact proteins, was demonstrated in [27]. Numerous studies suggest a benefit of partially hydrolyzed formulas in managing infantile colic, regurgitation, and constipation [28]. Unfortunately, the partial hydrolyzation of the protein is only one of several changes in formula composition in all these studies. Other changes include reduced lactose, change in lipid content, and the addition of a thickening agent, and, therefore, it is impossible to pinpoint the hydrolysate as the single influential factor.

4. Conclusions

The risks and benefits of choosing a partially hydrolyzed formula in non-exclusively breastfed infants should be discussed between the health care professional and the infant's caregivers. The current stage of knowledge leads to a philosophical discussion than to an evidence-guided information. While there is a high degree of certainty that partially hydrolyzed formulas are safe, substantial proof of their benefit has not been demonstrated. Regarding allergy prevention, studies showed either no benefit or some benefit. Most studies show benefits regarding the management and prevention of functional gastrointestinal disorders, although the hydrolyzed protein was always only one of the multiple changes introduced to the formula. A conservative, evidence-based analysis would conclude that there is insufficient evidence for an active recommendation. A more positive interpretation would be that, while there is no evidence to state that there is a benefit, the possibility of some benefit cannot be ruled out. Although the knowledge that a partial hydrolysate might be closer to the protein composition in human milk than intact cow's milk protein, and that in vitro and animal studies strongly indicate benefit might be decisive in this approach, today there is insufficient evidence to recommend their universal use. Last, but not least, clinical trials with different hydrolysates are needed.

Author Contributions: Conceptualization, Y.V.; writing–original draft preparation, Y.V.; writing—review and editing, J.K., M.S.L., N.M., J.-C.P., L.A.R., A.S., and M.W. All authors have read and agreed to the published version of the manuscript.

Funding: This research received no external funding.

Institutional Review Board Statement: Not applicable.

Informed Consent Statement: Not applicable.

Data Availability Statement: Not applicable.

Conflicts of Interest: J.K.: Lectures for: BBraun, Fresenius Kabi, Nestle, Nutricia; N.M.: participation as advisory board member for Nestlé Nutrition Institute; J.-C.P.: clinical investigator, and/or advisory board member, and/or speaker for Nestlé Research, Bledina, Nestlé Nutrition Institute, Medela; A.S.: research funding from Nestlé and Abbott Plc; and honoraria to give lectures and attend advisory boards for Nestlé Nutrition Institute, Danone, Wyeth Nutrition, Reckitt, Phillips, Abbott Nutrition and Academic Institutions; M.W.: NNI European Advisory Board; M.S.L.: Advisory Board from Nestle; L.A.R. and Y.V. declare no conflict of interest.

References

1. Nutten, S. Proteins, peptides and amino acids: Role in infant nutrition. *Nestle Nutr. Inst. Workshop Ser.* **2016**, *86*, 1–10. [PubMed]
2. Nutten, S.; Schuh, S.; Dutter, T.; Heine, R.G.; Kuslys, M. Design, quality, safety and efficacy of extensively hydrolysed formula for management of cow's milk protein allergy: What are the challenges? *Adv. Food Nutr. Res.* **2020**, *93*, 147–204. [PubMed]
3. Petrus, N.C.; Schoemaker, A.F.; van Hoek, M.W.; Jansen, L.; Jansen-van der Weide, M.C.; van Aalderen, W.M.; Sprikkelman, A.B. Remaining symptoms in half the children treated for milk allergy. *Eur J. Pediatr.* **2015**, *174*, 759–765. [CrossRef] [PubMed]
4. Bourdeau, T.; Affolter, M.; Dupuis, L.; Panchaud, A.; Lahrichi, S.; Merminod, L.; Martin-Paschoud, C.; Adams, R.; Nutten, S.; Blanchard, C. Peptide characterization and functional stability of a partially hydrolyzed whey-based formula over time. *Nutrients* **2021**, *13*, 3011. [CrossRef]
5. Victora, C.G.; Bahl, R.; Barros, A.J.; França, G.V.; Horton, S.; Krasevec, J.; Murch, S.; Sankar, M.J.; Walker, N.; Rollins, N.C.; et al. Breastfeeding in the 21st century: Epidemiology, mechanisms, and lifelong effect. *Lancet* **2016**, *387*, 475–490. [CrossRef]
6. Dallas, D.C.; Murray, N.M.; Gan, J. Proteolytic system in milk: Perspectives on the evolutionary function within the mammary gland and the infant. *J. Mammary Gland. Biol. Neoplasia* **2015**, *20*, 133–147. [CrossRef]
7. Nielsen, S.D.; Beverly, R.L.; Dallas, D.C. Milk proteins are predigested within the human mammary gland. *J. Mammary Gland Biol. Neoplasia* **2017**, *22*, 251–261. [CrossRef]
8. Greer, F.R.; Sicherer, S.H.; Burks, W.A.; Abrams, S.A.; Fuchs, G.J.; Kim, J.H. The effects of early nutritional interventions on the development of atopic disease in infants and children: The role of maternal dietary restriction, breastfeeding, hydrolyzed formulas, and timing of introduction of allergenic complementary foods. *Pediatrics* **2019**, *143*, e20190281. [CrossRef]
9. Boyle, R.J.; Ierodiakonou, D.; Khan, T.; Chivinge, J.; Robinson, Z.; Geoghegan, N.; Jarrold, K.; Afxentiou, T.; Reeves, T.; Cunha, S.; et al. Hydrolysed formula and risk of allergic or autoimmune disease: Systematic review and meta-analysis. *BMJ* **2016**, *352*, i974. [CrossRef]
10. Halken, S.; Muraro, A.; de Silva, D.; Khaleva, E.; Angier, E.; Arasi, S.; Arshad, H.; Bahnson, H.T.; Beyer, K.; Boyle, R.; et al. EAACI guideline: Preventing the development of food allergy in infants and young children (2020 update). *Pediatric Allergy Immunol.* **2021**, *32*, 843–858. [CrossRef]
11. American Academy of Pediatrics. Committee on Nutrition. Hypoallergenic infant formulae. *Pediatrics* **2000**, *106*, 346–349. [CrossRef]
12. Hochwallner, H.; Schulmeister, U.; Swoboda, I.; Focke-Tejkl, M.; Reininger, R.; Civai, V.; Campana, R.; Thalhamer, J.; Scheiblhofer, S.; Balic, N.; et al. Infant milk formulas differ regarding their allergenic activity and induction of T-cell and cytokine responses. *Allergy* **2017**, *72*, 416–424. [CrossRef] [PubMed]
13. Graversen, K.B.; Larsen, J.M.; Pedersen, S.S.; Sørensen, L.V.; Christoffersen, H.F.; Jacobsen, L.N.; Halken, S.; Licht, T.R.; Bahl, M.I.; Bøgh, K.L. Partially hydrolysed whey has superior allergy preventive capacity compared to intact whey regardless of amoxicillin administration in brown Norway rats. *Front. Immunol.* **2021**, *12*, 705543. [CrossRef] [PubMed]
14. Iwamoto, H.; Matsubara, T.; Okamoto, T.; Yoshikawa, M.; Matsumoto, T.; Kono, G.; Takeda, Y. Epicutaneous immunogenicity of partially hydrolyzed whey protein evaluated using tape-stripped mouse model. *Pediatric Allergy Immunol.* **2020**, *31*, 388–395. [CrossRef] [PubMed]
15. Holvoet, S.; Nutten, S.; Dupuis, L.; Donnicola, D.; Bourdeau, T.; Hughes-Formella, B.; Simon, D.; Simon, H.U.; Carvalho, R.S.; Spergel, J.M.; et al. Partially hydrolysed whey-based infant formula improves skin barrier function. *Nutrients* **2021**, *13*, 3113. [CrossRef] [PubMed]
16. von Berg, A.; Koletzko, S.; Filipiak-Pittroff, B.; Laubereau, B.; Grübl, A.; Wichmann, H.E.; Bauer, C.P.; Reinhardt, D.; Berdel, D.; German Infant Nutritional Intervention Study Group. Certain hydrolyzed formulas reduce the incidence of atopic dermatitis but not that of asthma: Three-year results of the German Infant Nutritional Intervention Study. *J. Allergy Clin. Immunol.* **2007**, *119*, 718–725. [CrossRef]
17. Gappa, M.; Filipiak-Pittroff, B.; Libuda, L.; von Berg, A.; Koletzko, S.; Bauer, C.P.; Heinrich, J.; Schikowski, T.; Berdel, D.; Standl, M. Long-term effects of hydrolyzed formulae on atopic diseases in the GINI study. *Allergy* **2021**, *76*, 1903–1907. [CrossRef]
18. Osborn, D.A.; Sinn, J.K.; Jones, L.J. Infant formulae containing hydrolysed protein for prevention of allergic disease. *Cochrane Database Syst. Rev.* **2018**, *10*, CD003664.
19. Szajewska, H.; Horvath, A. A partially hydrolyzed 100% whey formula and the risk of eczema and any allergy: An updated meta-analysis. *World Allergy Organ. J.* **2017**, *10*, 27. [CrossRef]
20. Worm, M.; Reese, I.; Ballmer-Weber, B.; Beyer, K.; Bischoff, S.C.; Bohle, B.; Brockow, K.; Claßen, M.; Fischer, P.J.; Hamelmann, E.; et al. Update of the S2k guideline on the management of IgE-mediated food allergies. *Allergol. Select* **2021**, *5*, 195–243. [CrossRef]
21. Australasian Society of Clinical Immunology and Allergy (ASCIA). ASCIA Guidelines—Infant Feeding and Allergy Prevention. Available online: https://www.allergy.org.au/hp/papers/infant-feeding-and-allergy-prevention (accessed on 24 March 2022).
22. Turner, P.J.; Feeney, M.; Meyer, R.; Perkin, M.R.; Fox, A.T. Implementing primary prevention of food allergy in infants: New BSACI guidance published. *Clin. Exp. Allergy* **2018**, *48*, 912–915. [CrossRef] [PubMed]
23. Davisse-Paturet, C.; Raherison, C.; Adel-Patient, K.; Divaret-Chauveau, A.; Bois, C.; Dufourg, M.N.; Lioret, S.; Charles, M.A.; de Lauzon-Guillain, B. Use of partially hydrolysed formula in infancy and incidence of eczema, respiratorysymptoms or food allergies in toddlers from the ELFE cohort. *Pediatr. Allergy Immunol.* **2019**, *30*, 614–623. [CrossRef] [PubMed]

24. Vandenplas, Y.; Meyer, R.; Chouraqui, J.P.; Dupont, C.; Fiocchi, A.; Salvatore, S.; Shamir, R.; Szajewska, H.; Thapar, N.; Venter, C.; et al. The role of milk feeds and other dietary supplementary interventions in preventing allergic disease in infants: Fact or fiction? *Clin. Nutr.* **2021**, *40*, 358–371. [CrossRef] [PubMed]
25. EFSA Panel on Dietetic Products, Nutrition and Allergies (NDA). Scientific Opinion on the essential composition of infant and follow-on formulae. *EFSA J.* **2014**, *12*, 3760. [CrossRef]
26. Billeaud, C.; Guillet, J.; Sandler, B. Gastric emptying in infants with or without gastro-oesophageal reflux according to the type of milk. *Eur. J. Clin. Nutr.* **1990**, *44*, 577–583. [PubMed]
27. Picaud, J.C.; Rigo, J.; Normand, S.; Lapillonne, A.; Reygrobellet, B.; Claris, O.; Salle, B.L. Nutritional efficacy of preterm formula with a partially hydrolyzed protein source: A randomized pilot study. *J. Pediatric Gastroenterol. Nutr.* **2001**, *32*, 555–561. [CrossRef]
28. Vandenplas, Y.; Salvatore, S. Infant formula with partially hydrolyzed proteins in functional gastrointestinal disorders. *Protein Neonatal Infant Nutr.* **2016**, *86*, 29–37.

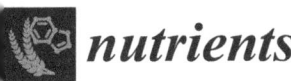

Systematic Review

Do Probiotics in Pregnancy Reduce Allergies and Asthma in Infancy and Childhood? A Systematic Review

Alexander S. Colquitt [1], Elizabeth A. Miles [1] and Philip C. Calder [1,2,*]

[1] School of Human Development and Health, Faculty of Medicine, University of Southampton, Southampton SO16 6YD, UK; asc2g19@soton.ac.uk (A.S.C.); e.a.miles@soton.ac.uk (E.A.M.)
[2] NIHR Southampton Biomedical Research Centre, University Hospital Southampton NHS Foundation Trust and University of Southampton, Southampton SO16 6YD, UK
* Correspondence: pcc@soton.ac.uk

Abstract: The maternal immune system is very important in the development of the foetal immune system. Probiotics have been shown to help regulate immune responses. Therefore, it is possible that the administration of probiotics to pregnant women could influence the development of the foetal immune system, reducing the likelihood of infants and children developing an allergic condition. The aim of this research was to conduct a systematic review to determine whether administering probiotics to pregnant women can reduce the incidence of allergic disease in their children. Medline, CINAHL and Embase databases were searched for randomised controlled trials (RCTs) that compared supplementation of probiotics to pregnant women to a placebo control and recorded the presentation of allergic conditions in their children. Data extracted from the study reports included their characteristics and findings. Study quality and risk of bias were assessed. From a total of 850 articles identified in the search, 6 were eligible for inclusion in this review. Two studies found no effect of maternal probiotics on the outcomes measured, two studies found that the incidence of eczema or atopic dermatitis (AD) was reduced by maternal probiotics, one study found no effect on the overall incidence of atopic sensitisation, but a reduction in a subgroup of children at high hereditary risk of allergic disease, and one study found no effect in an intention to treat analysis, but a reduction in AD in complete case analysis. The results of these studies are inconsistent but demonstrate that probiotics may have the potential to reduce infant allergies when administered prenatally, particularly in children at high risk of allergy development. There is a need for further larger-scale studies to be performed in order to provide a more definitive answer. Such studies should focus on at-risk groups.

Keywords: pregnancy; infancy; childhood; immune development; probiotic; microbiota; allergy; asthma; eczema; atopic dermatitis

1. Introduction

The incidence of allergic disorders such as atopic dermatitis (AD, also called atopic eczema), allergic rhinoconjunctivitis (ARC), food allergies and asthma has increased over the last decades in both developed and developing countries [1–5]. Allergy is caused when the immune system actively responds to otherwise harmless antigens [6], and these antigens are referred to as allergens. Allergic reactions can be categorised into two types: immunoglobulin E (IgE)-mediated and non-IgE-mediated. IgE-mediated reactions include ARC, food allergies and allergic asthma, and are generally characterised by the T helper 2 (Th2) cell inflammatory pathway [6,7]. The initial setting up of IgE-mediated allergic disease occurs when an infant is first sensitised to an allergen [6]. There is evidence that such predisposition to allergic disease occurs in foetal life, i.e., before birth [8,9]. Eczema (i.e., AD) is the first manifestation of allergic disease in infants, followed by food allergy, asthma and allergic rhinitis, and asthma may not manifest until 5 years of age and allergic

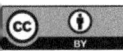

rhinitis until 7 years of age. This progressive development of allergic disease is referred to as the "atopic march" [10,11].

The gut microbiota is believed to be important in immune development and determining allergy risk [12]. It is widely considered that the human foetus is sterile when in utero, although recent studies have challenged this [13]. Nevertheless, neonates are exposed to microbes during and after the birthing process from their mother and surroundings [14]. The mode of delivery has a significant effect on the microbes that are able to colonise the gut, and microbes are also transferred from mother to infant via kissing, suckling and hugging directly after birth [14]. Post-partum, infants are exposed to new microbes via food (e.g., in mother's breastmilk) and by entering new environments. The infant microbiota seems to be essential in the development of a mature immune system, and its manipulation could alter the course of development of allergic disease [15]. Older studies identified that infants raised on farms had a lower risk of allergic disease [16,17], and these observations gave rise to the "hygiene hypothesis" [18] that linked early exposure to microbes to more optimal immune maturation and in turn to reduced allergy risk. Furthermore, infants who were born via a natural birth instead of caesarean section, exclusively breastfed or not exposed to antibiotic treatment had more diverse microbiota, which also correlated with a lower risk of developing allergic disease [19]. Together, these observations suggest that strategies to manipulate the gut microbiota may be a means for lowering the risk of allergic disease. In this context, probiotics are a way of manipulating the infant microbiota to increase its diversity for the purpose of preventing allergies [15,20]. There are many different probiotic species, but lactobacilli and bifidobacteria are amongst the most common [21]. Both have been studied extensively in the context of allergy and have been associated with reductions in rates of AD, food allergy, ARC and asthma [20,22]. These bacteria are shown to modulate the host's Th1/Th2 balance by producing cytokines that promote the Th1 pathway, therefore suppressing the Th2 pathway that is associated with allergy development [20,22].

Several studies have linked probiotics with the primary prevention of allergies and allergic diseases, especially when taken by the children themselves [23–25], but there are fewer studies that look into the effect of manipulation of the pregnant mother's microbiota and allergy risk of the child. Randomised controlled trials (RCTs) that have been conducted in the field have produced inconsistent results, and therefore systematic reviews are needed to summarise the evidence and try to arrive at a clearer view of the findings and to identify knowledge gaps and research priorities. One such review was recently published on this topic [25]. The authors concluded that some probiotic mixtures do "probably reduce the risk of developing atopic dermatitis compared with placebo" [25]; however, the review included many studies in which the probiotic was administered to both the mother and the infant, as well as focusing on AD as the primary outcome.

The aim of the current review is to assess the impact of prenatal probiotic use (i.e., administering probiotics to the mother only) on the development of a wider range of allergic conditions, including both AD and asthma.

2. Materials and Methods

2.1. Overview

This systematic review was conducted according to the "Preferred Reporting Items for Systematic review and Meta-Analysis" (PRISMA) guidelines [26] and the reporting herein is consistent with these. The review was not registered as it was performed for educational purposes and a formal protocol was not prepared. The PICO (Patient or population, Intervention, Comparison and Outcome) approach was utilised to identify search terms. The population group was pregnant women and their offspring, the intervention was any probiotic, the comparison was between groups of offspring of mothers who received probiotics or who received a control and the outcome measure was any outcome related to allergy, including asthma.

2.2. Literature Search

The following databases were searched for relevant literature: Ovid MEDLINE (1946 to week 2 of September 2021), EMBASE (1974 to 22 September 2021) and CINAHL. Free-text searches, using the terms: 'pregnan*', 'prenatal', 'pre-natal', 'pregnant women', 'mother', 'probiotic', 'allerg*', 'hypersensitiv*', 'dermatitis', 'asthma*', 'raised IgE', 'atop*', 'eczema', 'skin prick test', 'SPT', 'child*', 'offspring' and 'infan*', were used.

2.3. Study Selection

Studies were selected for this systematic review based on the following inclusion criteria: must be an RCT, must have compared a probiotic treatment to a control group, mothers must have received the probiotic during pregnancy or pregnancy and lactation, a measure of allergy must have been reported in the children, published as a full research paper and published in the English language. Exclusion criteria included: combined use of probiotics with another intervention, use of synbiotics and probiotics administered to the children.

2.4. Data Extraction

Data from the studies that were extracted included sample size, probiotic used, type of control, duration of treatment, outcomes measured, test results for those outcomes and the conclusions drawn from those results.

2.5. Quality Assessment

The studies included in this systematic review were assessed for bias using the Cochrane Risk of Bias 2 tool [27] and assessed for quality using the Jadad quality scale [28]. The Cochrane Risk of Bias tool is a system that assesses whether a study holds a high, medium or low risk of bias by asking a series of questions over 5 domains in which bias may arise. The Jadad quality scale is a 0–5-point scale (0 being lowest quality, 5 the highest quality) in which points are awarded or deducted for a study based on a series of 7 questions.

3. Results

3.1. Search Results

The search of 3 databases returned a total of 850 records, with no additional records found with a manual search (Figure 1). Of these records, 293 were duplicates, leaving 557 records. After screening by title, 498 of these records were removed, and a further 47 were removed after screening by abstract, leaving 12 records. The full articles were retrieved for these records and 6 were removed for the following reasons: administration of probiotics to the infants ($n = 3$) and no relevant outcome measured in infants ($n = 3$).

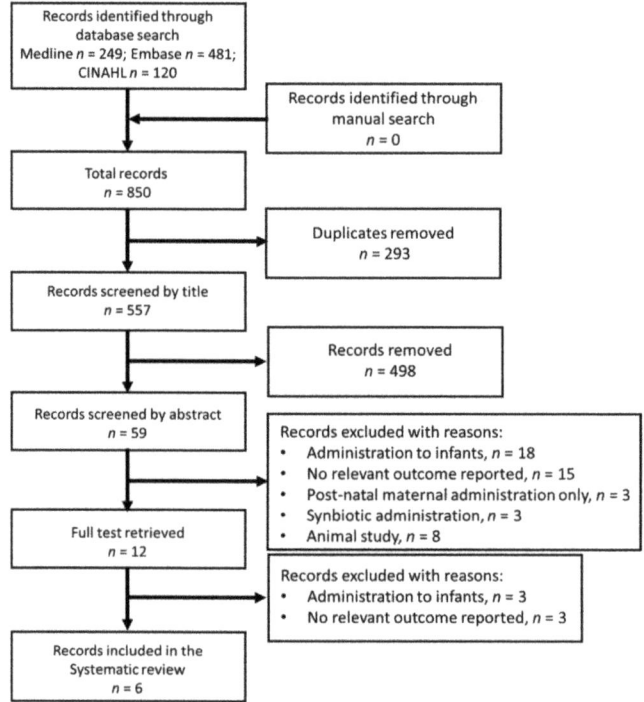

Figure 1. Flow diagram summarizing the identification and selection of articles for inclusion in the review.

3.2. Characteristics of the Included Studies

Six papers were included [29–34]. These represent five separate trials because two papers were published from the same trial but reporting outcomes at two different periods of follow-up [30,33]. Key characteristics of the trials included in this review are presented in Table 1. Initial points to note are that 3 out of the 5 trials (4 out of 6 included articles) involved the administration of a common probiotic species: *Lactobacillus rhamnosus* GG [29,31,33], 4 studies (5 articles) involved post-natal (as well as prenatal) administration of probiotics to the mother [30–34] and 1 study stopped the intervention at the time of delivery [29].

Boyle et al. [29] randomised 250 pregnant women (212 of whom completed the trial) to receive either *Lactobacillus rhamnosus* GG intervention or a maltodextrin placebo from 36 weeks of gestation to delivery. The children were assessed for eczema as the trial's primary outcome, along with eczema severity, whether IgE-associated, and also atopic sensitisation in the form of a skin prick test (SPT) at 3 follow-up sessions at ages 3, 6 and 12 months.

Dotterud et al. [30] randomised 415 women (278 of whom completed) to receive either a probiotic milk containing a mixture of *Lactobacillus rhamnosus* GG, *Bifidobacterium animalis* subsp. *lactis* BB12 and *Lactobacillus acidophilus* La-5, or a heat-treated sterile milk placebo. The treatment lasted from 36 weeks of gestation to 3 months post-natal. The primary outcome was the development of atopic disease within two years, so children were assessed for AD, asthma and ARC at a two-year follow-up session, and the children were also assessed for atopic sensitisation in the form of a SPT.

Huurre et al. [31] randomised 140 pregnant women to receive a probiotic mixture of *Lactobacillus rhamnosus* GG and *Bifidobacterium lactis* BB12, or a microcrystalline cellulose and dextrose anhydrate placebo from the 1st trimester until the end of exclusive breastfeeding.

The children were followed up 3 times at ages 1, 6 and 12 months and were assessed for atopic sensitisation by SPT.

Table 1. Characteristics of the studies included in the review.

Reference	Country Where Trial Conducted	Number of Mothers Randomised/ Completed	Probiotic Used	Control	Time of Treatment (Start, End)	Outcomes Assessed	Age at Follow-Up
Boyle et al. [29]	Australia	250/212	L. rhamnosus GG	Maltodextrin	36 weeks of gestation, delivery	Primary outcome: Eczema during 1st year Secondary outcomes: Allergic sensitisation, IgE-associated eczema, Eczema severity	3, 6, 12 months
Dotterud et al. [30]	Norway	415/278	Milk with: L. rhamnosus GG, B. animalis BB12 and L. acidophilus La-5	Heat-treated sterile milk	36 weeks of gestation, 3 months post-natal	Primary outcome: Atopic disease in first 2 years AD, Asthma, ARC Secondary outcome: Atopic sensitisation, IgE-associated AD, Non-IgE-associated AD	2 years
Huurre et al. [31]	Finland	140/NA	L. rhamnosus GG and B. animalis BB12	Microcrystalline cellulose and dextrose anhydrate	1st trimester, end of exclusive breastfeeding	Atopic sensitisation (skin prick test) at 12 months	1, 6, 12 months
Rautava et al. [32]	Finland	241/205	Multivitamin and mineral supplement + EITHER L. rhamnosus LPR and B. longum BL999 OR L. paracasei ST11 and B. longum BL999	Multivitamin and mineral supplement	2 months prenatal, 2 months post-natal	Primary outcome: Eczema by age 2 years Secondary outcome: Atopic sensitisation (skin prick test)	1, 3, 6, 12, 24 months
Simpson et al. [33]	Norway	415/281	Milk with: L. rhamnosus GG, B. animalis BB12 and L. acidophilus La-5	Heat-treated sterile milk	36 weeks of gestation, 3 months post-natal	Primary outcome: Atopic disease in first 6 years AD, Asthma, ARC Secondary outcome: Atopic sensitisation	6 years
Wickens et al. [34]	New Zealand	423/403	L. rhamnosus HN001	Maltodextrin	14–16 weeks of gestation, 6 months post-natal	Primary outcome: Eczema within 12 months Secondary outcomes: SCORAD ≥ 10, Wheeze, Atopic sensitisation	6, 12 months

NA indicates not available.

Rautava et al. [32] randomised 241 women into 3 groups—2 intervention groups and 1 placebo. The intervention groups received a probiotic mix of either *Lactobacillus rhamnosus* LPR and *Bifidobacterium longum* BL999 or *Lactobacillus paracasei* ST11 and *Bifidobacterium longum* BL999 in the form of a tablet which also contained vitamins and minerals. The placebo group received the same multi-vitamin and mineral tablet but without any probiotic bacteria. The intervention lasted from 2 months prenatal until 2 months post-natal. The children were assessed at 5 follow-up sessions at 1, 3, 6, 12 and 24 months, primarily for eczema, and a SPT was also performed to test for atopic sensitisation.

Simpson et al. [33] performed a 6-year follow-up of the Pro-PACT study completed by Dotterud et al. [26], where 281 participants completed the follow-up. The primary outcome was any atopic disease within 6 years, and the children were assessed for AD, asthma (within the last year), ARC as well as atopic sensitisation by SPT.

Wickens et al. [34] randomised 423 pregnant women to receive either *Lactobacillus rhamnosus* HN001 or a maltodextrin placebo. The intervention was administered from 14 to 16 weeks of gestation up until 6 months post-partum. The children were assessed at 6 and 12 months for eczema, and secondary outcomes were eczema severity on the SCORAD scale, wheeze and atopic sensitisation by SPT.

3.3. Effects of Probiotics on Infant Eczema and AD

A full description of the findings reported in the six included papers can be found in Table 2. A diagnosis of eczema or AD was reported in five of the six papers included [29,30,32–34] and was the primary outcome in three papers [29,32,34]. Boyle et al. [29] found that the probiotic intervention had no significant effect on eczema diagnosis at one year, including IgE-associated eczema, and had no effect on eczema severity. Dotterud et al. [30] reported a reduction in the overall incidence of AD at two years, and this effect was greatest in the non-IgE-associated AD subgroup, as there was no effect in the IgE-associated subgroup. Rautava et al. [32] found that both probiotic interventions had a very similar effect, and both significantly reduced the rate of eczema at two years in the children compared to the placebo. In their follow-up of the Pro-PACT study [30], Simpson et al. [33] found that there was no effect on AD at six years in the intention to treat analysis; however, there was a significant reduction in AD in the complete case analysis. Adjustment of the results for family history, child sex and siblings did not alter these findings [33]. Wickens et al. [34] found no effect on the incidence of eczema or its severity at one year.

Table 2. Findings of the studies included in the review.

Reference	Outcomes Assessed	Effect of Probiotic			Conclusion
Boyle et al. [29]	Primary outcome: Eczema during 1st year Secondary outcomes: Allergic sensitisation, IgE-associated eczema, Eczema severity	Risk difference: −4.7% (−16.9, 7.4) 0% (−12.7, 12.8) −1.1% (−11.6, 9.5) N/A			No effect for any outcome
Dotterud et al. [30]	Primary outcome: Atopic disease in first 2 years AD, Asthma, ARC Secondary outcome: Atopic sensitisation IgE-associated AD Non-IgE-associated AD	ITT analysis OR 0.51 (0.30, 0.87) 0.68 (0.26, 1.80) N/A 1.45 (0.46, 4.59) 0.90 (0.37, 2.17) 0.43 (0.23, 0.81)	Complete case series analysis OR 0.51 (0.30, 0.87) 0.66 (0.26, 1.66) N/A 1.19 (0.35, 4.01) 0.91 (0.36, 2.31) 0.43 (0.23, 0.83)	Per protocol analysis OR 0.47 (0.26, 0.85) N/A N/A N/A 0.92 (0.36, 2.36) 0.37 (0.18, 0.77)	Reduced incidence of AD. No effect on asthma or ARC. No effect on atopic sensitisation. Reduced incidence of non-IgE-associated AD
Huurre et al. [31]	Atopic sensitisation (skin prick test) at 12 months	All infants OR 0.92 (0.45, 1.0) Infants at high hereditary risk OR 0.34 (0.13, 0.88)			No effect on overall incidence of atopic sensitisation. Reduced incidence in infants at high hereditary risk
Rautava et al. [32]	Primary outcome: Eczema by age 2 years Secondary outcome: Atopic sensitisation (skin prick test)	OR LPR + BL999 0.17 (0.08, 0.35) ST11 + BL999 0.16 (0.08, 0.35) LPR + BL999 0.81 (0.36, 1.76) ST11 + BL999 0.99 (0.46, 2.13)			Reduce risk of eczema but no effect on sensitisation
Simpson et al. [33]	Primary outcome: Atopic disease in first 6 years AD, Asthma, ARC Secondary outcome: Atopic sensitisation	ITT analysis (OR) 0.64 (0.39, 1.07) 1.68 (0.21, 13.20) 1.19 (0.66, 2.16) 1.11 (0.62, 1.96)		Complete case analysis (OR) 0.48 (0.25, 0.92) 3.25 (0.33, 31.6) 1.22 (0.64, 2.37) 1.25 (0.62, 2.54)	No effect on AD in ITT analysis but less AD in complete case analysis. No effect on asthma, ARC or atopic sensitisation
Wickens et al. [34]	Primary outcome: Eczema within 12 months Secondary outcomes: SCORAD ≥ 10, Wheeze, Atopic sensitisation	Hazard ratio 0.83 (0.53, 1.29) 0.95 (0.69, 1.31) 0.89 (0.66, 1.20) 1.02 (0.63, 1.64)			No effect on any outcome

Figures in parentheses represent the 95% confidence interval. ITT, intention to treat; N/A not available; OR, odds ratio.

3.4. Effects of Probiotics on Infant Asthma

Asthma was reported in two papers [30,33], both from the same study, and wheeze was reported in one paper [34]. Dotterud et al. [30] reported that there was no effect on asthma in either intention to treat or complete case analysis. Simpson et al. [33] reported in their follow-up to Dotterud et al. [30] that the intervention had no effect on incidence of asthma. Wickens et al. [34] also reported that probiotic intervention had no effect on wheeze.

3.5. Effects of Probiotics on Infant Atopic Sensitisation

Atopic sensitisation determined by a positive SPT was assessed in all papers included and was the primary outcome of Huurre et al. [31]. In that study, there was no reduction in the overall incidence of atopic sensitisation; however, there was a reduction in a subgroup of children who were at a high hereditary risk of allergic disease (due to maternal sensitisation). There was no effect of probiotics in pregnancy on atopic sensitisation in any other paper [29,30,32–34].

3.6. Effects of Probiotics on Infant ARC

Incidence of ARC was measured in the Dotterud et al. Pro-PACT study [30] and the Simpson et al. six-year follow-up of this study [33]. Dotterud et al. [30] reported only one case in each group. Simpson et al. [33] reported no effect of maternal probiotics on ARC.

3.7. Quality and Risk of Bias Assessment

Five of the six included papers [29,30,32–34] were assessed as having a low risk of bias using the Cochrane risk of bias assessment (Table 3) and were awarded 5/5 on the Jadad quality scale (Table 4). The study by Huurre et al. [31] was given a high risk of bias due to the fact that the methods of randomisation and of group assignment concealment were not disclosed, and also because there was no explanation for the participants who dropped out of the trial or for variable sample sizes in the results. The same paper [31] was also given a score of 3 on the Jadad scale due to there being no description of the method of randomisation of dropouts/withdrawals.

Table 3. Bias assessment of included studies based upon the Cochrane risk of bias tool. Green indicates low risk, orange indicates moderate risk and red indicates high risk.

Reference	Domain 1: Randomisation Process	Domain 2: Deviations from Intended Interventions	Domain 3: Missing Outcome Data	Domain 4: Measurement of Outcome	Domain 5: Selection of Reported Result	Overall Risk of Bias
Boyle et al. [29]	Low	Low	Low	Low	Low	Low
Dotterud et al. [30]	Low	Low	Low	Low	Low	Low
Huurre et al. [31]	Moderate	Moderate/High	High	Low	Low	High
Rautava et al. [32]	Low	Low	Low	Low	Low	Low
Simpson et al. [33]	Low	Low	Low	Low	Low	Low
Wickens et al. [34]	Low	Low	Low	Low	Low	Low

Table 4. Quality assessment of included studies based on the Jadad quality assessment.

Reference	Was the Study Described as Randomised?	Was the Method Used to Generate the Sequence of Randomisation Described and Appropriate?	Was the Study Described as Double-Blind?	Was There a Description of the Withdrawals and Drop-Outs?	Deduct one Point If the Method Used to Generate the Sequence of Randomisation Was Described and It Was Inappropriate	Deduct One Point If the Study Was Described as Double-Blind but the Method Blinding Was Inappropriate	Jadad Score (1 to 5)
Boyle et al. [29]	1	1	1	1	0	0	5
Dotterud et al. [30]	1	1	1	1	0	0	5
Huurre et al. [31]	1	0	1	1	0	0	3
Rautava et al. [32]	1	1	1	1	0	0	5
Simpson et al. [33]	1	1	1	1	0	0	5
Wickens et al. [34]	1	1	1	1	0	0	5

4. Discussion

This systematic review found limited evidence in support of the hypothesis that probiotics in pregnancy will reduce risk of allergic disease in the children; however, some studies produced findings in support of this hypothesis. Therefore, overall, the findings are inconsistent. This may be due to differences among the studies, such as the probiotic used, when the intervention was started, the duration of the intervention and the risk of the child. For example, Huurre et al. [31] found that maternal probiotics caused a significant reduction in risk of AD at 12 months in infants at high hereditary risk due to maternal allergic sensitisation, but no effect of maternal probiotics in the cohort of infants as a whole. This systematic review included six papers from five randomised, double-blind, placebo-controlled trials of probiotic supplements administered to pregnant and nursing mothers for the prevention of atopic disease and allergy [29–34]. The studies assessed the use of seven different strains of probiotics (*Lactobacillus rhamnosus* GG, *Bifidobacterium animalis* subsp. lactis BB12, *Lactobacillus acidophilus* La-5, *Lactobacillus rhamnosus* LPR, *Bifidobacterium longum* BL999, *Lactobacillus paracasei* ST11, *Lactobacillus rhamnosus* HN001), which were used alone in two studies [29,34] and in combination in three [30–33]. Probiotics were administered from 36 weeks of gestation to delivery (approximately 4 weeks) [29], 36 weeks of gestation to 3 months post-natal (approximately 16 weeks) [30,33], 1st trimester to end of exclusive breastfeeding (approximately 50 weeks) [31], 2 months prenatal to 2 months post-natal (approximately 16 weeks) [32], or 14–16 weeks of gestation to 6 months post-partum (approximately 50 weeks) [34]. Studies reported on the presentation of AD/eczema [29,30,32–34], atopic sensitisation [29–34], asthma [30,33], wheeze [34] and ARC [30,33], and three studies followed up infants within one year [29,31,34], and two within two years [30,32]. Simpson et al.'s study [33] was a six-year follow-up of Dotterud et al.'s work [30]. None of the included studies reported any adverse effects experienced by mothers or infants during probiotic supplementation, which supports previous research into the safety of probiotic use during pregnancy and lactation [35].

Five of these papers [29–31,33,34] were included in a recently published systematic review and meta-analysis that included twenty-one studies of probiotics administered pre- or postnatally, including in infants [25], which concluded that "[certain probiotic preparations] probably reduce the risk of atopic dermatitis based on low-quality evidence compared with placebo when given to infants" [25]. Four of the papers [29,31–33] were also included in an earlier review which assessed a total of seventeen studies [23], concluding that "strain-specific sub-meta-analyses showed that probiotic mixtures were effective in reducing the incidence of eczema, while no effect was documented for products containing lactobacilli or bifidobacteria alone" [23]. The reason for the smaller number of included papers in the present review is that the focus was on the administration of probiotics to the mother only, whereas a large proportion of the current literature includes administration to infants, too. Despite the differences in these two previous reviews, the conclusion of this review remains qualitatively similar: that although the results of RCTs are inconsistent, some show that maternal probiotic supplementation can reduce the prevalence of infant AD and eczema, but that there is no effect on other atopic conditions such as asthma and ARC.

Three out of six studies concluded that the incidence of AD or eczema was reduced by maternal probiotics [30,32,33], but there were no effects reported on ARC or asthma. One study [31] described no overall effect on atopic sensitisation, but a reduction in risk among a subgroup of children at high hereditary risk of atopic disease. When analysing the results with regard to the species of probiotic used, in the two studies where lactobacilli were assessed alone [29,34], there were no effects found on infant atopic disease. There were no studies that administered bifidobacteria alone. Three studies (four papers) assessed the administration of different combinations of probiotics [30–33], all of which included both a lactobacillus and a bifidobacterium strain. All of these combinations showed some form of reduction in the rate of infant atopy—either in AD or atopic sensitisation—showing that perhaps bifidobacteria or a combination of probiotic species are more effective at preventing atopic disease than lactobacilli alone.

The studies included in this review were of varying duration: one of the trials administered probiotics from 36 weeks of gestation up until delivery [29]. This was the only study not to continue probiotic use after delivery and yielded no significant difference in the rates of eczema in infants between the probiotic and placebo groups. The study by Dotterud et al. [30] and it's follow-up by Simpson et al. [33] also administered a probiotic from 36 weeks of gestation, but continued administration until 3 months post-natal and found a reduction in AD. Two studies [31,34] started probiotic administration at the end of the first trimester: Huurre et al. [31] stopped administration at the end of exclusive breastfeeding (approximately six months) and Wickens et al. [34] stopped at six months post-natal. Rautava et al. [32] administered the probiotic formulas from two months prenatal to two months post-natal and reported that infants in both probiotic groups had significantly lower rates of atopic disease than the placebo groups. These results suggest that a supplementation period of approximately 16 weeks can be effective [30,32,33] and that the post-natal period, including the period of breastfeeding, may be essential to the effects of probiotics on allergy risk. When comparing the studies by duration of follow-up, the studies that reported results after two years [30,32] seemed to show a greater reduction in rates of atopic disease than those that reported after one year [29,31,34], although this may be due to differences in the probiotic species used and the duration of administration. Interestingly, the six-year follow-up [33] to Dotterud et al. [30] reported a less significant reduction in atopic disease between the treatment groups than the original two-year follow-up. This may be because other factors such as lifestyle begin to have a greater effect as the child gets older; in other words, the effect of the probiotic may wear-off over time.

The results of risk of bias and quality assessments showed that all but one of the included studies carried a low risk of bias. The study by Huurre et al. [31] was deemed to carry a high risk of bias due to the fact that the method of randomisation of mother/infant pairs to probiotic and placebo groups and the method of blinding were not disclosed and the number of participants who dropped out of the study was not clearly reported. The report by Huurre et al., was the smallest of the 6 included studies, with 140 mother/infant pairs being randomised, and it concluded that there was no overall effect of maternal probiotic supplementation on atopic sensitisation in their children; however, there was a reduced risk among a subgroup of children at high hereditary risk of atopic disease. This suggests that probiotics may have a greater effect in higher-risk than lower-risk infants/children.

The strength of this review is the inclusion of trials in which probiotics were administered only to pregnant mothers and not infants. This allowed the analysis of more homogeneous studies when compared to other reviews which included trials that administered probiotics, prebiotics and synbiotics to both mothers and their infants. Another strength of this review is the assessment of only double-blind RCTs, which minimised any bias that could arise during a study. This risk of bias was further minimised by the use of the Cochrane risk of bias tool and Jadad quality assessment to identify any errors in conducting or reporting the trials. One limitation of the review, however, comes from a potential for publication bias due to the fact that RCTs that were not published in the English language were excluded and so some relevant studies may have been missed. Inclusion of other studies was maximised by conducting a manual literature search of reference lists of included papers and other systematic reviews, which found no additional studies. There is potential that studies may have been completed within the field but not published, and so the data were not available. Other important limitations of this review are the relatively small number of studies available for analysis and that there were not any two studies that reported on the administration of the same probiotic. Finally, it is important to note that the studies included in this review were of modest sample size for reporting on clinical outcomes, although four out of the five studies (five out of the six papers) [29,30,32–34] performed sample size estimates and recruited women according to those.

The outcomes of this review show that there is some potential for probiotics to be used by mothers during pregnancy and after delivery as a preventative measure for AD in infants. The evidence suggests that the most effective method is to administer lactobacilli and bifidobacteria strains in combination for the months leading up to delivery and for 3–6 months post-partum. Future research should aim to compare the efficacies of different probiotic strains, as well as determine the optimal time to start the use of probiotic supplements and the duration of their use to achieve consistent long-term benefits. Finally, a comparison of effects of maternal probiotics between high- and low-risk groups should be performed.

5. Conclusions

The results from the five studies reported in the six papers were inconsistent but demonstrated that probiotics may have the potential to reduce the risk of infant AD or eczema when administered to mothers both during pregnancy and for a period of 3–6 months post-partum. In particular, treatment containing a combination of lactobacilli and bifidobacteria probiotic strains may be effective, especially if the child is at a high hereditary risk of developing an allergic condition. There is a need for further larger-scale studies to be performed in order to provide a more definitive answer. Such studies should focus on at-risk groups.

Author Contributions: Conceptualisation, A.S.C. and P.C.C.; investigation, A.S.C.; writing—original draft preparation, A.S.C.; writing—review and editing, E.A.M. and P.C.C.; supervision, P.C.C. All authors have read and agreed to the published version of the manuscript.

Funding: This research received no external funding.

Institutional Review Board Statement: Not applicable.

Informed Consent Statement: Not applicable.

Data Availability Statement: Not applicable.

Conflicts of Interest: A.S.C. and E.A.M. have no conflict of interest to declare. P.C.C. has acted as an adviser to, and has received study products from, Christian Hansen and DSM.

References

1. Katelaris, C.H.; Lee, B.W.; Potter, P.C.; Maspero, J.F.; Cingi, C.; Lopatin, A.; Saffer, M.; Xu, G.; Walters, R.D. Prevalence and diversity of allergic rhinitis in regions of the world beyond Europe and North America. *Clin. Exp. Allergy* **2012**, *42*, 186–207. [CrossRef] [PubMed]
2. Lundbäck, B.; Backman, H.; Lötvall, J.; Rönmark, E. Is asthma prevalence still increasing? *Expert Rev. Respir. Med.* **2016**, *10*, 39–51. [CrossRef] [PubMed]
3. Loh, W.; Tang, M.L.K. The Epidemiology of Food Allergy in the Global Context. *Int. J. Environ. Res. Public Health* **2018**, *15*, 2043. [CrossRef] [PubMed]
4. GBD 2019 Diseases and Injuries Collaborators. Global burden of 369 diseases and injuries in 204 countries and territories, 1990–2019: A systematic analysis for the Global Burden of Disease Study 2019. *Lancet* **2020**, *396*, 1204–1222.

5. Conrado, A.B.; Ierodiakonou, D.; Gowland, M.H.; Boyle, R.J.; Turner, P.J. Food anaphylaxis in the United Kingdom: Analysis of national data, 1998–2018. *BMJ* **2021**, *372*, n251. [CrossRef]
6. Averbeck, M.; Gebhardt, C.; Emmrich, F.; Treudler, R.; Simon, J.C. Immunologic Principles of Allergic Disease. *JDDG: Journal der Deutschen Dermatologischen Gesellschaft* **2007**, *5*, 1015–1027. [CrossRef]
7. Yang, Y.L.; Pan, Y.Q.; He, B.S.; Zhong, T.Y. Regulatory T cells and Th1/Th2 in peripheral blood and their roles in asthmatic children. *Transl. Pediatr.* **2013**, *2*, 27–33.
8. Warner, J.O. The early life origins of asthma and related allergic disorders. *Arch. Dis. Child.* **2004**, *89*, 97–102. [CrossRef]
9. Wegmann, T.; Lin, H.; Guilbert, L.; Mossman, T.R. Bi-directional cytokine interactions in the maternal fetal relationship: Is successful pregnancy a Th-2-like phenomenon? *Immunol. Today* **1993**, *14*, 353–356. [CrossRef]
10. Spergel, J.M.; Paller, A.S. Atopic dermatitis and the atopic march. *J. Allergy Clin. Immunol.* **2003**, *112*, s118–s127. [CrossRef]
11. Rhodes, H.L.; Sporik, R.; Thomas, P.; Holgate, S.T.; Cogswell, J.J. Early life risk factors for adult asthma: A birth cohort study of subjects at risk. *J. Allergy Clin. Immunol.* **2001**, *108*, 720–725. [CrossRef] [PubMed]
12. Milani, C.; Duranti, S.; Bottacini, F.; Casey, E.; Turroni, F.; Mahony, J.; Belzer, C.; Delgado Palacio, S.; Arboleya Montes, S.; Mancabelli, L.; et al. The First Microbial Colonizers of the Human Gut: Composition, Activities, and Health Implications of the Infant Gut Microbiota. *Microbiol. Mol. Biol. Rev.* **2017**, *81*, e00036-17. [CrossRef] [PubMed]
13. Stinson, L.F.; Boyce, M.C.; Payne, M.S.; Keelan, J.A. The Not-so-Sterile Womb: Evidence That the Human Fetus Is Exposed to Bacteria Prior to Birth. *Front. Microbiol.* **2019**, *10*, 1124. [CrossRef] [PubMed]
14. Mackie, R.I.; Sghir, A.; Gaskins, H.R. Developmental microbial ecology of the neonatal gastrointestinal tract. *Am. J. Clin. Nutr.* **1999**, *69*, 1035s–1045s. [CrossRef] [PubMed]
15. Cukrowska, B.; Bierła, J.B.; Zakrzewska, M.; Klukowski, M.; Maciorkowska, E. The relationship between the infant gut mi-crobiota and allergy. the role of Bifidobacterium breve and prebiotic oligosaccharides in the activation of anti-allergic mecha-nisms in early life. *Nutrients* **2020**, *12*, 946. [CrossRef]
16. Von Ehrenstein, O.S.; Von Mutius, E.; Illi, S.; Baumann, L.; Böhm, O.; Von Kries, R. Reduced risk of hay fever and asthma among children of farmers. *Clin. Exp. Allergy* **2000**, *30*, 187–193. [CrossRef]
17. Riedler, J.; Braun-Fahrländer, C.; Eder, W.; Schreuer, M.; Waser, M.; Maisch, S.; Carr, D.; Schierl, R.; Nowak, D.; von Mutius, E. ALEX Study Team Exposure to farming in early life and development of asthma and allergy: A cross-sectional survey. *Lancet* **2001**, *358*, 1129–1133. [CrossRef]
18. Strachen, D. Hay fever, hygiene, and household size. *Brit. Med. J.* **1989**, *299*, 1259–1260. [CrossRef]
19. Hu, T.; Dong, Y.; Yang, C.; Zhao, M.; He, Q. Pathogenesis of children's allergic diseases: Refocusing the role of the gut micro-biota. *Front. Physiol.* **2021**, *12*, 749544. [CrossRef]
20. Michail, S. The role of Probiotics in allergic diseases. *Allergy Asthma Clin. Immunol.* **2009**, *5*, 5. [CrossRef]
21. Hill, C.; Guarner, F.; Reid, G.; Gibson, G.R.; Merenstein, D.J.; Pot, B.; Morelli, L.; Canani, R.B.; Flint, H.J.; Salminen, S.; et al. Expert consensus document: The International Scientific Association for Probiotics and Prebiotics consensus statement on the scope and appropriate use of the term probiotic. *Nat. Rev. Gastroenterol. Hepatol.* **2014**, *11*, 506–514. [CrossRef] [PubMed]
22. Furrie, E. Probiotics and allergy. *Proc. Nutr. Soc.* **2005**, *64*, 465–469. [CrossRef] [PubMed]
23. Zuccotti, G.V.; Meneghin, F.; Aceti, A.; Barone, G.; Callegari, M.L.; Di Mauro, A.; Fantini, M.P.; Gori, D.; Indrio, F.; Maggio, L.; et al. Probiotics for prevention of atopic diseases in infants: Systematic review and meta-analysis. *Allergy* **2015**, *70*, 1356–1371. [CrossRef] [PubMed]
24. Sestito, S.; D'Auria, E.; Baldassarre, M.E.; Salvatore, S.; Tallarico, V.; Stefanelli, E.; Tarsitano, F.; Concolino, D.; Pensabene, L. The Role of Prebiotics and Probiotics in Prevention of Allergic Diseases in Infants. *Front. Pediatr.* **2020**, *8*, 870. [CrossRef] [PubMed]
25. Tan-Lim, C.S.C.; Esteban-Ipac, N.A.R.; Recto, M.S.T.; Castor, M.A.R.; Casis-Hao, R.J.; Nano, A.L.M. Comparative effectiveness of probiotic strains on the prevention of pediatric atopic dermatitis: A systematic review and network meta-analysis. *Pediatr. Allergy Immunol.* **2021**, *32*, 1255–1270. [CrossRef]
26. Moher, D.; Shamseer, L.; Clarke, M.; Ghersi, D.; Liberati, A.; Petticrew, M.; Shekelle, P.; Stewart, L.A. Preferred reporting items for systematic review and meta-analysis protocols (prisma-p) 2015 statement. *Syst. Rev.* **2015**, *4*, 1. [CrossRef]
27. Sterne, J.A.C.; Savović, J.; Page, M.J.; Elbers, R.G.; Blencowe, N.S.; Boutron, I.; Cates, C.J.; Cheng, H.Y.; Corbett, M.S.; Eldridge, S.M.; et al. RoB 2: A revised tool for assessing risk of bias in randomised trials. *BMJ* **2019**, *366*, l4898. [CrossRef]
28. Jadad, A.R.; Moore, R.A.; Carroll, D.; Jenkinson, C.; Reynolds, D.J.M.; Gavaghan, D.J.; McQuay, H.J. Assessing the quality of reports of randomized clinical trials: Is blinding necessary? *Control. Clin. Trials* **1996**, *17*, 1–12. [CrossRef]
29. Boyle, R.J.; Ismail, I.H.; Kivivuori, S.; Licciardi, P.V.; Robins-Browne, R.M.; Mah, L.-J.; Axelrad, C.; Moore, S.; Donath, S.; Carlin, J.B.; et al. Lactobacillus GG treatment during pregnancy for the prevention of eczema: A randomized controlled trial. *Allergy* **2010**, *66*, 509–516. [CrossRef]
30. Dotterud, C.K.; Storrø, O.; Johnsen, R.; Øien, T. Probiotics in pregnant women to prevent allergic disease: A randomized, double-blind trial. *Br. J. Dermatol.* **2010**, *163*, 616–623. [CrossRef]
31. Huurre, A.; Laitinen, K.; Rautava, S.; Korkeamaki, M.; Isolauri, E. Impact of maternal atopy and probiotic supplementation during pregnancy on infant sensitization: A double-blind placebo-controlled study. *Clin. Exp. Allergy* **2008**, *38*, 1342–1348. [CrossRef] [PubMed]
32. Rautava, S.; Kainonen, E.; Salminen, S.; Isolauri, E. Maternal probiotic supplementation during pregnancy and breast-feeding reduces the risk of eczema in the infant. *J. Allergy Clin. Immunol.* **2021**, *130*, 1355–1360. [CrossRef] [PubMed]

33. Simpson, M.R.; Dotterud, C.K.; Storrø, O.; Johnsen, R.; Øien, T. Perinatal probiotic supplementation in the prevention of allergy related disease: 6 year follow up of a randomised controlled trial. *BMC Dermatol.* **2015**, *15*, 13. [CrossRef] [PubMed]
34. Wickens, K.; Barthow, C.; Mitchell, E.A.; Stanley, T.V.; Purdie, G.; Rowden, J.; Kang, J.; Hood, F.; van den Elsen, L.; Forbes-Blom, E.; et al. Maternal sup-plementation alone with Lactobacillus rhamnosus HN001 during pregnancy and breastfeeding does not reduce infant eczema. *Pediatr. Allergy Immunol.* **2018**, *29*, 296–302. [CrossRef] [PubMed]
35. Dugoua, J.-J.; Machado, M.; Zhu, X.; Chen, X.; Koren, G.; Einarson, T.R. Probiotic Safety in Pregnancy: A Systematic Review and Meta-analysis of Randomized Controlled Trials of Lactobacillus, Bifidobacterium, and Saccharomyces spp. *J. Obstet. Gynaecol. Can.* **2009**, *31*, 542–552. [CrossRef]

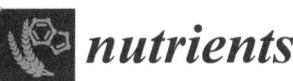

Review

Breastfeeding and Allergy Effect Modified by Genetic, Environmental, Dietary, and Immunological Factors

Hanna Danielewicz

1st Clinical Department of Pediatrics, Allergology and Cardiology, Wroclaw Medical University, ul. Chałubińskiego 2a, 50-368 Wrocław, Poland; hanna.danielewicz@umed.wroc.pl

Abstract: Breastfeeding (BF) is the most natural mode of nutrition. Its beneficial effect has been revealed in terms of both the neonatal period and those of lifelong effects. However, as for protection against allergy, there is not enough data. In the current narrative review, the literature within the last five years from clinical trials and population-based studies on breastfeeding and allergy from different aspects was explored. The aim of this review was to explain how different factors could contribute to the overall effect of BF. Special consideration was given to accompanying exposure to cow milk, supplement use, the introduction of solid foods, microbiota changes, and the epigenetic function of BF. Those factors seem to be modifying the impact of BF. We also identified studies regarding BF in atopic mothers, with SCFA as a main player explaining differences according to this status. Conclusion: Based on the population-based studies, breastfeeding could be protective against some allergic phenotypes, but the results differ within different study groups. According to the new research in that matter, the effect of BF could be modified by different genetic (HMO composition), environmental (cesarean section, allergen exposure), dietary (SCFA, introduction of solid food), and immunologic factors (IgG, IgE), thus partially explaining the variance.

Keywords: breastfeeding; maternal atopy; epigenetics; food allergy

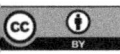

1. Introduction

Breastfeeding is the most natural mode of nutrition in the first months of life. Its beneficial effect has been elucidated, not only in the neonatal period but also in terms of lifelong impacts. Recent large meta-analyses on this style of feeding have revealed protection against metabolic conditions, such as overweight and diabetes, as well as against early childhood infections. However, no evidence, little evidence, or inconclusive results has been indicated for breastfeeding and different allergy phenotypes [1]. In earlier studies, some protective effect was visible for atopic dermatitis in infancy [2]. In the context of developing allergies early in life, two main types of interventions have been studied over the last few years. The first was exclusive breastfeeding in the first 4 to 6 months of life in comparison to formula feeding; the second was the early introduction of allergenic foods. The second aspect has emerged since the publication of the LEAP study results showing a protective effect of the early introduction of peanuts on the prevention of peanut allergy [3]. Nevertheless, this intervention did not affect in any way sensitization to other food allergens.

The LEAP study was one of the first studies investigating the early introduction of solid food, similar to the EAT study [4] that introduced egg, peanut, sesame, cod fish, and wheat [5], the STAR and HealthyNuts studies that introduced egg, and PreventADALL [6]. In spite of early promising results, some of these studies showed no protective effect [7].

The main mechanism discussed in the context of the protective performance of breast milk is epigenetic imprinting. This phenomenon could explain long-lasting health benefits. It has been speculated that breastfeeding impacts epigenetic processes both by the direct effect of bio-compounds present in human milk and indirect effects depending on the shaping of the microbiome in the neonatal gut and the related presence of bacteria metabolites such as butyrate and propionate, which operate as active compounds. The active bio-compounds in breast milk could work at different levels of epigenetic imprinting. These active elements are mainly dendritic cells containing live maternal gut bacteria, prostaglandin J and PUFA exhibiting metabolic effects, lactoferrin with its ability to bind bacterial CpG thus preventing the NFκB response against flora, microvesicles with the demonstrated effect of inhibiting atopic sensitization, fat globules containing microRNA, which target several infant genes, and multipotential stem cells [1,8].

Due to existing controversies on the subject regarding the protection of BF against allergy, we have searched the most recent literature through the two databases: PubMed and Embase, with the search term: "breastfeeding and allergy" for any new findings in the last 5 years, within the matter including clinical trials, randomized clinical trials, and population-based studies, with the respect of the sub-population of atopic mothers. We have included in this narrative review all the studies identified if they were related to BF and allergy or immune outcomes. The aim of this review was to explain how different factors could contribute to the overall effect of BF. The summary of the studies is presented in Table 1.

Table 1. Summary of the recent literature regarding breastfeeding (BF) and allergy outcomes.

	Intervention or Observation	Age of Intervention or Observation	Type of Study	Outcome	Age of Outcome	Number of Participants	Effect of BF on Outcome	Limitations	Conclusion
	Cow milk exposure								
Urashima M, 2019 [9]	Avoiding supplementation with cow milk	1 day–5 months	RCT	Sensitization to cow milk Food allergy (including CMA and anaphylaxis)	2 years	312	RR 0.52 (0.34–0.81)	Amino acid formula in avoiding CM arm and switching to CM arm after 3 days	Sensitization to cow milk is preventable by avoiding CMF for at least 3 days of life
Sakihara T, 2021 [10]	Early introduction and daily infant CMF	1–2 months	RCT	CMA by OFC	6 months	504	RR 0.12 (0.01–0.5)	Soya-based formula in no CMF arm	Daily ingestion of CMF prevents CMA development
	BF effect as only exposure								
Ek WE, 2018 [11]	BF yes or not	time of BF	Cohort Born 1937–1969	Self-reported asthma hay fever eczema	38–73 years	336,364	Asthma OR 0.99 (0.96–1.02) hay fever/eczema OR 1.06 (1.03–1.08)	Wide time interval, population with different environmental exposure and cultural behaviors	BF is associated with an increased risk for hay fever and eczema, no effect on asthma
Flohr C, 2018 [12]	BF promotion	birth	Cluster RT	Spirometry Eczema Asthma Wheezing	16 years	17,046	Eczema OR 0.46 (0.25–0.83)	Allocation was not blinded	BF reduces eczema risk but not asthma
Filipiak-Pirttroff B, 2018 [13]	Exclusive BF for 4 month or supplementation with randomized formula Non-intervention group—no recommendations	birth	RCT	Asthma Eczema Allergic rhinitis	1, 2, 3, 4, 6, 10, and 15 years	5991	non-risk non-intervention allergic rhinitis OR 0.65 (0.42–0.99)	Recall bias in non-intervention group	In the non-intervention non-risk cohort—BF showed no effect on eczema and asthma, but a risk reduction for allergic rhinitis
Hu Y, 2021 [14]	Duration of BF	6–11 years	Population based	Asthma Allergic rhinitis Urticaria Food allergy Drug allergy	6–11 years	10,464	Asthma (and vaginal delivery) OR 0.78 (0.66–0.92)	Self-reported allergy Recall bias	BF > 6 months is inversely associated with childhood asthma and allergic diseases and modifies the risks of parental allergy and Cesarean section
	BF and microbiome composition								
Sordillo JE, 2017 [15]	Infant gut microbiome VDAART study (supplementation with low and high vitamin D at pregnancy) High-risk infants (atopic mother or father)	Pregnancy—vitamin D Infancy BF	RCT	Gut microbiome composition	3–6 months stool	333	beta −0.45 p < 0.001	High-risk infants, No allergy phenotype was studied at that point	Ethnicity, mode of delivery, BF, and cord blood vitamin D levels are associated with infant gut microbiome composition
Savage JH, 2018 [16]	Intestinal microbiome in breastfed high-risk infants (atopic mother or father) VDAART study (supplementation with low and high vitamin D at pregnancy)	pregnancy	RCT	Microbial composition	3–6 months	323	Bifidobacterium beta 0.56 (0.12, 1.00) Lactobacillus beta 3.50 (2.14, 4.86)	Included only high-risk infants	BF is dietary factor independently associated with microbiome composition
Korpela K, 2018 [17]	Probiotic supplementation with BF High-risk infants	pregnancy and infancy until 6 month	RCT	Intestinal microbiota composition	3 months	428	NA	Studying microbiota only, not proving any impact on allergy risk	At least partial breastfeeding together with probiotic supplementation might correct unfavorable changes in microbiota composition (possibly related to allergy risk) caused by antibiotics and cesarean birth

Table 1. Cont.

	Intervention or Observation	Age of Intervention or Observation	Type of Study	Outcome	Age of Outcome	Number of Participants	Effect of BF on Outcome	Limitations	Conclusion
Lee-Sarwar KA, 2019 [18]	Intestinal microbiome VDAART study	pregnancy	RCT	Asthma at 3 y	3 years	361	beta 0.02 (0.01–0.03)	Parent reported asthma Not all metabolites were included Only high-risk children	Asthma-associated intestinal metabolites are significant mediators of the inverse relationship between exclusive breastfeeding for the first 4 months of life and asthma
	Supplement use with BF								
Sprenger N, 2017 [19]	FUT2-HMO measurement in the placebo group from supplementation with probiotics and prebiotics trial high-risk infants	Mean 2.6 day	RCT	Allergy IgE-allergy Eczema IgE-eczema	2 years 5 years	266	beta −2.14 SE 1.23 $p = 0.083$	High-risk infants Trend only	A lower risk of manifesting IgE-associated eczema at 2 years, but not 5 years, when fed breast milk with FUT2-HMO
Wickens K, 2018 [20]	Supplementation with either Lactobacillus rhamnosus HN001 Lactobacillus rhamnosus HN001 or Bifidobacterium lactis HN019	Mothers from 35 weeks of pregnancy—6 month Postpartum; children 1 day–2 year	RCT	Eczema Asthma Wheeze Rhinitis	10 years	298	12 months prevalence eczema RR 0.46 (0.25–0.86) hay fever RR = 0.73 (0.53–1.00) Lifelong prevalence atopic sensitization HR = 0.71 (0.51–1.00) eczema HR = 0.58 (0.41–0.82) wheeze HR = 0.76 (0.57–0.99)	Study not directed at BF, mixed effect of maternal and child's diet supplementation	HN001 supplementation is associated with a significant reduction in hay fever, eczema, wheeze, and atopic sensitization
Henrick BM, 2021 [21]	Supplementation with B.infantis EVC001 Metagenomics profiling of BF infants	7–28 day $n = 60$	CT	Metagenomics profile $n = 288$ Galectin-1 Th2 Th17 $n = 60$	1–6 month	208 Sweden 60 U.S.	NA	No intestinal tissue studied	Infants colonized early in life with Bifidobacterium species are less likely to develop immune-mediated diseases
Pitt TJ, 2018 [22]	Peanut introduction before 12 month	Infancy and time of BF	Cohort	Peanut sensitization	7 years	545	OR 0.08 (0.01–0.85)	No data on environmental peanut exposure and peanut exposure during pregnancy	Maternal peanut consumption while breastfeeding paired with direct introduction is associated with a lower risk of peanut sensitization
Marrs T, 2021 [23]	Solid food regular consumption of 6 allergenic foods from 3 months alongside continued BF or EBF until 6 month	3 months	RCT	Intestinal microbiota Allergen-specific IgE Atopic dermatitis	6 months 12 months	288	NA	No data before 3 month	Introduction of allergenic solids from age 3 months alongside breastfeeding is associated with maturation of the gut microbiota
	Epigenetic effect of BF								
Mallisetty Y, 2020 [24]	Epigenetics of BF	Time of BF	Cohort IOWBC	Methylation in blood Lung function Serum IgE	birth 10 years 18 years	201	NA	Relatively small sample size	87 CpGs were identified as DM, the methylation pattern in EFF group was more stable from birth to 10 years and significantly lower cg25458520 (MAPK13 gene) is related to an increase in FEV1/FVC in EBF
	Atopic mothers								
Stinson LF, 2020 [25]	SCFA composition measurement in BM from atopic and non-atopic mothers	1 month	Cohort	SCFA composition	1 month	109	NA	No allergy phenotype in children studied	Atopic mothers had significantly lower concentrations of acetate and butyrate than non-atopic mothers

The table contains data from clinical trials (CT), randomized clinical trials (RCT), and population-based (cohort) studies. RR—relative risk, OR—odds ratio, beta—estimate in the regression model, BM—breast milk, CMF—cow milk formula, CM—cow milk, CMA—cow milk allergy, OFC—oral food challenge, SCFA—short fatty chain acids, EBF—exclusively breastfed, EFF—exclusively formula fed, VDAART—Vitamin D Atenatal Asthma Reduction Trial, FUT2—Fucosyltransferase 2 gene, IOWBC—The Isle Of Wight Whole Population Birth Cohort, HMO—human milk oligosaccharides, DM—differentially methylated NA—not applicable.

2. The Effect of Breastfeeding as an Only Exposure

Few studies have considered the protective effect of breastfeeding by itself, with emerging contraindicative results. Breastfeeding seemed to increase the risk of allergic rhinitis and allergic sensitization [11] and decrease the risk of asthma [18]. In the first study, the population born from 1937 to 1969 in the U.K. was examined with self-reported allergic outcomes. Since nowadays we observe an increase in allergies in the younger population (10–30 years), there is doubt as to whether we can extrapolate the results from the older group with different environmental exposures in the first years of life. As the authors concluded, the year of birth, socioeconomic status, and smoking status had high confounding power in the analysis, which confirms that lifestyle factors modify the effect of breastfeeding.

The second study showed an association between exclusive breastfeeding in the first 4 months of life and the composition of the intestinal metabolome at 3 years of age. This relation seemed to further mediate the association between protection against asthma and breastfeeding. From other possible predictors of a child's intestinal metabolome, such as antibiotic use, cesarean section, having siblings, or dog ownership, only breastfeeding was an independent factor affecting the metabolome at 3 years.

Contrary to these results, the promotion of breastfeeding, i.e., prolonged duration and exclusivity for infants born in 1996–1997 in Belarus, has been shown to reduce the risk of flexural atopic dermatitis but had no impact on spirometry at 16 years [12]. Another large study in China has shown a protective effect against different allergic conditions. More than 10,000 children aged 6–11 years were evaluated for the reported diagnosis of asthma and other allergic conditions. Factors such as male sex, high socioeconomic status, cesarean section, being an only child, and a family history of allergy were associated with an increased risk for having asthma and other allergic conditions at that age, while prolonged (>6 months) breastfeeding was related to a decreased risk. In addition, breastfeeding attenuated the risk connected to other factors [14]. In GINI (German Infant Nutritional Intervention) study, full breastfeeding showed no effect on eczema and asthma, but a risk reduction for allergic rhinitis was observed [13].

These opposing results could be the effect of the complex nature of different exposures in the first years of life. Including all of them could bring some explanation, so if one is missing, controversies emerge.

3. Exposure to Cow Milk

One of the factors that could modify the effect of BF is cow milk exposure. Two contradictory study results have been published regarding early exposure to cow milk in breastfed infants. In the first ABC trial (Atopy induced by Breastfeeding or Cow's milk formula), introducing milk formula at the earliest in the first 3 days of life was found to increase the risk of further allergy to not only cow milk but also other food allergens. In this trial, neonates received either breast milk and an amino acid formula as supplementation if necessary or breast milk and cow milk formula. Sensitization to cow milk and other secondary outcomes such as anaphylaxis and food allergy were estimated in the second year of life [9]. In the second study (SPADE—Strategy for Prevention of milk Allergy by Daily ingestion of infant formula in Early infancy), avoiding cow milk formula in comparison to feeding with at least 10 mL in the period between 1 and 2 months of life increased the risk of having an allergy, measured by OFC (oral food challenge) and sIgE and SPT (skin prick test) at the age of 6 months [10]. In both trials, infants in the cow milk avoidance arm received an alternative formula containing amino acids in the first case and soy formula in the second, so the results could have been affected by the impact of these formulas on the outcomes. The question is what was really studied: cow milk formula vs. soy/amino acid formula or avoiding cow milk allergens versus exposure. In addition, timing could make a huge difference here since the first days of life could be a very sensitive period for allergy development.

4. Breastfeeding and Changes in the Microbiota

Another factor that could both reflect and modify the effect of BF is microbiota composition. As changes in the gut microbiota are believed to be the main factor responsible for the immunomodulatory effect of breast milk, some studies have focused solely on this parameter. Surprisingly, breastfed children have shown lover diversity levels in comparison to formula-fed children. Despite having lower biodiversity, breastfed infants had more beneficial genera such as *Bifidobacterium* and *Lactobacillus*. This pattern appears to be beneficial according to the immaturity of the neonatal immune system. Apart from breastfeeding, ethnicity and maternal diet during pregnancy have some effect on stool microbiota at the age of 3–6 months, but not as strong as human milk [16]. A similar effect regarding microbiome diversity was confirmed in another study at different time points, i.e., 3, 6, 9, and 12 months of life [26]. In a large meta-analysis of seven microbiome studies, five cohorts, and 684 infants, the differences in the microbiome in relation to the mode of feeding were visible and persisted after 6 months of life (up to 2 years). Both diversity and the age of the microbiome were lower in breastfed infants in comparison to formula-fed infants. These differences were observed for composition and functional pathways, and the mode of delivery was a factor modifying the difference [27].

Children born by cesarean section can have more *Clostridium* in the gut microbiome [17]. *Clostridium* colonization is believed to be the main effector of harmful effects on different aspects of human health, as it has been revealed that it has an impact on microbiome composition, only in exclusively breast infants but not in formula-fed infants, suggesting an already changed microbiome in the latter. *Clostridium* is believed to induce gut inflammation and disrupt the intestinal epithelial barrier, thereby further promoting colonization by non-commensal pathogens [28]. The changes in the microbiota of 3- to 6-month-old infants have been shown to not only rely on feeding mode and delivery type but also depend on some other independent factors such as race/ethnicity and the cord blood vitamin D level. As an example, Caucasian infants have a less diverse microbiome but more *Bacteroides* in comparison to African American, while cesarean section causes an increase in diversity but decreases in *Bacteroides*, and formula-fed infants have increased levels of *Clostridium* [15]. However, in another study, the mode of delivery did not affect the diversity or the level of *Bifidobacteria*, but there were some differences in the abundance of the phyla Bacteroidetes and Verrucomicrobia, in the genera *Bacteroides*, *Akkermansia*, and *Kluyvera*, and in the species *B. longum*. In this specific study, only mothers with the Se+ phenotype were included, which could impact the results. Se+ means that they had an active FUT2 enzyme and produced high amounts of α1-2 fucosylated HMO (human oligosaccharides), such as 2′FL and lacto-N-fucopentaose I (LNFP I) in breast milk. This biocomponent is believed to be beneficial for the proper development of the infant microbiota [29].

HMOs are oligosaccharides with individual diversity and composition. So far, 200 types are known. They function not only as prebiotics but also impact epithelial barrier function, serving as a decoy to block the attachment of bacteria. A decrease in specifically one type, i.e., LNFPIII, has been indicated to be linked to cow milk food allergy in infants fed by mothers with low amounts of this HMO in breast milk [30]. To make the case more complicated, the introduction of solid food is an independent factor changing microbiota diversity in breastfed infants. The early life gut microbiota become more diverse when allergenic foods are introduced and mature toward a *Bacteroides*-rich community at the age of 12 months. Significant changes have been observed at a younger age in infants with early introduction of allergenic solids, beginning from 3 months of life [23]. It appears that this kind of intervention has the potential to change the distinct characteristics of the breastfed and formula-fed microbiome [31].

Another factor that could influence the infant's intestinal microbiome is maternal metabolic status. Since there is a link connecting maternal obesity to allergy in offspring [32], this factor seems to affect the child's gut microbiome primarily, both in utero and at birth, resulting later in dysbiosis and the development of unfavorable outcomes such as obesity [33,34] or allergy [35]. Maternal obesity also modifies breast milk composition resulting in low n-3 and elevated n-6 PUFA levels, with its further consequences [36].

In summary, breastfed infants present with lower diversity of the gut microbiota, breastfeeding (BF) is a strong predictor of the gut microbiota, and the cessation of BF is associated with a shift toward an adult-type microbiota. The predominant genus in the gut of BF infants is *Bifidobacterium*, with less abundance reported for *Firmicutes* and *Bacteroides* [37].

5. Supplements and Breastfeeding

Some supplements have been shown recently as possible modifiers of BF effect, with the main impact on microbial composition. The introduction of the supplement EVC001 (*Bifidobacterium infantis*), which utilizes HMO, a biocomponent of human milk that cannot be digested but act as a nutrient for bacteria only, was found to switch the immune response with a decrease in pro-allergy Th2 and pro-inflammatory Th17 response and an increase in INF-β. These events indicate the induction of tolerance to the intestinal microbiota, a crucial process for the healthy development of the immune system. *Bifidobacterium infantis* was discovered recently in the microbiota of infants from developing countries. This bacteria co-evolved with humans but is rare in the "modern" countries of Europe and North America. Studies performed in Sweden confirmed the absence of the gene for processing HMO in the bacteria metagenome profile of breastfed infants born in that country. *Bifidobacterium infantis* expresses all the genes necessary to utilize HMO [21]. In addition, HMO added to formula starting at 0–14 days and continuing up to 6 months had the effect of fewer infections and more *Bifidobacteria* in the gut, an effect similar to that of breastfeeding [38]. Similarly, *Lactobacillus rhamnosus* supplementation in breastfed infants from birth up to the second year of life, together with supplementation in mothers from 35 weeks of gestation up to 6 months after birth or until the end of breastfeeding, decreased the risk of atopic dermatitis at 11 years, and a lifetime decrease in the prevalence of eczema, atopic sensitization and wheeze [20]; such supplementation during pregnancy only did not have such an effect [39]. Another intervention based on the introduction of the oligosaccharide FUT2 in breastfed infants showed a reduced risk of atopic dermatitis at 2 years old. FUT2 is genetically polymorphic in mothers and determines the breast milk glycan composition and the variation of specific human milk oligosaccharides, which act as prebiotics. Thus, this factor seemed to impact the microbiota composition, also explaining the differences between human milk from different subjects. Non-secretor mothers, who lack a functional FUT2 enzyme, characterize approximately 15–25% of mothers depending on ethnic background. The presence of FUT2-dependent oligosaccharides is associated with the establishment of a *Bifidobacteria*-loaded microbiota [19]. Probiotics consisting of *Bifidobacterium breve* Bb99 (Bp99 2×10^8 cfu) *Propionibacterium freudenreichii* subsp. shermanii JS (2×10^9 cfu), *Lactobacillus rhamnosus* Lc705 (5×10^9 cfu), and *Lactobacillus rhamnosus* GG (5×10^9 cfu) given to both mothers and infants have been shown to modify the risk associated with cesarean section and the use of antibiotics early in life, by impacting the microbiota up to the third month of life, but only in breastfed infants. Breastfed infants also showed the expected increase in *Bifidobacteria* and a reduction in *Proteobacteria* and *Clostridium* [17].

Supplementation with different types of probiotics is showing promising results as a method of prevention against allergy. However, more caution is necessary with the way how the microbiota is being changed, specifically if one single component is modified. Possibly more natural, diet-driven interventions will be studied in the future.

6. Introduction of Solid Foods

Another factor that plays a major role in the development of allergic phenotype is an allergenic foods introduction. The early or late exposure could change the direction of immune events, inducing sensitization or tolerance. Additionally, BF seems to be impacting this specific effect. Allergenic foods play different roles depending on the timing of introduction but also the interaction of the intervention in both lactating mothers and children. Only the introduction of peanuts to both the mother during lactation and the child before 12 months of life resulted in a reduction in peanut allergy at 7 years old. Peanut antigens, given through breast milk, are distributed to the infant together with multiple bioactive factors, including maternal immunoglobulins, cytokines, microbiota, and immune cells, which possibly prime the infant's immune system to develop tolerance when peanut is consumed a few months later by the child [22].

Since the 1990s, national societies have recommended delaying the introduction of common allergenic foods, including peanuts, until 2 or 3 years of age. However, despite these recommendations, the prevalence of food allergy increased over the following decades, leading to skepticism regarding delayed introduction as an effective prevention measure. Recent studies mentioned earlier in this review suggest that early introduction of allergenic food may rather reduce the risk of developing food allergy. In addition, studies in animal models have shown that maternal milk factors such as TGF-β, vitamin A and maternal OVA-specific IgG are required for the induction of oral tolerance when OVA is transmitted through the breast milk [40,41].

In contrast, the presence of aeroallergens in breast milk seemed to have the opposite effect in the case of dust mite allergens in a mouse model. Most inhaled proteins are likely ingested due to respiratory tract mucociliary clearance and go the same way in breast milk as food antigens. This theory was confirmed by finding the presence of *D. pteronyssinus* allergen in human digestive fluids. The presence of *D. pteronyssinus* in human milk has been shown to be associated with allergic sensitization, allergic rhinitis, and asthma in children [42]. *D. pteronyssinus* in breast milk seems to have the effect of priming the allergic response in adulthood, both in mice and humans and may interfere with the induction of oral tolerance to other food antigens. In a mouse model, *D. pteronyssinus* increased epithelial permeability, IL-33 expression, as well as ILC2 and Th2 differentiation while blocking the formation of Treg, processes related to allergic reactions [43].

The significance of allergen presence in breast milk and the early introduction of allergenic foods to infant diet for allergy development stays controversial for decades. It is not clear the way some allergens seem to be inducing tolerance when others have the opposite effect. The explanation emerging from discussed studies points to the immune status of lactating mothers as a key player.

7. Mechanism of the Effect of Breastfeeding

As epigenetics translates the environmental influence on genetic risk, feeding mode has been shown to impact methylation, with stable changes up to 10 years of life and a lowered global methylation profile in formula-fed infants. One study analyzed the methylome that formed on the Isle of Wight in children born in 1989 and 1990. In total, 87 CpGs were associated with the feeding mode, with 27 distinctly related to exclusive breastfeeding. The described effect could be caused by the bio-compounds present in the human milk and indirectly caused by changes in the microbiota, with known SCFAs (short-chain fatty acids) role as epigenetic modifiers [24]. Another study revealed changes in the methylation of DMs (differentially methylated site) at SNH25, which is related to the regulation of TGF-β and further production of IgA, and DMR (differentially methylated region) at FDFT1, related to hyperlipidemia, as a marker of breastfeeding duration and methylation at 10 years of age [44]. An EWAS (epigenetic wide association study) study on the ALSPAC (Avon Longitudinal Study of Parents And Children) cohort assessed the long-term effect of breastfeeding but revealed differences in methylation at only two DM sites and 12 DMRs related to breastfeeding (markers present at 7 and 15–17 years but not at birth) with a small global effect and absent dose-response relationship [45].

Nevertheless, within the same cohort, another study showed that DNA methylation was associated with 3 to 5 months of exclusive breastfeeding and slower BMI increase in the first 6 years of life in a dose-response manner with exclusive breastfeeding duration [46]. Another study identified six novel CpG sites associated with breastfeeding duration using an EWAS approach. One DM presented consistent associations with breastfeeding (cg00574958, CPT1A) in infancy and childhood but not at birth, while two differentially methylated sites in infancy (cg19693031, TXNIP; cg23307264, KHSRP) were not present at birth but did not persist into childhood [47]. In the past, some candidate gene studies have been evaluated with significant results for NPY, LEP, and Slc2a4 [48].

Other epigenetic mechanisms apart from DNA methylation have been taken into account, such as histone modifications, known for the possible epigenetic effect of dietary

PUFA (polyunsaturated fatty acids) and the expression of PRKC2, FOXP3, IL10RA, and IL7R [49]. Moreover, epigenetic modifications are believed to be transgenerational via piRNA and miRNA. For the latter, there are interesting findings in animal studies indicating epigenetic modifications by the abnormality rates in milk siblings [50]. These may have further consequences in terms of milk biobanking. Although nursing by adoptive mothers has been performed for centuries, the exact consequences of such an action have never been considered. Breast milk seems to be infant-specific, and the composition is modified by both fetus-mother and later infant-mother interplay [51,52]. Even though pasteurization of donor milk is mandatory in order to destroy high-risk viruses and non-spore-forming bacteria, studies investigating the HoP (Holder pasteurization) process (62.5 for 30 min) reported conflicting results, with one reporting no change in selected miRNAs and the other showing substantial degradation [53]. Some important miRNA affecting different developmental properties in a child are *miR-148a-3p, miR-182-5p, let 7f-5p, miR-21* and *let7-c* [51]. The scheme presenting the effect of BF on allergy phenotypes is presented in Figure 1.

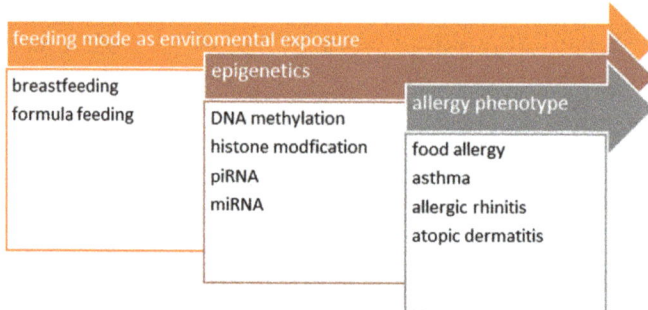

Figure 1. The figure illustrates the epigenetic effect of BF.

The epigenetic effect relies on the direct action of breast milk bio-compounds such as PUFA, miRNA, and piRNA, but also on indirect effects dependable on the microbiota composition. Both PUFA and microbiome variations provide some opportunity for future interventions.

8. Breastfeeding in Atopic Mothers

A possible confounder considering BF effect could be maternal atopy. Atopic mothers have less SCFA in their milk, which has been shown to be responsible for less protective effects in terms of allergy. SCFAs (formate, acetate, propionate, butyrate, and valerate) are interim and final products of alimentary carbohydrate fermentation by gut bacteria [25]. The controversy around breast milk from atopic mothers was indicted before, but only one large study showed that exclusive breastfeeding by atopic mothers for 3 months was associated with an increased risk of asthma at 7 years of life. The reverse relationship may exist before this time point, as shown in a study conducted in Tasmania estimating the risk of having asthma in relation to the mode of feeding in subjects 14–44 years old [54]. In another study, among children with a parental history of atopy (more maternal than paternal), breastfeeding added an additional risk of having allergic outcomes later in life. This association was further modified by the sex of children [55]. This finding is consistent with the speculation that the milk of mothers with atopy or asthma may differ with regard to immunologically active substances. It has been shown that the maternal IgE level is associated with IgE in the child only if the child is breastfed, and further, that prolonged breastfeeding among children whose mothers had high IgE was associated with high IgE in the child. This was further confirmed by observations in mice born to non-allergic mothers that were then breastfed by asthmatic foster mothers, which later developed increased airway hyperresponsiveness and eosinophilic airway inflammation [56]. However, somehow contrary to previous results in established risk/protection factors related to BF, this mode of feeding and vaginal delivery seems to modify the risk connected to maternal atopy [57] and asthma [58,59].

Another factor largely modifying the risk of allergic sensitization in children is the presence of allergen-specific IgG derived from mothers during pregnancy and lactation. It has been shown that the levels of these immunoglobulins are comparable in different sources, e.g., cord blood, the serum of mothers, and breast milk. The higher the concentration of allergen-specific IgG, the lowest the risk of IgE sensitization to the same allergen. Even though these levels could vary according to maternal allergy status, a protective effect has been shown to be present for both sensitized and non-sensitized mothers [60].

Based on the discussed studies, it is reasonable to say that atopy in pregnant and lactating mothers could modify the definitive effect of BF on allergy development in children, depending on the SCFA concentration and the immune status of mothers.

9. Conclusions

Breastfeeding is still the most recommended mode of feeding in infancy for its benefits to general health. However, with regard to allergy risk, the results of population-based studies in the last years are still inconclusive. According to the new research in that matter, based mainly on clinical trials, the effect could be modified by different genetic (HMO composition), environmental (cesarean section, allergen exposure), dietary (SCFA, introduction of solid food), and immunologic factors (IgG, IgE), thus explaining partially the differences observed in the population studies.

Funding: This research received no external funding.

Institutional Review Board Statement: Not applicable.

Informed Consent Statement: Not applicable.

Data Availability Statement: Not applicable.

Conflicts of Interest: Danielewicz H reports grant and personal fees from the National Science Center, Poland, and lecturer fees from Mead Johnson Nutrition and Takeda outside submitted work.

Abbreviations

BF	breastfeeding
SCFA	short-chain fatty acids
HMO	human oligosaccharide
OVA	ovalbumin
ILC2	innate lymphoid cell type 2

References

1. Victora, C.G.; Bahl, R.; Barros, A.J.D.; França, V.A.; Horton, S.; Krasevec, J.; Murch, S.; Sankar, M.J.; Walker, N.; Rollins, N.C. Breastfeeding 1 Breastfeeding in the 21st century: Epidemiology, mechanisms, and lifelong effect. *Lancet* **2016**, *387*, 475. [CrossRef]
2. Kramer, M.S. Breastfeeding and Allergy: The Evidence. *Ann. Nutr. Metab.* **2007**, *335*, 20–26. [CrossRef]
3. Du Toit, G.; Roberts, G.; Sayre, P.H.; Bahnson, H.T.; Radulovic, S.; Santos, A.F.; Brough, H.A.; Phippard, D.; Basting, M.; Feeney, M.; et al. Randomized trial of peanut consumption in infants at risk for peanut allergy. *N. Engl. J. Med.* **2015**, *372*, 803–813. [CrossRef]
4. Wei-Liang Tan, J.; Valerio, C.; Barnes, E.H.; Turner, P.J.; Van Asperen, P.A.; Kakakios, A.M.; Campbell, D.E. A randomized trial of egg introduction from 4 months of age in infants at risk for egg allergy. *J. Allergy Clin. Immunol.* **2017**, *139*, 1621–1628.e8. [CrossRef]
5. Perkin, M.R.; Logan, K.; Marrs, T.; Radulovic, S.; Craven, J.; Flohr, C.; Lack, G.; EAT Study Team, E.S. Enquiring About Tolerance (EAT) study: Feasibility of an early allergenic food introduction regimen. *J. Allergy Clin. Immunol.* **2016**, *137*, 1477–1486.e8. [CrossRef]
6. Lødrup Carlsen, K.C.; Rehbinder, E.M.; Skjerven, H.O.; Carlsen, M.H.; Fatnes, T.A.; Fugelli, P.; Granum, B.; Haugen, G.; Hedlin, G.; Jonassen, C.M.; et al. Preventing Atopic Dermatitis and ALLergies in Children—the PreventADALL study. *Allergy* **2018**, *73*, 2063–2070. [CrossRef]

7. Perkin, M.R.; Logan, K.; Tseng, A.; Raji, B.; Ayis, S.; Peacock, J.; Brough, H.; Marrs, T.; Radulovic, S.; Craven, J.; et al. Randomized Trial of Introduction of Allergenic Foods in Breast-Fed Infants. *N. Engl. J. Med.* **2016**, *374*, 1733–1743. [CrossRef]
8. Annesi-Maesano, I.; Fleddermann, M.; Hornef, M.; Von Mutius, E.; Pabst, O.; Schaubeck, M.; Fiocchi, A. Allergic diseases in infancy: I—Epidemiology and current interpretation. *World Allergy Organ. J.* **2021**, *14*, 100591. [CrossRef]
9. Urashima, M.; Urashima, M.; Mezawa, H.; Okuyama, M.; Urashima, T.; Hirano, D.; Gocho, N.; Tachimoto, H. Primary Prevention of Cow's Milk Sensitization and Food Allergy by Avoiding Supplementation With Cow's Milk Formula at Birth: A Randomized Clinical Trial. *JAMA Pediatr.* **2019**, *173*, 1137–1145. [CrossRef]
10. Sakihara, T.; Otsuji, K.; Arakaki, Y.; Hamada, K.; Sugiura, S.; Ito, K.; Aichi, J. Randomized trial of early infant formula introduction to prevent cow's milk allergy. *J. Allergy Clin. Immunol.* **2021**, *147*, 224–232.e8. [CrossRef]
11. Ek, W.E.; Karlsson, T.; Hernándes, C.A.; Rask-Andersen, M.; Johansson, Å. Breast-feeding and risk of asthma, hay fever, and eczema. *J. Allergy Clin. Immunol.* **2018**, *141*, 1157–1159.e9. [CrossRef] [PubMed]
12. Flohr, C.; John Henderson, A.; Kramer, M.S.; Patel, R.; Thompson, J.; Rifas-Shiman, S.L.; Yang, S.; Vilchuck, K.; Bogdanovich, N.; Hameza, M.; et al. Effect of an Intervention to Promote Breastfeeding on Asthma, Lung Function, and Atopic Eczema at Age 16 Years: Follow-up of the PROBIT Randomized Trial. *JAMA Pediatr.* **2018**, *172*, e174064. [CrossRef] [PubMed]
13. Filipiak-Pittroff, B.; Koletzko, S.; Krämer, U.; Standl, M.; Bauer, C.P.; Berdel, D.; von Berg, A. Full breastfeeding and allergies from infancy until adolescence in the GINIplus cohort. *Pediatr. Allergy Immunol.* **2018**, *29*, 96–101. [CrossRef]
14. Hu, Y.; Chen, Y.; Liu, S.; Jiang, F.; Wu, M.; Yan, C.; Tan, J.; Yu, G.; Hu, Y.; Yin, Y.; et al. Breastfeeding duration modified the effects of neonatal and familial risk factors on childhood asthma and allergy: A population-based study. *Respir. Res.* **2021**, *22*, 41. [CrossRef]
15. Sordillo, J.E.; Zhou, Y.; McGeachie, M.J.; Ziniti, J.; Lange, N.; Laranjo, N.; Savage, J.R.; Carey, V.; O'Connor, G.; Sandel, M.; et al. Factors Influencing the Infant Gut Microbiome at Age 3–6 months: Findings from the ethnically diverse Vitamin D Antenatal Asthma Reduction Trial (VDAART). *J. Allergy Clin. Immunol.* **2017**, *139*, 482. [CrossRef]
16. Savage, J.H.; Lee-Sarwar, K.A.; Sordillo, J.E.; Lange, N.E.; Zhou, Y.; O'Connor, G.T.; Sandel, M.; Bacharier, L.B.; Zeiger, R.; Sodergren, E.; et al. Diet during Pregnancy and Infancy and the Infant Intestinal Microbiome. *J. Pediatr.* **2018**, *203*, 47. [CrossRef]
17. Korpela, K.; Salonen, A.; Vepsäläinen, O.; Suomalainen, M.; Kolmeder, C.; Varjosalo, M.; Miettinen, S.; Kukkonen, K.; Savilahti, E.; Kuitunen, M.; et al. Probiotic supplementation restores normal microbiota composition and function in antibiotic-treated and in caesarean-born infants. *Microbiome* **2018**, *6*, 182. [CrossRef]
18. Lee-Sarwar, K.A.; Kelly, R.S.; Lasky-Su, J.; Zeiger, R.S.; O'Connor, G.T.; Sandel, M.T.; Bacharier, L.B.; Beigelman, A.; Laranjo, N.; Gold, D.R.; et al. Integrative analysis of the intestinal metabolome of childhood asthma. *J. Allergy Clin. Immunol.* **2019**, *144*, 442–454. [CrossRef]
19. Sprenger, N.; Odenwald, H.; Kukkonen, A.K.; Kuitunen, M.; Savilahti, E.; Kunz, C. FUT2-dependent breast milk oligosaccharides and allergy at 2 and 5 years of age in infants with high hereditary allergy risk. *Eur. J. Nutr.* **2017**, *56*, 1293–1301. [CrossRef]
20. Wickens, K.; Barthow, C.; Mitchell, E.A.; Kang, J.; van Zyl, N.; Purdie, G.; Stanley, T.; Fitzharris, P.; Murphy, R.; Crane, J. Effects of Lactobacillus rhamnosus HN001 in early life on the cumulative prevalence of allergic disease to 11 years. *Pediatr. Allergy Immunol.* **2018**, *29*, 808–814. [CrossRef]
21. Henrick, B.M.; Rodriguez, L.; Lakshmikanth, T.; Pou, C.; Henckel, E.; Arzoomand, A.; Olin, A.; Wang, J.; Mikes, J.; Tan, Z.; et al. Bifidobacteria-mediated immune system imprinting early in life. *Cell* **2021**, *184*, 3884–3898.e11. [CrossRef] [PubMed]
22. Pitt, T.J.; Becker, A.B.; Chan-Yeung, M.; Chan, E.S.; Watson, W.T.A.; Chooniedass, R.; Azad, M.B. Reduced risk of peanut sensitization following exposure through breast-feeding and early peanut introduction. *J. Allergy Clin. Immunol.* **2018**, *141*, 620–625.e1. [CrossRef] [PubMed]
23. Marrs, T.; Jo, J.H.; Perkin, M.R.; Rivett, D.W.; Witney, A.A.; Bruce, K.D.; Logan, K.; Craven, J.; Radulovic, S.; Versteeg, S.A.; et al. Gut microbiota development during infancy: Impact of introducing allergenic foods. *J. Allergy Clin. Immunol.* **2021**, *147*, 613–621.e9. [CrossRef] [PubMed]
24. Mallisetty, Y.; Mukherjee, N.; Jiang, Y.; Chen, S.; Ewart, S.; Hasan Arshad, S.; Holloway, J.W.; Zhang, H.; Karmaus, W. Epigenome-Wide Association of Infant Feeding and Changes in DNA Methylation from Birth to 10 Years. *Nutrients* **2020**, *13*, 99. [CrossRef] [PubMed]
25. Stinson, L.F.; Gay, M.C.L.; Koleva, P.T.; Eggesbø, M.; Johnson, C.C.; Wegienka, G.; du Toit, E.; Shimojo, N.; Munblit, D.; Campbell, D.E.; et al. Human Milk From Atopic Mothers Has Lower Levels of Short Chain Fatty Acids. *Front. Immunol.* **2020**, *11*, 1427. [CrossRef]
26. Brink, L.R.; Mercer, K.E.; Piccolo, B.D.; Chintapalli, S.V.; Elolimy, A.; Bowlin, A.K.; Matazel, K.S.; Pack, L.; Adams, S.H.; Shankar, K.; et al. Neonatal diet alters fecal microbiota and metabolome profiles at different ages in infants fed breast milk or formula. *Am. J. Clin. Nutr.* **2020**, *111*, 1190–1202. [CrossRef]
27. Ho, N.T.; Li, F.; Lee-Sarwar, K.A.; Tun, H.M.; Brown, B.P.; Pannaraj, P.S.; Bender, J.M.; Azad, M.B.; Thompson, A.L.; Weiss, S.T.; et al. Meta-analysis of effects of exclusive breastfeeding on infant gut microbiota across populations. *Nat. Commun.* **2018**, *9*, 4169. [CrossRef]
28. Drall, K.M.; Tun, H.M.; Morales-Lizcano, N.P.; Konya, T.B.; Guttman, D.S.; Field, C.J.; Mandal, R.; Wishart, D.S.; Becker, A.B.; Azad, M.B.; et al. Clostridioides difficile Colonization Is Differentially Associated With Gut Microbiome Profiles by Infant Feeding Modality at 3-4 Months of Age. *Front. Immunol.* **2019**, *10*, 2866. [CrossRef]

29. Tonon, K.M.; Morais, T.B.; Taddei, C.R.; Araújo-Filho, H.B.; Abrão, A.C.F.V.; Miranda, A.; De Morais, M.B. Gut microbiota comparison of vaginally and cesarean born infants exclusively breastfed by mothers secreting α1-2 fucosylated oligosaccharides in breast milk. *PLoS ONE* **2021**, *16*, e0246839. [CrossRef]
30. Seppo, A.E.; Autran, C.A.; Bode, L.; Järvinen, K.M. Human milk oligosaccharides and development of cow's milk allergy in infants. *J. Allergy Clin. Immunol.* **2017**, *139*, 708. [CrossRef]
31. He, X.; Parenti, M.; Grip, T.; Lönnerdal, B.; Timby, N.; Domellöf, M.; Hernell, O.; Slupsky, C.M. Fecal microbiome and metabolome of infants fed bovine MFGM supplemented formula or standard formula with breast-fed infants as reference: A randomized controlled trial. *Sci. Rep.* **2019**, *9*, 11589. [CrossRef] [PubMed]
32. Dow, M.L.; Szymanski, L.M. Effects of Overweight and Obesity in Pregnancy on Health of the Offspring. *Endocrinol. Metab. Clin. N. Am.* **2020**, *49*, 251–263. [CrossRef] [PubMed]
33. Walker, W.A. The importance of appropriate initial bacterial colonization of the intestine in newborn, child and adult health. *Pediatr. Res.* **2017**, *82*, 387. [CrossRef] [PubMed]
34. Galley, J.D.; Bailey, M.; Dush, C.K.; Schoppe-Sullivan, S.; Christian, L.M. Maternal Obesity Is Associated with Alterations in the Gut Microbiome in Toddlers. *PLoS ONE* **2014**, *9*, 113026. [CrossRef]
35. Stiemsma, L.T.; Michels, K.B. The Role of the Microbiome in the Developmental Origins of Health and Disease. *Pediatrics* **2018**, *141*, e20172437. [CrossRef]
36. Álvarez, D.; Muñoz, Y.; Ortiz, M.; Maliqueo, M.; Chouinard-Watkins, R.; Valenzuela, R. Impact of Maternal Obesity on the Metabolism and Bioavailability of Polyunsaturated Fatty Acids during Pregnancy and Breastfeeding. *Nutrients* **2020**, *13*, 19. [CrossRef]
37. Kim, H.; Sitarik, A.R.; Woodcroft, K.; Johnson, C.C.; Zoratti, E. Birth Mode, Breastfeeding, Pet Exposure, and Antibiotic Use: Associations With the Gut Microbiome and Sensitization in Children. *Curr. Allergy Asthma Rep.* **2019**, *19*, 22. [CrossRef]
38. Berger, B.; Porta, N.; Foata, F.; Grathwohl, D.; Delley, M.; Moine, D.; Charpagne, A.; Siegwald, L.; Descombes, P.; Alliet, P.; et al. Linking Human Milk Oligosaccharides, Infant Fecal Community Types, and Later Risk To Require Antibiotics. *MBio* **2020**, *11*, e03196-19. [CrossRef]
39. Wickens, K.; Barthow, C.; Mitchell, E.A.; Stanley, T.V.; Purdie, G.; Rowden, J.; Kang, J.; Hood, F.; van den Elsen, L.; Forbes-Blom, E.; et al. Maternal supplementation alone with Lactobacillus rhamnosus HN001 during pregnancy and breastfeeding does not reduce infant eczema. *Pediatr. Allergy Immunol.* **2018**, *29*, 296–302. [CrossRef]
40. Turfkruyer, M.; Rekima, A.; Macchiaverni, P.; Le Bourhis, L.; Muncan, V.; Van Den Brink, G.R.; Tulic, M.K.; Verhasselt, V. Oral tolerance is inefficient in neonatal mice due to a physiological vitamin A deficiency. *Mucosal Immunol.* **2015**, *9*, 479–491. [CrossRef]
41. Rekima, A.; Macchiaverni, P.; Turfkruyer, M.; Holvoet, S.; Dupuis, L.; Baiz, N.; Annesi-Maesano, I.; Mercenier, A.; Nutten, S.; Verhasselt, V. Long-term reduction in food allergy susceptibility in mice by combining breastfeeding-induced tolerance and TGF-β-enriched formula after weaning. *Clin. Exp. Allergy* **2017**, *47*, 565–576. [CrossRef] [PubMed]
42. Schweitzer, M.; Macchiaverni, P.; Tulic, M.K.; Rekima, A.; Annesi-Maesano, I.; Verhasselt, V.; Bernard, J.Y.; Botton, J.; Charles, M.A.; Dargent-Molina, P.; et al. Early oral exposure to house dust mite allergen through breast milk: A potential risk factor for allergic sensitization and respiratory allergies in children. *J. Allergy Clin. Immunol.* **2017**, *139*, 369–372.e10. [CrossRef]
43. Rekima, A.; Bonnart, C.; Macchiaverni, P.; Metcalfe, J.; Tulic, M.K.; Halloin, N.; Rekima, S.; Genuneit, J.; Zanelli, S.; Medeiros, S.; et al. A role for early oral exposure to house dust mite allergens through breast milk in IgE-mediated food allergy susceptibility. *J. Allergy Clin. Immunol.* **2020**, *145*, 1416–1429.e11. [CrossRef] [PubMed]
44. Sherwood, W.B.; Kothalawala, D.M.; Kadalayil, L.; Ewart, S.; Zhang, H.; Karmaus, W.; Hasan Arshad, S.; Holloway, J.W.; Rezwan, F.I. Epigenome-Wide Association Study Reveals Duration of Breastfeeding Is Associated with Epigenetic Differences in Children. *Int. J. Environ. Res. Public Health* **2020**, *17*, 3569. [CrossRef]
45. Hartwig, F.P.; Davey Smith, G.; Simpkin, A.J.; Victora, C.G.; Relton, C.L.; Caramaschi, D. Association between Breastfeeding and DNA Methylation over the Life Course: Findings from the Avon Longitudinal Study of Parents and Children (ALSPAC). *Nutrients* **2020**, *12*, 3309. [CrossRef]
46. Briollais, L.; Rustand, D.; Allard, C.; Wu, Y.; Xu, J.; Rajan, S.G.; Hivert, M.F.; Doyon, M.; Bouchard, L.; McGowan, P.O.; et al. DNA methylation mediates the association between breastfeeding and early-life growth trajectories. *Clin. Epigenet.* **2021**, *13*, 231. [CrossRef]
47. Walker-Short, E.; Buckner, T.; Vigers, T.; Carry, P.; Vanderlinden, L.A.; Dong, F.; Johnson, R.K.; Yang, I.V.; Kechris, K.; Rewers, M.; et al. Epigenome-Wide Association Study of Infant Feeding and DNA Methylation in Infancy and Childhood in a Population at Increased Risk for Type 1 Diabetes. *Nutrients* **2021**, *13*, 4057. [CrossRef]
48. Hartwig, F.P.; De Mola, C.L.; Davies, N.M.; Victora, C.G.; Relton, C.L. Breastfeeding effects on DNA methylation in the offspring: A systematic literature review. *PLoS ONE* **2017**, *12*, e0173070. [CrossRef]
49. Acevedo, N.; Alhamwe, B.A.; Caraballo, L.; Ding, M.; Ferrante, A.; Garn, H.; Garssen, J.; Hii, C.S.; Irvine, J.; Llinás-Caballero, K.; et al. Perinatal and Early-Life Nutrition, Epigenetics, and Allergy. *Nutrients* **2021**, *13*, 724. [CrossRef]
50. Ozkan, H.; Tuzun, F.; Taheri, S.; Korhan, P.; Akokay, P.; Yılmaz, O.; Duman, N.; Özer, E.; Tufan, E.; Kumral, A.; et al. Epigenetic Programming Through Breast Milk and Its Impact on Milk-Siblings Mating. *Front. Genet.* **2020**, *11*, 569232. [CrossRef]
51. Leroux, C.; Chervet, M.L.; German, J.B. Perspective: Milk microRNAs as Important Players in Infant Physiology and Development. *Adv. Nutr. Int. Rev. J.* **2021**, *12*, 1625–1635. [CrossRef] [PubMed]

52. Bozack, A.K.; Colicino, E.; Rodosthenous, R.; Bloomquist, T.R.; Baccarelli, A.A.; Wright, R.O.; Wright, R.J.; Lee, A.G. Associations between maternal lifetime stressors and negative events in pregnancy and breast milk-derived extracellular vesicle microRNAs in the programming of intergenerational stress mechanisms (PRISM) pregnancy cohort. *Epigenetics* **2021**, *16*, 389–404. [CrossRef] [PubMed]
53. Tingö, L.; Ahlberg, E.; Johansson, L.; Pedersen, S.A.; Chawla, K.; Sætrom, P.; Cione, E.; Simpson, M.R. Non-Coding RNAs in Human Breast Milk: A Systematic Review. *Front. Immunol.* **2021**, *12*, 725323. [CrossRef]
54. Matheson, M.C.; Erbas, B.; Balasuriya, A.; Jenkins, M.A.; Wharton, C.L.; Tang, M.L.-K.; Abramson, M.J.; Walters, E.H.; Hopper, J.L.; Dharmage, S.C. Breast-feeding and atopic disease: A cohort study from childhood to middle age. *J. Allergy Clin. Immunol.* **2007**, *120*, 1051–1057. [CrossRef]
55. Mandhane, P.J.; Greene, J.M. Original articles Interactions between breast-feeding, specific parental atopy, and sex on development of asthma and atopy. *J. Allergy Clin. Immunol.* **2007**, *119*, 1359–1366. [CrossRef] [PubMed]
56. Guilbert, T.W.; Stern, D.A.; Morgan, W.J.; Martinez, F.D.; Wright, A.L. Effect of Breastfeeding on Lung Function in Childhood and Modulation by Maternal Asthma and Atopy. *Am. J. Respir. Crit. Care Med.* **2007**, *176*, 843–848. [CrossRef]
57. Sitarik, A.R.; Kasmikha, N.S.; Kim, H.; Wegienka, G.; Havstad, S.; Ownby, D.; Zoratti, E.; Johnson, C.C. Breastfeeding and Delivery Mode Modify the Association between Maternal Atopy and Childhood Allergic Outcomes. *J. Allergy Clin. Immunol.* **2018**, *142*, 2002. [CrossRef]
58. Harvey, S.M.; Murphy, V.E.; Gibson, P.G.; Collison, A.; Robinson, P.; Sly, P.D.; Mattes, J.; Jensen, M.E. Maternal asthma, breastfeeding, and respiratory outcomes in the first year of life. *Pediatr. Pulmonol.* **2020**, *55*, 1690–1696. [CrossRef]
59. Azad, M.B.; Vehling, L.; Lu, Z.; Dai, D.; Subbarao, P.; Becker, A.B.; Mandhane, P.J.; Turvey, S.E.; Lefebvre, D.L.; Sears, M.R.; et al. Breastfeeding, maternal asthma and wheezing in the first year of life: A longitudinal birth cohort study. *Eur. Respir. J.* **2017**, *49*, 1602019. [CrossRef]
60. Lupinek, C.; Hochwallner, H.; Johansson, C.; Mie, A.; Rigler, E.; Scheynius, A.; Alm, J.; Valenta, R. Maternal allergen-specific IgG might protect the child against allergic sensitization. *J. Allergy Clin. Immunol.* **2019**, *144*, 536–548. [CrossRef]

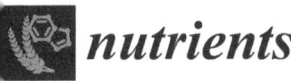

Article

Extensively Hydrolyzed Hypoallergenic Infant Formula with Retained T Cell Reactivity

Raphaela Freidl [1], Victoria Garib [1,2], Birgit Linhart [1], Elisabeth M. Haberl [3], Isabelle Mader [3], Zsolt Szépfalusi [4], Klara Schmidthaler [4], Nikos Douladiris [5], Alexander Pampura [6], Evgeniy Varlamov [6], Tatiana Lepeshkova [7], Evgeny Beltyukov [7], Veronika Naumova [7], Styliani Taka [5], Dina Nosova [8], Olga Guliashko [8], Michael Kundi [9], Alina Kiyamova [2], Stefani Katsamaki [2] and Rudolf Valenta [1,10,11,12,*]

[1] Center for Pathophysiology, Infectiology and Immunology, Institute of Pathophysiology and Allergy Research, Medical University of Vienna, A-1090 Vienna, Austria
[2] International Center of Molecular Allergology, Ministry of Innovation Development, Tashkent 100174, Uzbekistan
[3] HiPP GmbH & Co. Vertrieb KG, 85276 Pfaffenhofen, Germany
[4] Department of Pediatrics and Adolescent Medicine, Division of Pediatric Pulmonology, Allergy and Endocrinology, Comprehensive Center of Pediatrics, Medical University Vienna, A-1090 Vienna, Austria
[5] Allergy Department, 2nd Pediatric Clinic, National & Kapodistrian University of Athens, 11527 Athens, Greece
[6] Department of Allergology and Clinical Immunology, Research and Clinical Institute for Pediatrics Named after Yuri Veltischev at the Pirogov Russian National Research Medical University of the Russian Ministry of Health, 117997 Moscow, Russia
[7] Department of Faculty Therapy, Endocrinology, Allergology and Immunology, Ural State Medical University, 620014 Ekaterinburg, Russia
[8] Allergy Department, UNIMED Laboratories, 119049 Moscow, Russia
[9] Department for Environmental Heath, Center for Public Health, Medical University of Vienna, A-1090 Vienna, Austria
[10] NRC Institute of Immunology FMBA of Russia, 119049 Moscow, Russia
[11] Laboratory of Immunopathology, Department of Clinical Immunology and Allergy, Sechenov First Moscow State Medical University, 119049 Moscow, Russia
[12] Karl Landsteiner University for Health Sciences, 3500 Krems, Austria
* Correspondence: rudolf.valenta@meduniwien.ac.at; Tel.: +43-1-40400-50420

Citation: Freidl, R.; Garib, V.; Linhart, B.; Haberl, E.M.; Mader, I.; Szépfalusi, Z.; Schmidthaler, K.; Douladiris, N.; Pampura, A.; Varlamov, E.; et al. Extensively Hydrolyzed Hypoallergenic Infant Formula with Retained T Cell Reactivity. *Nutrients* 2023, 15, 111. https://doi.org/10.3390/nu15010111

Academic Editors: RJ Joost Van Neerven and Janneke Ruinemans-Koerts

Received: 3 October 2022
Revised: 29 November 2022
Accepted: 7 December 2022
Published: 26 December 2022

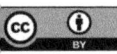

Copyright: © 2022 by the authors. Licensee MDPI, Basel, Switzerland. This article is an open access article distributed under the terms and conditions of the Creative Commons Attribution (CC BY) license (https://creativecommons.org/licenses/by/4.0/).

Abstract: Background: Immunoglobulin E (IgE)-mediated cow's milk allergy (CMA) can be life-threatening and affects up to 3% of children. Hypoallergenic infant formulas based on hydrolyzed cow's milk protein are increasingly considered for therapy and prevention of cow's milk allergy. The aim of this study was to investigate the allergenic activity and ability to induce T cell and cytokine responses of an infant formula based on extensively hydrolyzed cow's milk protein (whey) (eHF, extensively hydrolyzed formula) supplemented with Galactooligosaccharides (GOS) and *Limosilactobacillus fermentum* CECT5716 (LF) to determine its suitability for treatment and prevention of CMA. Methods: eHF and standard protein formula based on intact cow's milk proteins (iPF) with or without Galactooligosaccharide (GOS) and *Limosilactobacillus fermentum* CECT5716 (LF) were investigated with allergen-specific antibodies and tested for IgE reactivity and allergenic activity in basophil degranulation assays with sera from cow's milk (CM)-allergic infants/children. Their ability to stimulate T cell proliferation and cytokine secretion in cultured peripheral blood mononuclear cells (PBMC) from CM-allergic infants and children was studied with a FACS-based carboxyfluorescein diacetate succinimidyl ester (CFSE) dilution assay and xMAP Luminex fluorescent bead-based technology, respectively. Results: An eHF supplemented with GOS and LF exhibiting almost no IgE reactivity and allergenic activity was identified. This eHF induced significantly lower inflammatory cytokine secretion as compared to an intact protein-based infant formula but retained T cell reactivity. Conclusions: Due to strongly reduced allergenic activity and induction of inflammatory cytokine secretion but retained T cell reactivity, the identified eHF may be used for treatment and prevention of CMA by induction of specific T cell tolerance.

Keywords: allergy; cow's milk allergy; allergen; hypoallergenic infant formula

1. Introduction

Immunoglobulin E (IgE)-mediated cow's milk allergy (CMA) affects approximately 3% of children, and manifestations usually occur early in children who receive cow's milk in their diet early in life [1,2]. Patients with an IgE sensitization to cow's milk may suffer from a broad spectrum of allergic symptoms that may affect the gastrointestinal tract as well as other organs like the skin, the respiratory tract and the cardiovascular system (e.g., life-threatening anaphylaxis) [3].

Interestingly, certain subjects with IgE sensitization to cow's milk may also remain asymptomatic [4]. The severity of allergic symptoms in subjects with IgE sensitization to cow's milk depends on several factors. For example, subjects with high levels of cow's milk-specific IgE antibodies were reported to suffer from more severe and systemic symptoms as compared to subjects with lower IgE levels [5].

Cow's milk contains several different allergen molecules that differ regarding their concentrations, allergenic activity and resistance to digestion and heating [6]. Accordingly, individuals with high levels of IgE antibodies against digestion-resistant and heat-stable milk allergens such as caseins may suffer from more severe symptoms. By contrast, subjects with an IgE sensitization to bovine serum albumin, which occurs in rather low levels in cow's milk and is easily digested, often have no symptoms of cow's milk allergy [7]. Additionally, other factors such as epithelial barrier function and the presence of neutralizing IgA antibodies that bind harmful antigens or allergen-specific IgG antibodies that block IgE binding to the allergens may influence the extent and quality of cow's milk-related allergic symptoms [8].

IgE-mediated allergic sensitization is the major risk factor for severe and life-threatening anaphylactic reactions to cow's milk. It is, therefore, important to determine if an individual carries IgE antibodies against cow's milk allergens or suffers from other forms of intolerance such as lactose intolerance, which is very common [3]. For other forms of immunologically mediated hypersensitivity reactions to cow's milk, there are currently no reliable diagnostic tests available that are based on the measurement of cow's milk-specific antibodies, other than IgE or cellular tests, and, therefore, such tests are not recommended [3,9].

In the first months after birth, breastfeeding is the ideal nutrition. For patients with confirmed IgE sensitization to cow's milk, standard treatment recommendations are: (i) cow's milk avoidance by strict diet, or (ii) consumption of extensively hydrolyzed hypoallergenic infant formulas or amino acid-based infant formulas [10,11]. For children 4 years and older with persistent cow's milk allergy, EAACI guidelines recommend allergen immunotherapy (AIT), although no uniform AIT protocols have been established yet [12]. Hypoallergenic formulas are especially important in early life when breastfeeding is not possible and are a suitable substitute for infant feeding provided the formula is hypoallergenic and safe [13]. This is usually the case for extensively hydrolyzed and amino acid-based formulas due to the destruction of IgE epitopes.

Another property, especially of partially hydrolyzed, hypoallergenic infant formulas, is the possibility of inducing immunological tolerance against cow's milk proteins, which requires the presence of cow's milk allergen-derived intact T cell epitopes to induce either clonal deletion or anergy in specific T cells or regulatory T cell responses [8]. Hypoallergenic formulas with such properties could, therefore, not only be used for treatment of established cow's milk allergy but also for prevention of the development of cow's milk allergy, not only by avoiding the induction of IgE sensitization but also by the induction of specific tolerance [14].

However, it has been reported that the degree of hydrolysis differently affects the presence of IgE and T cell epitopes in formulas, and it is, therefore, necessary to characterize formulas regarding their immunological properties [15].

Whether the induction of cow's milk allergen-specific tolerance is possible is a controversial issue because certain studies performed in animal models [16] suggest that the induction of tolerance is not likely [17]. Another recent study using an extensively hydrolyzed whey fraction indicates that tolerance induction can be achieved [18]. Here, we studied such an extensively hydrolyzed whey fraction regarding its allergenic properties and effects on T cell proliferation and cytokine production in the blood of cow's milk-allergic infants and children. We identified an extensively hydrolyzed whey fraction that had greatly reduced allergenic activity and induced significantly less production of inflammatory cytokines but at the same time retained allergen-specific epitopes recognized by human T cells. Our findings suggest that this formula combines the features of reduced allergenic activity required for treatment and maintains T cell epitopes for possible tolerance induction.

2. Materials and Methods

2.1. Cow's Milk-Allergic Patients, Sera, PBMC Samples

A demographic and clinical description of individuals analyzed in this study is provided in Table 1. In total, 59 individuals were analyzed in the study, of whom 49 had reported symptoms upon cow's milk consumption (Table 1). Ten control individuals were included, of whom seven had other allergies but not cow's milk allergy (NCMA 48, 49, 50, 51, 53, 55 and 56, Table 1), and three were non-allergic subjects (NA1–NA3, Table 1).

Table 1. Demographic and clinical characteristics of allergic patients and of non-allergic individuals.

Number	Age Years	Sex F/M	CMP-Related Clinical Symptoms	SPT CMP	Allergy to Other Food Allergen Sources
1	0.9	M	A, AD	pos	no
2	12.0	M	A, AD	pos	lentil
3	5.0	M	A, AD	pos	egg, wheat, walnut
4	2.4	F	A, AD	pos	egg
5	8.0	M	A	pos	egg
6	0.5	M	AD	pos	wheat, fish
7	4.0	M	AD	n.d.	peach, apricot
8	8.0	F	A, AD	n.d.	beef, egg
9	4.1	M	A, AD	n.d.	beef, pork, egg, wheat
10	1.9	F	AD	pos	egg, potato, wheat
11	3.4	M	AD	n.d.	egg
12	3.0	F	AD	n.d.	beef, egg
13	1.3	M	AD	n.d.	egg
14	6.1	M	A, AD	n.d.	egg
15	4.5	F	AD	pos	egg
16	1.6	M	AD	n.d.	no
17	8.0	F	A, AD	n.d.	no
18	10	F	AD	n.d.	egg, fruits, vegetables, cereals, fish, meat
19	6.0	M	AD	n.d.	fish, egg, meat, potato
20	1.1	M	A, AD	pos	wheat, fish
21	8.0	M	A, AD	pos	egg, walnut
22	2.9	F	A, GI	pos	no
23	2.9	F	A, GI	n.d.	egg
24	7.2	M	AD, GI	pos	peanut
25	3.7	M	A, AD, GI	n.d.	egg
26	5.0	F	A, AD, GI	pos	egg, nuts, caviar
27	2.9	F	A, AD, GI	n.d.	no
28	2.5	F	A, AD, GI	n.d.	no
29	4.1	M	AD, GI	n.d.	no
30	11.2	M	A, GI	pos	no

Table 1. *Cont.*

Number	Age Years	Sex F/M	CMP-Related Clinical Symptoms	SPT CMP	Allergy to Other Food Allergen Sources
31	6.0	M	AD, GI	n.d.	egg
32	6.1	F	A, GI	pos	egg
33	4.2	M	A, AD, GI	n.d.	no
34	1.3	M	AD, GI	pos	egg, cereals, fish
35	10.6	M	A, AD, GI	pos	egg
36	7.3	F	AD, GI	n.d.	egg, oat
37	3.4	M	A, GI	n.d.	egg
38	1.4	M	A, AD, GI	n.d.	egg, cereals
39	5.6	M	AD, GI	n.d.	egg, wheat, caviar
40	6.6	M	AD, GI	n.d.	egg, wheat, caviar
41	1.8	M	A, AD, GI	n.d.	egg, wheat, walnut
42	4.8	M	A, AD, GI	n.d.	egg, walnut, peanut, soy
43	10.9	M	A, AD, GI	pos	no
44	3.2	M	A, AD, GI	n.d.	egg, wheat, nuts, soy
45	2.5	M	A, AD, GI	n.d.	egg
46	2.3	M	A, AD, GI	n.d.	egg
47	10.8	M	A, AD, GI	n.d.	peanut, soy, walnut
52	1.7	M	AD, GI	n.d.	egg, salmon, codfish
54	2.5	M	A	n.d.	egg, walnut
NCMA 48	1.7	M	no	n.d.	peanut
NCMA 49	11.3	M	no	n.d.	hazelnut, codfish
NCMA 50	11.1	M	no	n.d.	no
NCMA 51	8.2	M	no	n.d.	no
NCMA 53	1.5	M	no	n.d.	egg
NCMA 55	5.3	M	no	n.d.	peanut
NCMA 56	9.4	M	no	n.d.	peanut
NA1	3.0	F	no	neg	no
NA2	2.1	M	no	neg	no
NA3	0.7	F	no	neg	no

F, female; M, male; CMP, cow milk proteins; SPT, skin prick test (wheal area); A, anaphylaxis; AD, atopic dermatitis; GI, gastrointestinal symptoms; NCMA, non-cow's milk allergic; NA, non-allergic; no, no symptoms to other food allergen sources; n.d., not done; pos, positive; neg, negative.

The patients were from the Department of Pediatrics and Adolescent Medicine, Medical University Vienna, Vienna, Austria, the Allergy Department, 2nd Pediatric Clinic University of Athens, Greece, the Department of Allergology and Clinical Immunology, Research and Clinical Institute for Pediatrics named after Yuri Veltischev at the Pirogov Russian National Research Medical University, Moscow, Russia and from the Department of Faculty Therapy, Endocrinology, Allergology and Immunology, Ural State Medical University, Ekaterinburg, Russia. Written informed consent was obtained from their parents, and blood sampling/analysis was performed under pseudonymized conditions with approval by the local ethics committees in Greece and Russia (N10/15.12.2017, N12/20.12.2017) and the ethics committee of the Medical University of Vienna, Austria (EK1641/2014). The analyses of patients' sera and blood samples were performed in an anonymized manner.

The diagnosis of CMA was based on the presence of clinical symptoms of CMA that could be unambiguously attributed to cow's milk consumption, and/or a positive skin prick test reaction to cow's milk, results from an open food challenge and/or detection of specific IgE to CM allergens as measured by ImmunoCAP or ImmunoCAP ISAC (Thermo Fisher

Scientific, Uppsala, Sweden). The cow's milk-related allergic symptoms of patients (mean age: 4.9 years; median age: 4.1 years) are summarized in Table 1 and included anaphylaxis as graded by Sampson [19], atopic dermatitis and/or gastrointestinal symptoms such as abdominal pain, vomiting, diarrhea, and blood in stool. Most of the CMA patients had allergic symptoms to other food allergen sources such as egg, peanut, wheat, nuts, soy, cereals, fish, and caviar (Table 1).

2.2. Allergens, Materials, Infant Formulas, Antibodies, SDS-PAGE

Purified natural cow's milk allergens, skim milk powder and human serum albumin (HSA) were purchased from Sigma Aldrich (St. Louis, Missouri, #9045-23-2, 9048-46-8, 9000-71-9, 9000-71-9, 9000-71-9, BCR685, 70024-90-7). Extensively hydrolyzed formula (eHF) with Galactooligosaccharides (GOS), intact protein formula (iPF) (i.e., cow´s milk protein that has not been hydrolyzed) with and without Galactooligosaccharides (GOS), *Limosilactobacillus fermentum* CECT5716 (LF), and extensively hydrolyzed whey protein (raw material Peptigen® IF-3080, eH_raw) were provided by HiPP GmbH & Co. Vertrieb KG (Pfaffenhofen, Germany) and Arla Foods Ingredients (Videbæk, Denmark), respectively (Table 2). In more detail, HiPP HA infant formula was manufactured from Peptigen® IF-3080 (supplied by Arla Foods Ingredients, Videbæk, Denmark). Peptigen® IF-3080 is an extensive whey protein hydrolysate suitable as the sole protein source in infant formula. It consists of short-chain peptides, obtained by a controlled enzymatic degradation of whey proteins. Hydrolysis is performed with food grade enzymes that are heat-inactivated upon termination of hydrolysis. Subsequently, the hydrolysate is filtered by ultrafiltration in order to remove larger peptides and aggregates thereof. Peptigen® IF-3080 has a degree of hydrolysis of up to 30%. The degree of hydrolysis is defined as the percentage of peptide bonds cleaved by hydrolysis and determined according to Adler-Nissen and Nielsen et al. [20,21].

Table 2. Description of investigated materials.

No.	Abbreviation	Description	BCA mg/mL	BCA Peptide mg/mL
1	eH_raw	Raw material: extensively hydrolyzed whey protein	n.a.	93.29
2	iPF	HiPP standard cow's milk infant formula (HiPP Pre BIO, powder) w/o synbiotics	25.45	n.a.
3	LF	*Limosilactobacillus fermentum* CECT5716 (originally obtained from human milk)	2.26	n.a.
4	eHF + GOS	HiPP HA infant formula (HiPP Pre HA Combiotik®, liquid)	n.a.	20.92
5	eHF + GOS + LF	HiPP HA infant formula (HiPP Pre HA Combiotik®, liquid) + *L. ferm.* CECT5716	n.d.	n.d.
6	iPF + GOS	HiPP standard cow's milk infant formula (HiPP Pre Bio Combiotik®, liquid)	22.64	n.a.
7	iPF + GOS + LF	HiPP standard cow's milk infant formula (HiPP Pre Bio Combiotik®, liquid) + *L. ferm.* CECT5716	n.d.	n.d.
8	dig_eH_raw	In vitro-digested raw material: extensively hydrolyzed whey protein	n.a.	5.27
9	dig_eHF + GOS	In vitro-digested HiPP HA infant formula (HiPP Pre HA Combiotik®, liquid)	n.a.	6.30
10	dig_eHF + GOS + LF	In vitro-digested HiPP HA infant formula (HiPP Pre HA Combiotik®, liquid) + *L. ferm.* CECT5716	n.a.	8.94
11	dig_iPF + GOS	In vitro-digested HiPP standard cow's milk infant formula (HiPP Pre Bio Combiotik®, liquid)	8.66	n.a.
12	dig_iPF + GOS + LF	In vitro-digested HiPP standard cow's milk infant formula (HiPP Pre Bio Combiotik®, liquid) + *L. ferm.* CECT5716	8.97	n.a.
13	HSA	Human serum albumin (neg. ctl.)	1	n.a.
14	Skim milk powder	Commercial cow's milk powder, Sigma Aldrich (pos. ctl.)	1	n.a.

eHF, extensively hydrolyzed formula; iPF, intact protein formula; GOS, Galactooligosaccharides; *L. ferm*, *L. fermentum* CECT5716; dig, digested (in-vitro infant SHIME® model, Prodigest BV). HA infant formula is based on extensively hydrolyzed cow's milk (whey) protein (eH_raw; Peptigen® IF-3080, Arla Foods Ingredients). Intact protein formula is based on intact cow's milk protein; BCA, bicinchoninic acid assay; n.a., not applicable; n.d., not done.

Freeze-dried *Limosilactobacillus fermentum* CECT5716 (LF) was added without further culture or passage to certain formulas/materials in a final concentration of 1.5×10^6 CFU/1 mL (CFU, colony forming unit) before experiments or tested as such. This concentration corresponded to that of the marketed HiPP infant formula and meets the amount of bacteria observed in human milk samples [22].

Customized in-vitro digestion simulating full passage through the oral, gastric and small intestinal phase was performed in a SHIME® model by ProDigest BV (Ghent, Belgium). In vitro digested samples were consistently labeled dig_ (Table 2, samples 8–12).

CM allergen-specific rabbit anti had been raised against the purified CM allergens, and normal rabbit serum (nrs) was used as control [6].

Proteins, materials and formulas were analyzed by 12% SDS-PAGE by loading aliquots of 1 µg natural CM allergens (α-casein, β-casein, κ-casein, α-lactalbumin, β-lactoglobulin) or 20 µL of infant formulas/materials (eHF + GOS, iPF + GOS, eH_raw, iPF). The SDS-PAGE was then stained with Coomassie-Brilliant Blue R250 or blotted onto nitrocellulose and reacted with CM-allergen-specific antisera as previously described [6]. The concentrations of proteins and peptides in the investigated materials were determined by bicinchoninic acid assays for proteins or peptides (BCA Protein and Peptide Assay Kits, Thermo Scientific, # 23225, 23275).

2.3. Immune Dot Blot

Immune dot blots were performed as previously described [14]. Briefly, aliquots of 1 µg of materials (i.e., extensively hydrolyzed infant formulas, digested infant formulas, intact cow's milk protein-based formulas, probiotic *L. fermentum* CECT5716, HSA or skim milk) were dotted on nitrocellulose membranes (Whatman Protran; Sigma-Aldrich) and dried. After blocking, stripes were incubated with CM allergen-specific rabbit antisera that had been raised against the purified CM allergens [6], and bound allergen-specific rabbit antibodies were detected with ^{125}I-labeled goat anti-rabbit antibodies (Perkin Elmer, Waltham, MA, USA) and visualized by autoradiography. Likewise, stripes were incubated with sera from cow's milk allergic patients or, for control purposes, with sera from non-allergic subjects (diluted 1:10) overnight (typically for 15–16 h) at 4 °C, before bound IgE antibodies were detected with 1:10 diluted ^{125}I-labeled anti-human IgE antibodies and visualized by autoradiography [14]. Buffer control (BC) without addition of primary antibodies (i.e., allergen-specific rabbit antisera or human sera) was performed with PBS containing 0.1% Tween for experiments performed with allergen-specific rabbit antibodies and with PBS containing 0.5% Tween and 0.5% BSA for experiments performed with human sera.

Signals obtained by autoradiography were obtained at identical exposure times to allow a comparison of signal intensities, which were arbitrarily compared and termed as lacking, weak, distinct = medium or strong.

2.4. Basophil Degranulation Assays

Basophil degranulation assays were performed with rat basophil leukemia (RBL) cells expressing the human high-affinity receptor for IgE as previously described [23].

In brief, RBL cells cultured in duplicates expressing the human FcεRI α/β/γ subunits were loaded with 1:10 diluted sera from 20 CM-sensitized patients from whom sufficient amounts of serum were available (#1, 3, 5, 6, 14, 16, 17, 21, 22, 25, 27, 28, 29, 35, 36, 37, 38, 46, 47, 54, Table 1) overnight, and degranulation was induced by adding antigens in a concentration of 10 ng/mL. The concentration 10 ng/mL was determined in pilot experiments to be representative for the increasing part of the bell-shaped curve of basophil degranulation by testing concentrations of 100, 10, 1 or 0.1 ng/mL (Figure S1). A concentration of 10 ng/mL of different allergen molecules was also identified in earlier work to represent the increasing part of the bell-shaped basophil degranulation curve using the RBL cell line [23]. The release of β-hexosaminidase supernatants was analyzed by incubating culture supernatants with 80 µmol/L 4-methylumbelliferyl -N-acetyl-β-D-glucosaminide (Sigma-Aldrich) in citrate buffer (0.1 mol/L, pH 4.5) for 1 h at 37 °C. The reaction was stopped by addition of 100 µL of glycine buffer (0.2 mol/L glycine and 0.2 mol/L NaCl, pH 10.7), and fluorescence was measured at an extinction wavelength of 360 nm to the emission wavelength of 465 nm by using a fluorescence microplate reader (CYTO FLUOR 2350; Millipore, Billerica, MA, USA). Results are reported as the percentage of total β-hexosaminidase released after complete cell lysis achieved by addition of 10% Triton X-100 (Merck, Darmstadt, Germany).

Results represent the average of duplicates with deviations of less than 10% and background (i.e., incubation with HSA was subtracted). The mean percentages +/− SEM were calculated for the group of 20 patients, and statistical analysis was performed as indicated in the section "Statistical analysis".

2.5. FACS-Based Analysis of the Proliferation of $CD4^+$ and $CD8^+$ T Cells in Response to Antigens by CFSE Dilution

Peripheral blood mononuclear cells (PBMCs) were isolated from heparinized blood samples of nine patients/subjects (Table 1: patients/subjects 48–56) using Ficoll density gradient centrifugation (Amersham Biosciences, Uppsala, Sweden). Aliquots of 200,000 PBMCs in 200 µL were stained with carboxyfluorescein diacetate succinimidyl ester (CFSE) dye, which distributes among dividing cells [24]. Gating was performed on $CD3^+$ and $CD4^+$ and $CD3^+$ and $CD8^+$ cells, respectively [25]. The cells were incubated in triplicate for 7 days at 37 °C in a humidified atmosphere with 5% CO_2 in 96-well plates (Nunclone; Nalgen Nunc International, Roskilde, Denmark) in Ultra Culture medium (BioWhittaker, Rockland, ME, USA) supplemented with 2 mM L-glutamine (Gibco, Carlsbad, CA, USA) and 50 µM beta-mercaptoethanol (Gibco) to prevent free radical build-up, and 0.1 mg gentamicin per 500 mL (Gibco) in the presence of allergens Bos d 4 (natural α-lactalbumin, nALA), Bos d 5 (natural β-lactoglobulin, nBLG), Bos d 8 (natural casein, ncasein), and infant formulas (10 µg protein/well) in triplicates. As positive control, T cell activator (1 µL/well) (Dynabeads Human T-Activator CD3/CD28; Thermo Fisher Scientific/Invitrogen) was used. Medium alone and 10 µg protein/well HSA served as a negative control [25]. For each of the 20 patients, cultivation with the different antigens was performed in triplicate. For each of the triplicates, the median of the medium-only wells was subtracted. For further statistical analysis, the mean of the three medium-corrected proliferation values was used.

2.6. Measurement of Cytokine Levels

Cytokine levels (IL-1b, IL-2, IL-4, IL-5, IL-6, IL-10, IL-12, IL-13, IL-17, IFN-g, GM-CSF; interleukin, IL; interferon-gamma, IFN-g, granulocyte-macrophage colony-stimulating factor, GM-CSF) were measured in supernatants collected from PBMC cultures at day 7 of culture using xMAP Luminex fluorescent bead-based technology according to the manufacturer's instructions (R&D Systems, Wiesbaden, Germany) [24]. The fluorescent signals were read on a Luminex 100 system (Luminex Corp., Austin, TX, USA). The limits of detection were 0.28 pg/mL for IL-1b, 1.7 pg/mL for IL-2, 0.2 pg/mL for IL-4, 5.6 pg/mL for IL-5, 0.45 pg/mL for IL-6, 0.81 pg/mL for IL-10, 2.01 pg/mL for IL-12, 0.36 pg/mL for IL-13, 2.74 pg/mL for IL-17, 1.67 pg/mL for IFN-g, and 0.43 pg/mL for GM-CSF. Results were analyzed as described for the analysis of T cell proliferations.

2.7. Statistical Analysis

Before evaluation, all variables were subjected to a distribution analysis of residuals after subtracting the estimated means. Except for results of the basophil degranulation assay that did not significantly deviate from a normal distribution, all variables were best fitted by a log-normal distribution and, therefore, log-transformed for subsequent statistical tests. For graphical presentation, means and ±SEM (standard error of mean) were back-transformed to express results on the original scale. Statistical comparisons were based on a generalized estimating equations (GEE) model with an unstructured correlation matrix to account for the fact that the same blood specimens were used for all formulas. Comparisons between formulas were restricted to pre-specified contrasts.

For cytokines and T-cell proliferation, only eHF and iPF were compared. For the specific basophil degranulation formulas, eHF + GOS, iPF + GOS, eHF + GOS + LF, and iPF + GOS + LF were compared against skim milk, and eHF + GOS as well as iPF + GOS formulas with and without LF were compared by linear contrast with Bonferroni correction. The hypothesis test applied was Wald's chi-square test. Correction was determined by the number of comparisons that were not orthogonal.

All statistical tests were performed by Stata 13.0 (StataSoft). Figures were generated by Statistica 10.0 (StatSoft) (*) p-value < 0.05, (**) p-value < 0.01, (***) p-value < 0.001.

3. Results

3.1. Extensively Hydrolyzed Infant Formulas Lack Intact Cow's Milk Allergens

Figure 1A shows the analysis of the extensively hydrolyzed formula with GOS (eHF + GOS), intact protein formula (iPF + GOS, iPF) with and without Galactooligosaccharide (GOS), as well as of the extensively hydrolyzed whey protein (eH_raw) in comparison with purified natural CM allergens (α-casein, β-casein, κ-casein, α-lactalbumin, β-lactoglobulin) by SDS-PAGE and Coomassie Brilliant Blue staining. We found that neither the raw material (eH_raw), which builds the protein basis for the extensively hydrolyzed formula eHF + GOS, nor the extensively hydrolyzed formula eHF + GOS itself contained intact proteins. By contrast, bands corresponding to the caseins, alpha-lactalbumin and ß-lactoglobulin were found in the intact protein formula with and without GOS (iPF + GOS, iPF).

After this analysis, we tested the different formulas, raw materials and purified cow's milk allergens for reactivity with rabbit antisera raised against purified cow's milk allergens (i.e., α-S1-casein, α-S2-casein, α-β-casein, α-κ-casein, α-lactalbumin, αβ-lactoglobulin, and α-lactoferrin) (Figure 1B,C). αS1/S2-casein, ß-casein, κ-casein, α-lactalbumin and ß-lactoglobulin but not lactoferrin were detected in skim milk and in undigested intact protein formula (iPF) with and without Galactooligosaccharides (GOS) (Figure 1C), but not in intact protein formulas that had been subjected to in vitro gastrointestinal digestion (dig_IPF + GOS, dig_iPF + GOS + LF, Figure 1B). None of the cow's milk allergens were detected in the raw material (eH_raw) for the extensively hydrolyzed formula eHF + GOS, or in the extensively hydrolyzed formula eHF + GOS regardless of whether they were digested or not (Figure 1B). A weak signal was observed when the anti-ß-casein antiserum was tested with *Limosilactobacillus fermentum* CECT5716 (*LF*) (Figure 1C) or with formulas containing *Limosilactobacillus fermentum* CECT5716 (*LF*) (Figure 1B). Weak signals were observed when the undigested extensively hydrolyzed formulas were tested with antisera specific for kappa casein, alpha-lactalbumin and ß-lactoglobulin (Figure 1B). No signal was observed when samples were tested with normal rabbit serum or buffer without addition of rabbit antibodies (negative controls) (Figure 1B,C). No reaction of any of the antisera with HSA was observed (Figure 1B,C).

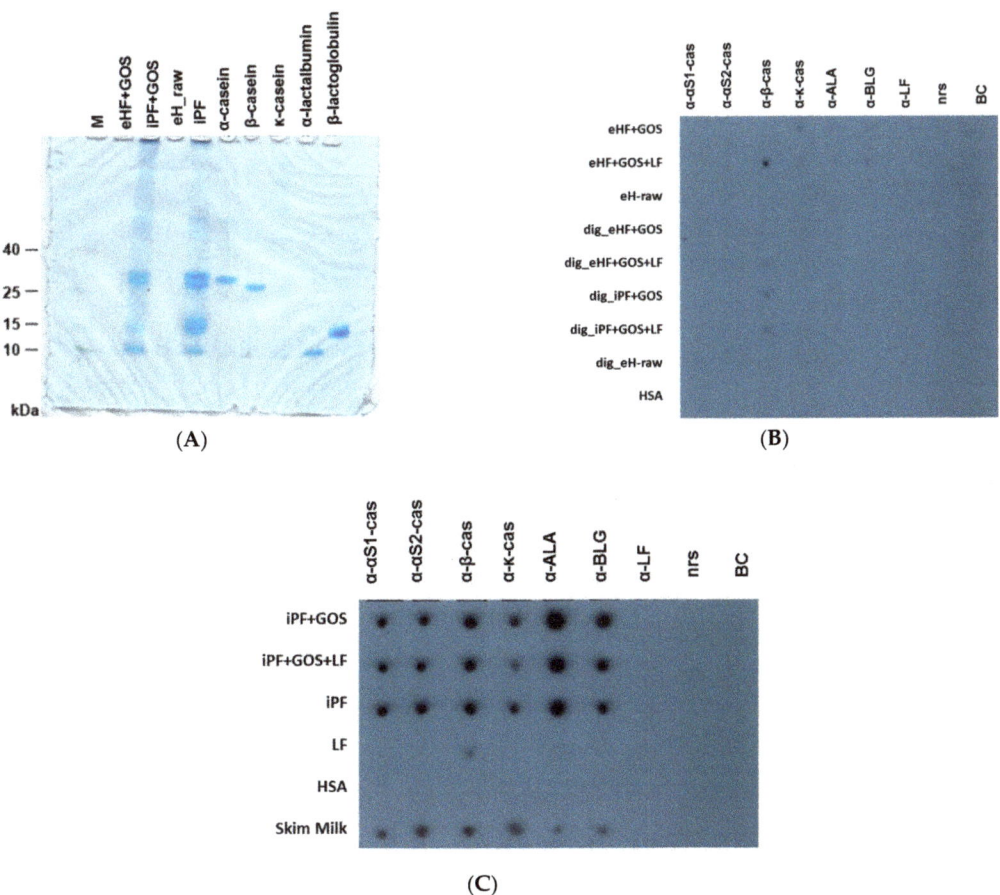

Figure 1. Analysis of materials by SDS-PAGE and dot blotting. (**A**) Infant formulas and milk allergens as indicated on the top (details described in Table 2) were separated by SDS-PAGE and stained with Coomassie Brilliant Blue. A molecular weight marker (lane M) was included, and molecular weights are indicated on the left margin. (**B,C**) Infant formulas, materials and proteins as indicated on the left margin were dotted onto nitrocellulose and then probed with rabbit antisera raised against milk allergens (α-S1-cas, α-S2-cas, α-β-casein, α-κ-casein, α-lactalbumin, α-β-lactoglobulin, and α-lactoferrin), a normal rabbit serum (nrs), or only buffer (**B,C**). Bound rabbit antibodies were detected with ^{125}I-labeled antibodies and visualized by autoradiography.

3.2. Extensively Hydrolyzed Formulas and In Vitro Digested Intact Protein Formulas Show Strongly Reduced IgE Reactivity

In the next set of experiments, we investigated the IgE reactivity of infant formulas, raw materials and skim milk using sera from cow's milk-allergic patients and, for control purposes, with sera from non-allergic subjects (Table 1) (Figure 2A–D).

The majority of cow's milk-allergic patients (i.e., patients 1, 2, 3, 5, 6, 8, 9, 10, 12, 14, 17, 18, 19, 21, 22, 24, 25, 26, 27, 28, 29, 35, 37, 39, 42, 44, 46, 47, 54) showed distinct = medium to strong IgE reactivity to dot-blotted intact milk (skim milk) and intact protein formulas (i.e., iPF, iPF + GOS, iPF + GOS + LF) (Figure 2C,D).

Some cow's milk-allergic patients showed weak (i.e., patients 7, 13, 15, 16, 20, 31, 36, 40, 45) or no (i.e., patients 4, 11, 23, 30, 32, 33, 34, 38, 41, 43, 48–53, 55, 56) IgE reactivity to the aforementioned intact protein formulas (Figure 1C,D).

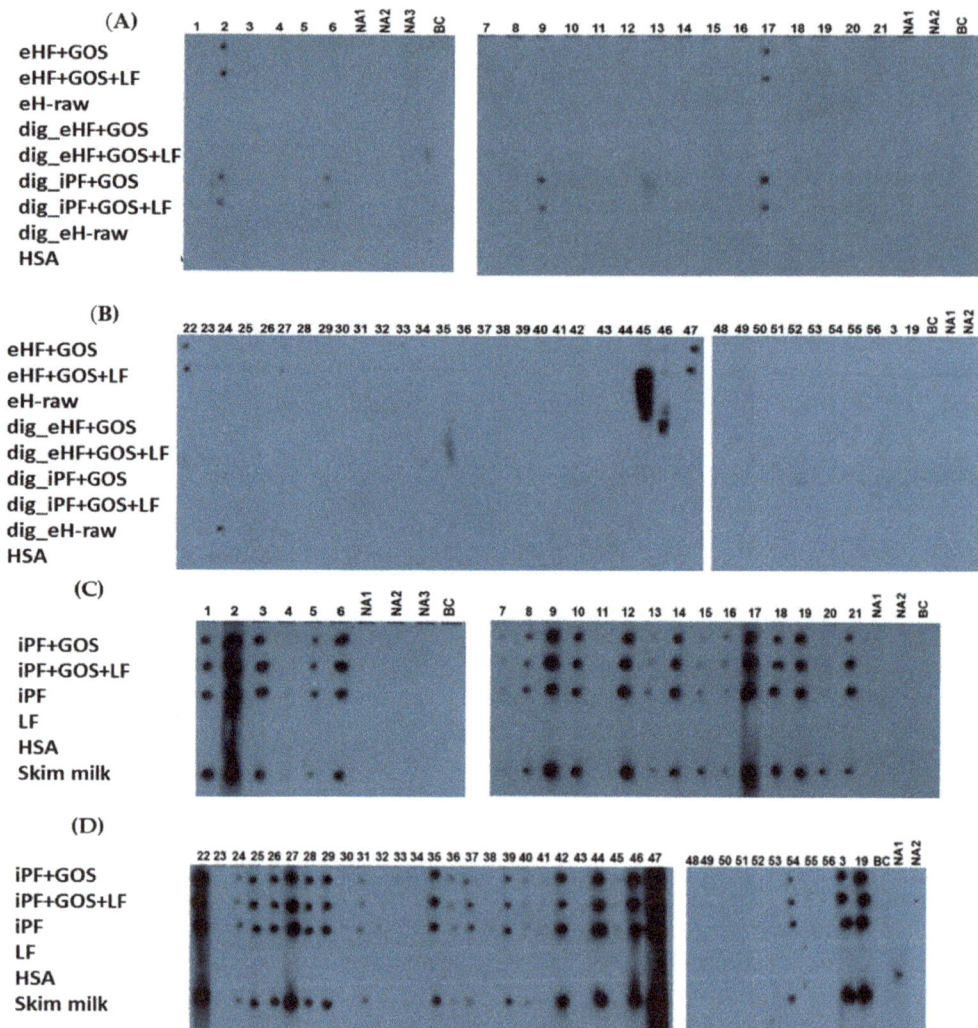

Figure 2. IgE reactivity to dot-blotted infant formulas or materials. (**A–D**) Dot-blotted infant formulas or materials (left; details described in Table 2) were exposed to sera from cow's milk-allergic patients (1–56), sera from non-allergic subjects (NA1, NA2), or buffer alone (**B,C**). Bound IgE antibodies were detected with ^{125}I-labeled anti-human IgE antibodies and visualized by autoradiography.

No IgE reactivity was observed for non-allergic subjects (NA1, NA2) or when buffer without addition of serum was tested with any of the dotted samples (Figure 1A–D). Sera that had shown distinct or strong IgE reactivity to intact protein formulas showed no or weak IgE reactivity to extensively hydrolyzed raw material, to undigested as well as to digested extensively hydrolyzed formulas, and digested intact protein formulas. Of note, patients 22 and 27 showed residual IgE reactivity to extensively hydrolyzed formulas but not to digested intact formulas, whereas patient 9 showed residual IgE reactivity to digested intact protein formulas but not to extensively hydrolyzed formulas (Figure 2A,B). No IgE reactivity to HSA or *Limosilactobacillus fermentum (LF)* was observed (Figure 2A–D).

3.3. Limosilactobacillus fermentum CECT5716 (LF)-Containing Extensively Hydrolyzed Formula Shows the Strongest Reduction of Allergenic Activity

In order to determine the allergenic activity of the tested formulas, basophil activation experiments were performed. For this purpose, we used rat basophil leukemia (RBL) cells that express the human high-affinity receptor for IgE and hence can be loaded with serum IgE from cow's milk-allergic patients, and then allergen-specific and IgE-mediated degranulation can be induced by the addition of allergens. Allergen-induced and IgE-mediated basophil degranulation is dose-dependent but results in a bell-shaped activation curve because excess of allergen will result in a lower rate of IgE cross-linking. Therefore, we determined in a pilot experiment the dose, which yielded degranulation in the increasing part of the bell-shaped curve (Supplemental Figure S1), and then performed basophil degranulation with this dose. Figure 3 displays the mean percentages of ß-hexosaminidase release for 20 cow's milk-allergic patients who had shown IgE reactivity to cow's milk allergens (i.e., skim milk) and extensively hydrolyzed and intact protein formulas with and without *Limosilactobacillus fermentum* CECT5716 (LF). The strongest basophil degranulation was obtained with skim milk, which was significantly stronger than that observed for the intact protein formula and the extensively hydrolyzed formula (Figure 3). ß-hexosaminidase release induced by the extensively hydrolyzed formula was significantly lower than that induced by the intact protein formula. Interestingly, the extensively hydrolyzed formula containing *Limosilactobacillus fermentum* CECT5716 (LF) (eHF + GOS + LF) showed almost no degranulation and induced significantly lower induction of basophil degranulation than the extensively hydrolyzed formula without *Limosilactobacillus fermentum* CECT5716 (LF) (eHF + GOS), whereas this effect of LF was not found for the intact protein formulas (Figure 3).

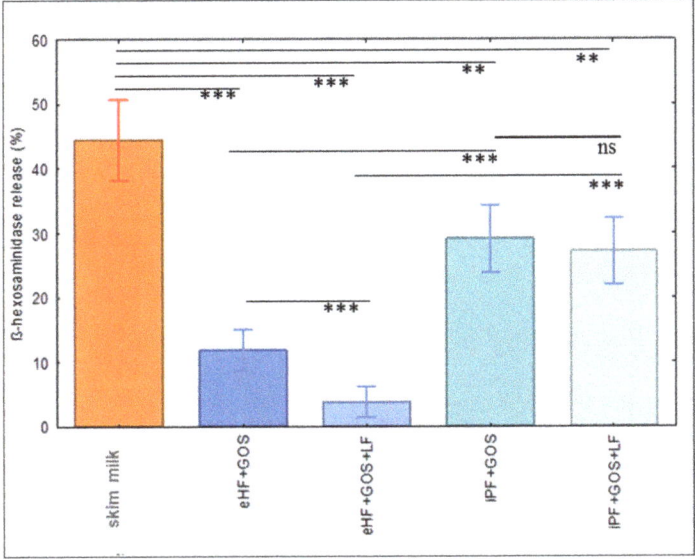

Figure 3. Specific basophil degranulation induced with milk products. Shown are the mean (n = 20) +/− SEM percentages of ß-hexosaminidase releases (*y*-axis) induced by a concentration of 10 ng/mL of different milk products or infant formula (*x*-axis; Table 2) from human FcεRI-expressing rat basophils that had been loaded with serum IgE from 20 different cow's milk-allergic patients. Significant differences in mediator release induced by the milk products or infant formula are indicated. ** $p \leq 0.01$, *** $p \leq 0.001$, ns, not significant.

3.4. Extensively Hydrolyzed GOS-Containing Infant Formula Induces T Cell Proliferation Similarly to GOS-Containing Intact Protein Formula

After having studied the allergenic activity of infant formulas, we investigated their ability to induce specific T cell proliferation. Figure 4 shows the median percentages +/− SEM of proliferated CD4$^+$ (left part of the figure) and CD8$^+$ T cells (right part of figure) in PBMC from subjects 48–56 (Table 1) stimulated with a mix of natural caseins (ncasein), ß-lactoglobulin (nBLG), alpha-lactalbumin (nALA), extensively hydrolyzed infant formula or intact protein GOS-containing formula (eHF + GOS, iPF + GOS). The casein mix induced the strongest milk-specific CD4$^+$ and CD8$^+$ T cell proliferation, whereas the proliferation induced by whey allergens (ß-lactoglobulin, alpha-lactalbumin) was comparable to that induced by the extensively hydrolyzed formula. Specifically, there was no significant difference between the CD4$^+$ and CD8$^+$ T cell proliferation induced by extensively hydrolyzed and intact protein formulas (Figure 4, right parts). Stimulation with anti-CD3 and anti-CD28 antibodies (i.e., positive control) induced strong CD4$^+$ and CD8$^+$ T cell proliferation.

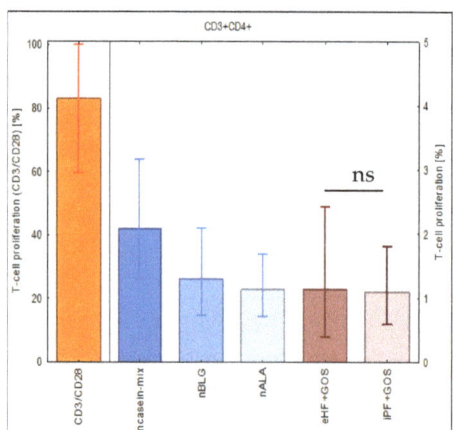 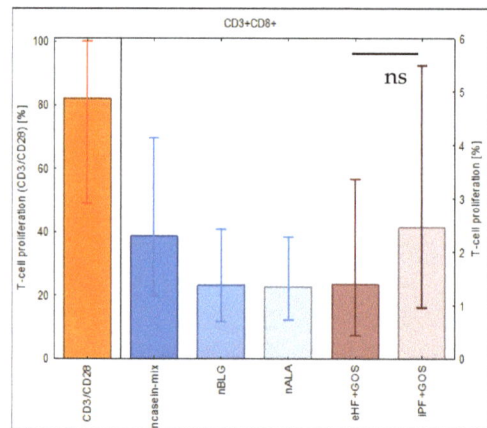

Figure 4. T cell proliferation specific for milk allergens, eHF + GOS and iPF + GOS. Shown are the back-transformed mean percentages +/− SEM of proliferated CD4$^+$ (left part) and CD8$^+$ T cells (right part) measured in PBMC samples from subjects 48–56 (Table 1) that had been stimulated with anti-CD3 and anti-CD28 (positive control), milk allergens or two milk products (x-axis; Table 2). Only eHF and iPF were compared statistically (ns, not significant).

3.5. Extensively Hydrolyzed GOS-Containing Infant Formula Induces Lower Secretion of Inflammatory Cytokines than GOS-Containing Intact Protein Formula

We then investigated the ability of cow's milk allergens and infant formulas to induce the secretion of cytokines in cultured PBMC samples from subjects 48–56 (Figure 5, Table 1). The extensively hydrolyzed GOS-containing infant formula (eHF + GOS) induced the secretion of lower levels of inflammatory cytokines than the intact GOS-containing formula (iPF + GOS), and this difference was significant for TNF-alpha, IL-1b, IL-2, IL-17, IL-4, IL-5, IL-13, IL-6 (data not shown) and GM-CSF (Figure 5). There was no significant difference regarding the levels of the tolerogenic cytokine IL-10 in cultures stimulated with eHF + GOS and iPF + GOS (Figure 5). We noted that except for MCP-1, whey allergens (i.e., ß-lactoglobulin, alpha-lactalbumin) induced higher levels of cytokines than caseins, although caseins had induced stronger T cell proliferation than whey allergens (Figure 4). Stimulation with anti-CD3 and anti-CD28 induced the production of each of the investigated cytokines in cultured PBMCs (Figure 5).

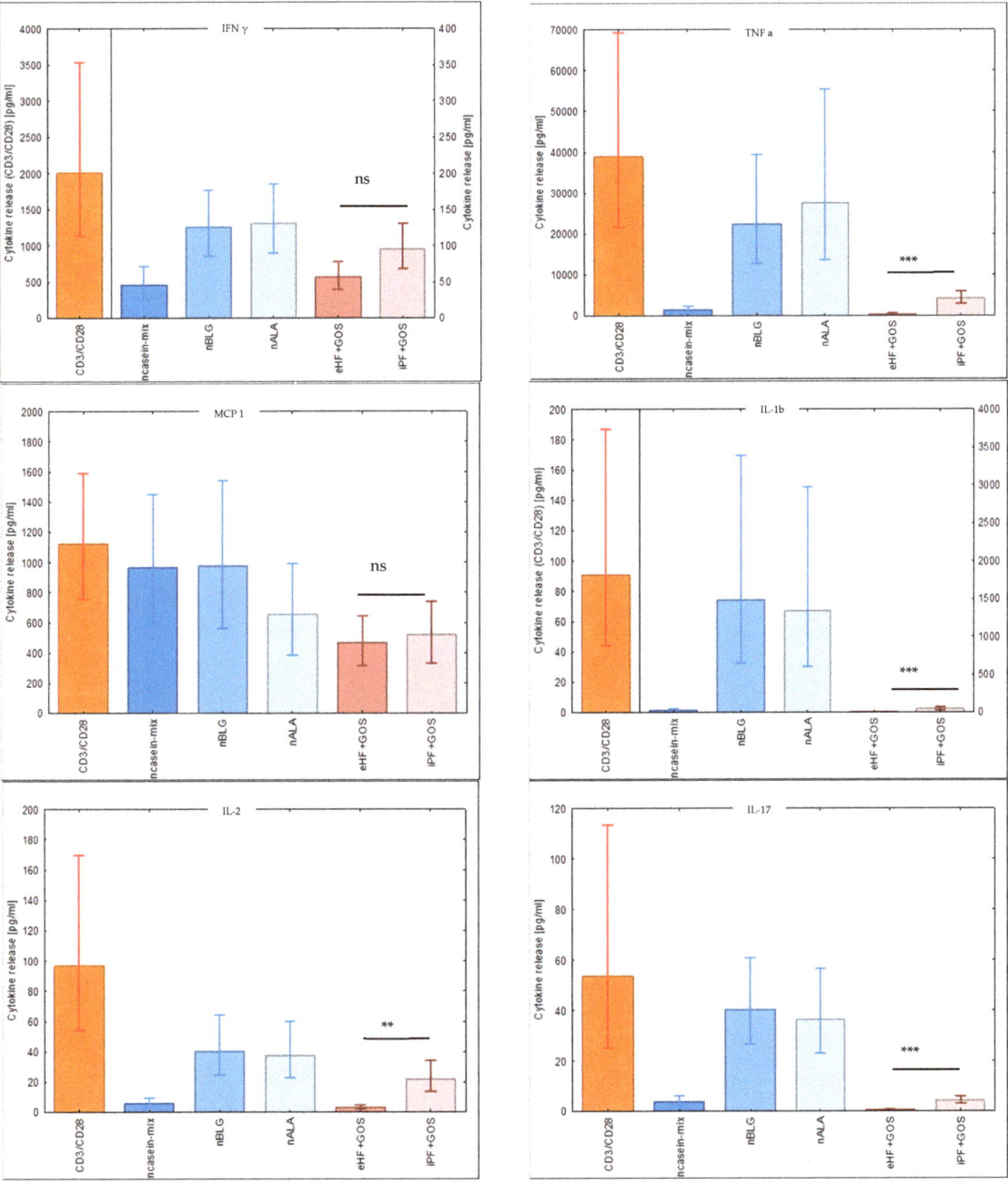

Figure 5. *Cont.*

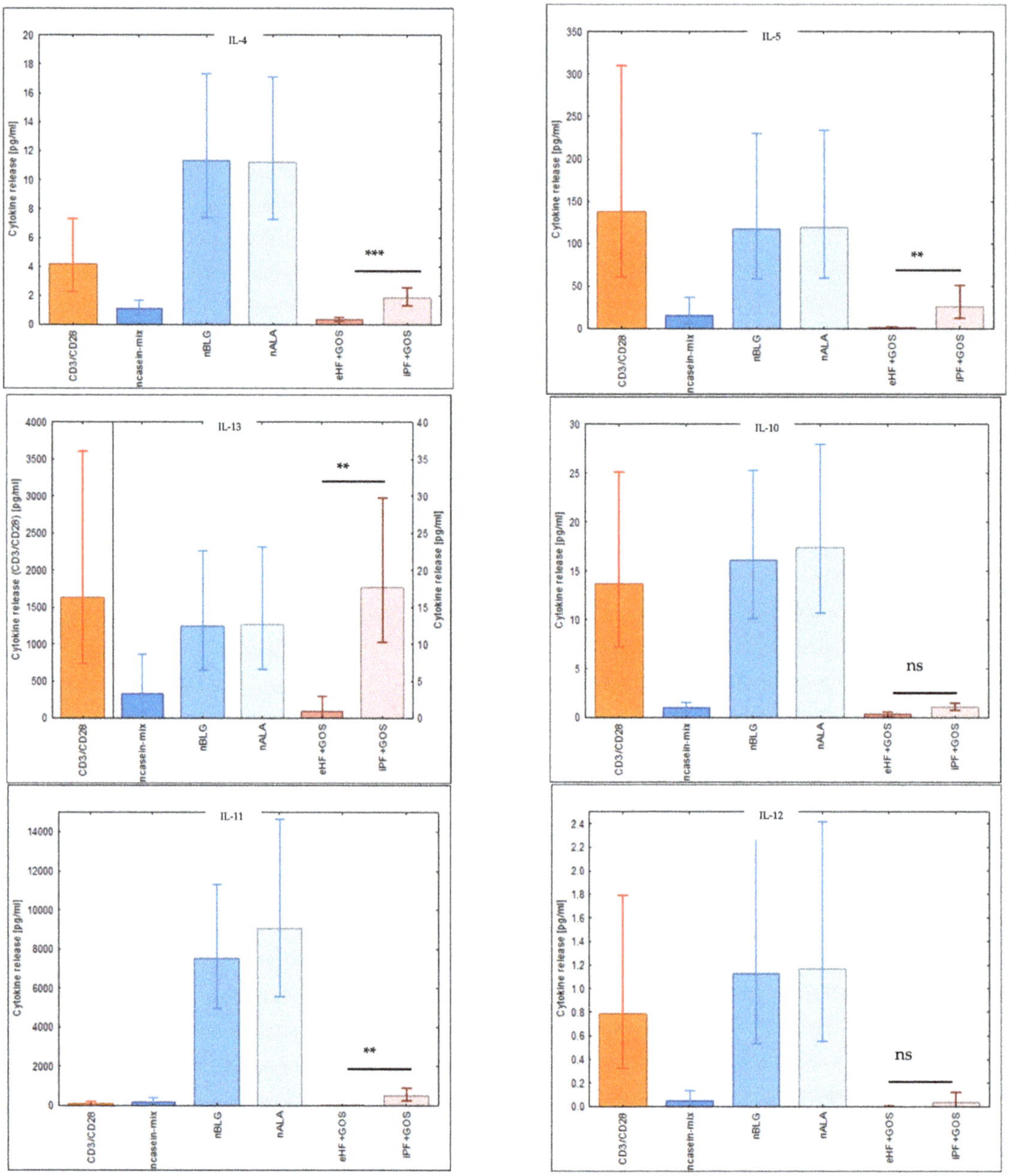

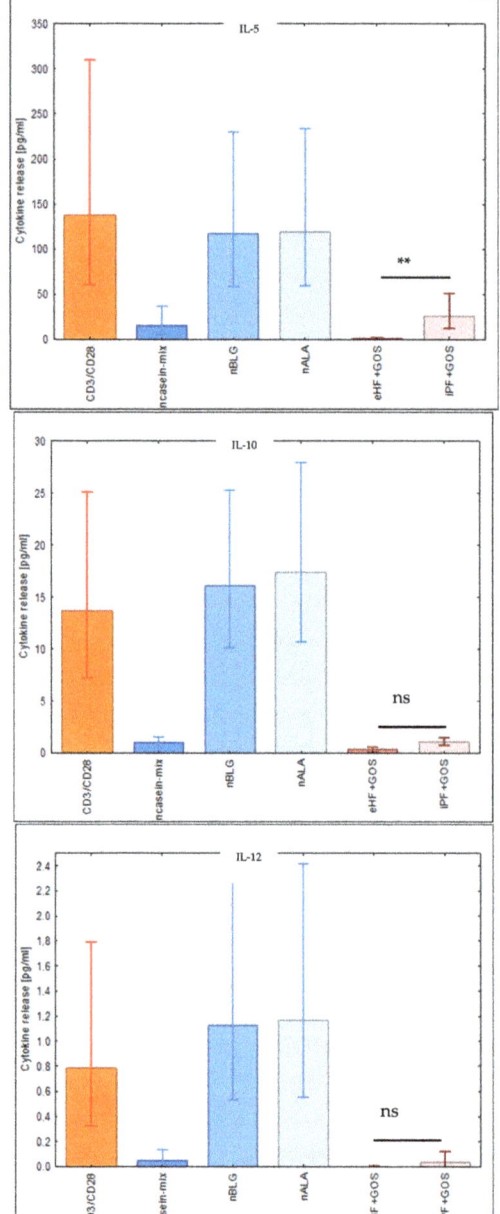

Figure 5. *Cont.*

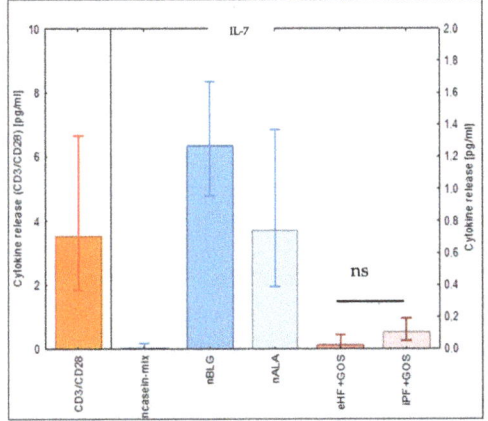
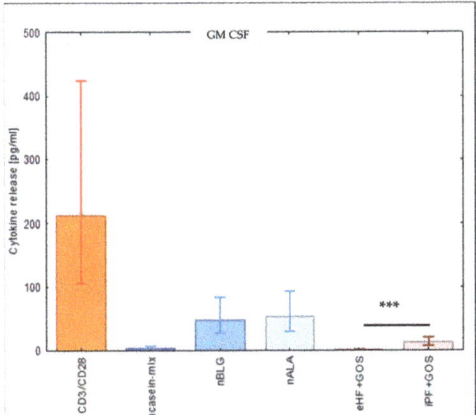

Figure 5. Cytokine responses specific for milk allergens and milk products. Shown are the back-transformed means +/− SEM of cytokines (as indicated on top of each figure) measured in supernatants of cultured PBMC samples from subjects 48–56 (Table 1) that had been stimulated with anti-CD3 and anti-CD28 (positive control), milk allergens, eHF + GOS and iPF + GOS (x-axis; Table 2). Only eHF and iPF were compared statistically (ns, not significant, ** $p \leq 0.01$, *** $p \leq 0.001$).

4. Discussion

Hydrolyzed formulas are obtained by enzymatic degradation of cow's milk or fractions thereof [8]. Depending on the degree of hydrolysis, IgE epitopes and T cell epitopes can be differently affected [14]. The reduction of IgE reactivity serves the purpose of reducing the allergenic activity of the formula so that it can be consumed by cow's milk-allergic infants and children without inducing IgE-mediated allergic inflammation. Accordingly, such formulas are suitable as nutrition for of cow's milk-allergic infants and children, in particular when they cannot be breast-fed. The more a particular formula is hydrolyzed, the lower is its risk of inducing IgE-mediated allergic inflammation, but at the same time also, allergen-specific T cell epitopes are destroyed [10]. However, maintained T cell epitopes are important for the induction of preventive T cell-mediated tolerance. Basically three T cell-mediated mechanisms are thought to be involved in the preventive induction of specific immunological tolerance [8]. They comprise the induction of regulatory T cells (Tregs) usually at lower antigen doses [26] and clonal deletion or clonal anergy at higher antigen doses [27]. While studies have identified hydrolyzed formulas with reduced allergenic activity and reduced ability to induce specific T cell and cytokine responses in cow's milk-allergic patients [13,14], studies performed in animals have yielded controversial results regarding whether hydrolyzed formulas can induce allergen-specific preventive tolerance. For example, one study demonstrated that the administration of extensive hydrolysates from caseins and *Lactobacillus rhamnosus* GG probiotic did not prevent cow's milk protein allergy in a mouse model [17], whereas another study performed in rats showed that partially hydrolyzed whey had allergy-preventive capacity [18].

In this study, we investigated an extensively hydrolyzed infant formula and compared it with an intact protein formula regarding IgE reactivity, allergenic activity, and induction of specific T cell and cytokine responses in cow's milk-allergic patients. We found that the eHF + GOS + LF lacked intact cow's milk allergens as compared to iPF + GOS + LF and accordingly showed almost no IgE reactivity even when tested with sera from highly cow's milk-allergic patients. We then studied the allergenic activity of the infant formulas using basophil degranulation experiments performed with rat basophilic leukemia cells that expressed the human FcεRI and hence could be loaded with serum IgE from cow's milk-allergic patients. This experiment was of particular importance because it examines whether hydrolyzed allergens can cross-link IgE on effector cells and thus induce immediate allergic inflammation. The basophil activation test based on rat basophilic leukemia cells expressing the human FcεRI was used because these cells can be loaded with serum IgE from cow's milk-allergic patients in a highly controlled manner, and the test is not influenced by the presence of allergen-specific IgG, as it occurs in whole blood samples and may affect basophil activation. Therefore, this assay seems to be better suited than a whole blood assay because the possible influence of blocking allergen-specific IgG on basophil activation can be excluded and the results truly reflect the allergenic activity of tested allergens/formulas. Furthermore, it would have been difficult to obtain fresh blood samples from a representative number of cow's milk-allergic children.

In these experiments, it was demonstrated that eHF + GOS and eHF + GOS + LF had significantly reduced allergenic activity as compared to iPF + GOS and iPF + GOS + LF, respectively. However, in these experiments, it turned out that the allergenic activity of eHF + GOS + LF was even significantly lower than that of eHF + GOS and thus almost completely abolished, whereas no significant difference was observed when iPF + GOS was compared with iPF + GOS + LF. This finding may be explained by a down-regulation of inflammatory responses by *Limosilactobacillus fermentum* CECT5716 that was attributed to a reduction of TLR2/TLR4 expression in a murine model of allergic asthma in a recent study [28]. This anti-inflammatory effect of *Limosilactobacillus fermentum* CECT 5716 may be more pronounced when inflammatory cell activation is already reduced due to already reduced IgE cross-linking. Regardless of what the specific mechanism behind the almost completely abolished allergenic activity of the eHF + GOS + LF formula is, it clearly identified this formula as the least allergenic formula among those investigated in our study, which should be useful for the treatment of cow's milk-allergic infants/children.

Usually, extensive hydrolysis destroys not only IgE epitopes but also T cell epitopes and, therefore, may render an extensively hydrolyzed formula not useful for the induction of T cell-mediated tolerance and hence the prevention of allergen-specific IgE sensitization. According to the manufacturer's information, the degree of hydrolysis of the eHF was up to 30%, which was confirmed by our SDS-PAGE analysis showing that eHF + GOS and eH_raw did not contain any visible protein bands even below 10 kDa. Nevertheless, eHF + GOS induced specific proliferation of $CD4^+$ and $CD8^+$ T cells and thus seems to contain peptides that are in the size of 9aa or at least long enough to fit and activate MHC class I and MHC class II.

In fact, we observed that there was no significant difference regarding the induction of T cell proliferation between eHF and iPF, suggesting that most of the allergen-specific T cell epitopes are preserved in eHF and that, therefore, this infant formula may indeed be used for preventive tolerance induction, similarly as reported for an extensively hydrolyzed whey product in earlier animal experiments [18]. Moreover, eHF, despite preservation of allergen-specific T cell epitopes, induced significantly lower amounts of inflammatory cytokines (i.e., TNF alpha, IL-1ß, IL-2, IL-17, IL-4, IL-5, IL-13, IL-6 and GM-CSF) in PBMC cultures of CMA patients and thus induced also lower inflammatory responses in addition to reduced mast cell activation. Although the eHF + GOS and eHF + GOS + LF infant formulas showed strongly reduced allergenic activity in vitro, it must be borne in mind that the strength of allergic reactions may vary in patients. Accordingly, in vivo testing, for example by provocation testing, will be necessary to confirm our results. It may be considered as a limitation of our study that we did not investigate IgG and IgG_1 subclass reactivity of the formulas due to the fact that international guidelines recommend against IgG testing [29]. Should clinical relevance of IgG_1 reactivity be confirmed in the future, the testing of formulas for IgG_1 reactivity may be considered.

In summary, from a preclinical point of view our study identified eHF as a hypoallergenic formula and gives a first promising hint that it may be safely used for the treatment of cow's milk allergy in already-sensitized infants and children. The formula hydrolysate also may be used for the specific primary prevention of cow's milk allergy in not-yet sensitized children. Noteworthy, from a clinical and preclinical point of view both possibilities must be investigated in additional clinical trials. Despite the fact that efficacy in regard to preventing and treating CMA still needs to be demonstrated in infants, a recent clinical trial demonstrated nutritional safety and suitability in terms of growth (EFSA opinion: https://www.efsa.europa.eu/de/efsajournal/pub/7141; assessed on 10 December 2022). It is thus obvious that more extensive clinical data are needed to support our promising preclinical results.

Supplementary Materials: The following supporting information can be downloaded at: https://www.mdpi.com/article/10.3390/nu15010111/s1, Figure S1: Pilot experiments determining the allergen dose inducing increasing basophil degranulation. Figure S2: Original autoradiographs from Figure 2 without cropping.

Author Contributions: R.F., V.G. and B.L., investigation, software, validation, analysis, writing—original draft preparation, review and editing; E.M.H. and I.M., funding acquisition, data curation; Z.S., K.S., N.D., A.P., E.V., T.L., E.B., V.N., S.T., D.N., O.G., A.K. and S.K., clinical investigation, sample collection, clinical data curation, writing—editing; M.K., software, statistical analysis, validation, writing—editing; R.V., conceptualization, methodology, project administration, supervision, writing—original draft preparation, review and editing. All authors have read and agreed to the published version of the manuscript.

Funding: This research was funded by HiPP GmbH & Co. Vertrieb KG, Pfaffenhofen, Germany and in part by the DANUBE Allergy Research Program of the Country of Lower Austria.

Institutional Review Board Statement: The study was conducted in accordance with the Declaration of Helsinki, and approved by Ethics Committee of Veltischev Research and Clinical Institute for Pediatrics of the Pirogov Russian National Research Medical University (protocol code 12/20.12.2017), Ural State Medical University, Ekaterinburg, Russia (protocol code 10/15.12.2017), and Vienna Medical University (protocol code EK1641/2014).

Informed Consent Statement: Written informed consent was obtained from all subjects or parents of subjects involved in the study.

Data Availability Statement: Data will be made available by the authors upon reasonable request.

Acknowledgments: This study was supported by a research grant from HiPP GmbH & Co. Vertrieb KG, Pfaffenhofen, Germany and in part by the DANUBE Allergy Research Program of the Country of Lower Austria. The funders had no influence on the writing of the paper, its contents and where it was submitted.

Conflicts of Interest: E.M.H. and I.M. are employed at HiPP GmbH & Co. Vertrieb KG, Pfaffenhofen, Germany, A.P. received personnel fees from LLC "Nutricia" and Friesland Campina, R.V. has received research grants from HiPP GmbH & Co. Vertrieb KG, Pfaffenhofen, Germany, Worg Pharmaceuticals, Hangzhou, China, HVD Biotech, Vienna, Austria and Viravaxx, Vienna, Austria. He serves as consultant for Viravaxx and Worg. The other authors declare no conflict of interest. The funders had no role in the design of the study; in the collection, analyses, or interpretation of data; or in the decision to publish the results.

References

1. Arasi, S.; Cafarotti, A.; Fiocchi, A. Cow's milk allergy. *Curr. Opin. Allergy Clin. Immunol.* **2022**, *22*, 181–187. [CrossRef] [PubMed]
2. Ostblom, E.; Lilja, G.; Pershagen, G.; van Hage, M.; Wickman, M. Phenotypes of food hypersensitivity and development of allergic diseases during the first 8 years of life. *Clin. Exp. Allergy* **2008**, *38*, 1325–1332. [CrossRef] [PubMed]
3. Valenta, R.; Hochwallner, H.; Linhart, B.; Pahr, S. Food allergies: The basics. *Gastroenterology* **2015**, *148*, 1120–1131. [CrossRef] [PubMed]
4. Karsonova, A.V.; Riabova, K.A.; Khaitov, M.R.; Elisyutina, O.G.; Ilina, N.; Fedenko, E.S.; Fomina, D.S.; Beltyukov, E.; Bondarenko, N.L.; Evsegneeva, I.V.; et al. Milk-Specific IgE Reactivity without Symptoms in Albumin-Sensitized Cat Allergic Patients. *Allergy Asthma Immunol. Res.* **2021**, *13*, 668–670. [CrossRef]

5. Sampson, H.A.; Ho, D.G. Relationship between food-specific IgE concentrations and the risk of positive food challenges in children and adolescents. *J. Allergy Clin. Immunol.* **1997**, *100*, 444–451. [CrossRef]
6. Hochwallner, H.; Schulmeister, U.; Swoboda, I.; Balic, N.; Geller, B.; Nystrand, M.; Härlin, A.; Thalhamer, J.; Scheiblhofer, S.; Niggemann, B.; et al. Microarray and allergenic activity assessment of milk allergens. *Clin. Exp. Allergy* **2010**, *40*, 1809–1818. [CrossRef]
7. Matricardi, P.M.; Kleine-Tebbe, J.; Hoffmann, H.J.; Valenta, R.; Hilger, C.; Hofmaier, S.; Aalberse, R.C.; Agache, I.; Asero, R.; Ballmer-Weber, B.; et al. EAACI Molecular Allergology User's Guide. *Pediatr. Allergy Immunol.* **2016**, *27*, 1–250. [CrossRef]
8. Kiewiet, M.B.G.; Gros, M.; van Neerven, R.J.J.; Faas, M.M.; de Vos, P. Immunomodulating properties of protein hydrolysates for application in cow's milk allergy. *Pediatr. Allergy Immunol.* **2015**, *26*, 206–217. [CrossRef]
9. Calvani, M.; Anania, C.; Cuomo, B.; D'Auria, E.; Decimo, F.; Indirli, G.C.; Marseglia, G.; Mastrorilli, V.; Sartorio, M.U.A.; Santoro, A.; et al. Non-IgE- or Mixed IgE/Non-IgE-Mediated Gastrointestinal Food Allergies in the First Years of Life: Old and New Tools for Diagnosis. *Nutrients* **2021**, *13*, 226. [CrossRef]
10. Linhart, B.; Freidl, R.; Elisyutina, O.; Khaitov, M.; Karaulov, A.; Valenta, R. Molecular Approaches for Diagnosis, Therapy and Prevention of Cows Milk Allergy. *Nutrients* **2019**, *11*, 1492. [CrossRef]
11. Zepeda-Ortega, B.; Goh, A.; Xepapadaki, P.; Sprikkelman, A.; Nicolaou, N.; Hernandez, R.E.H.; Latiff, A.H.A.; Yat, M.T.; Diab, M.; Hussaini, B.A.; et al. Strategies and Future Opportunities for the Prevention, Diagnosis, and Management of Cow Milk Allergy. *Front. Immunol.* **2021**, *10*, 608372. [CrossRef] [PubMed]
12. Nurmatov, U.; Dhami, S.; Arasi, S.; Pajno, G.B.; Fernandez-Rivas, M.; Muraro, A.; Roberts, G.; Akdis, C.; Alvaro-Lozano, M.; Beyer, K.; et al. Allergen immunotherapy for IgE-mediated food allergy: A systematic review and meta-analysis. *Allergy* **2017**, *72*, 1133. [CrossRef] [PubMed]
13. Martin, C.R.; Ling, P.R.; Blackburn, G.L. Review of Infant Feeding: Key Features of Breast Milk and Infant Formula. *Nutrients* **2016**, *8*, 279. [CrossRef]
14. Hochwallner, H.; Schulmeister, U.; Swoboda, I.; Focke-Tejkl, M.; Reininger, R.; Civaj, V.; Campana, R.; Thalhamer, J.; Scheiblhofer, S.; Balic, N.; et al. Infant milk formulas differ regarding their allergenic activity and induction of T-cell and cytokine responses. *Allergy* **2017**, *72*, 416–424. [CrossRef]
15. Meulenbroek, L.A.; Oliveira, S.; den Hartog Jager, C.F.; Klemans, R.J.; Lebens, A.F.; van Baalen, T.; Knulst, A.C.; Bruijnzeel-Koomen, C.A.; Garssen, J.; Knippels, L.M.; et al. The degree of whey hydrolysis does not uniformly affect in vitro basophil and T cell responses of cow's milk-allergic patients. *Clin. Exp. Allergy* **2014**, *44*, 529–539. [CrossRef]
16. Fritsché, R. Animal models in food allergy: Assessment of allergenicity and preventive activity of infant formulas. *Toxicol. Lett.* **2003**, *140–141*, 303–309. [CrossRef]
17. Adel-Patient, K.; Guinot, M.; Guillon, B.; Bernard, H.; Chikhi, A.; Hazebrouck, S.; Junot, C. Administration of extensive hydrolysates from caseins and *Lactobacillus rhamnosus* GG probiotic does not prevent cow's milk proteins allergy in a mouse model. *Front. Immunol.* **2020**, *11*, 1700. [CrossRef]
18. Graversen, K.B.; Larsen, J.M.; Pedersen, S.S.; Sørensen, L.V.; Christoffersen, H.F.; Jacobsen, L.N.; Halken, S.; Licht, T.R.; Bahl, M.I.; Bøgh, K.L. Partially Hydrolysed Whey Has Superior Allergy Preventive Capacity Compared to Intact Whey Regardless of Amoxicillin Administration in Brown Norway Rats. *Front. Immunol.* **2021**, *12*, 705543. [CrossRef]
19. Sampson, H.A.; Muñoz-Furlong, A.; Campbell, R.L.; Adkinson, N.F.; Bock, S.A.; Branum, A.; Brown, S.G.; Camargo, C.A.; Cydulka, R.; Galli, S.J.; et al. Second symposium on the definition and 15 management of ana-phylaxis: Summary report–Second National Institute of Allergy and 16 Infectious Dis-ease/Food Allergy and Anaphylaxis Network symposium. *J. Allergy Clin. Immunol.* **2006**, *117*, 391–397. [CrossRef]
20. Adler-Nissen, J. Determination of the degree of hydrolysis of food protein hydrolysates by trinitrobenzenesulfonic acid. *J. Agric. Food Chem.* **1979**, *27*, 1256–1262. [CrossRef]
21. Nielsen, P.M.; Petersen, D.; Dambmann, C. Improved method for determining food protein degree of hydrolysis. *J. Food Sci.* **2001**, *66*, 642–646. [CrossRef]
22. Sakwinska, O.; Moine, D.; Delley, M.; Combremont, S.; Rezzonico, E.; Descombes, P.; Vinyes-Pares, G.; Zhang, Y.; Wang, P.; Thakkar, S.K. Microbiota in Breast Milk of Chinese Lactating Mothers. *PLoS ONE* **2016**, *11*, e0160856. [CrossRef]
23. Garib, V.; Ben-Ali, M.; Kundi, M.; Curin, M.; Yaakoubi, R.; Ben-Mustapha, I.; Mekki, N.; Froeschl, R.; Perkmann, T.; Valenta, R.; et al. Profound differences in IgE and IgG recognition of micro-arrayed allergens in hyper-IgE syndromes. *Allergy* **2022**, *77*, 1761–1771. [CrossRef] [PubMed]
24. Eckl-Dorna, J.; Campana, R.; Valenta, R.; Niederberger, V. Poor association of allergen-specific antibody, T- and B-cell responses revealed with recombinant allergens and a CFSE dilution-based assay. *Allergy* **2015**, *70*, 1222–1229. [CrossRef] [PubMed]
25. Huang, H.J.; Curin, M.; Banerjee, S.; Chen, K.W.; Garmatiuk, T.; Resch-Marat, Y.; Carvalho-Queiroz, C.; Blatt, K.; Gafvelin, G.; Grönlund, H.; et al. A hypoallergenic peptide mix containing T cell epitopes of the clinically relevant house dust mite allergens. *Allergy* **2019**, *74*, 2461–2478. [CrossRef] [PubMed]
26. Weiner, H.L.; da Cunha, A.P.; Quintana, F.; Wu, H. Oral tolerance. *Immunol. Rev.* **2011**, *241*, 241–259. [CrossRef]

27. Strobel, S. Immunity induced after a feed of antigen during early life: Oral tolerance v. sensitisation. *Proc. Nutr. Soc.* **2001**, *60*, 437–442. [CrossRef] [PubMed]
28. Wang, W.; Li, Y.; Han, G.; Li, A.; Kong, X. Lactobacillus fermentum CECT5716 Alleviates the Inflammatory Response in Asthma by Regulating TLR2/TLR4 Expression. *Front. Nutr.* **2022**, *9*, 931427. [CrossRef]
29. Stapel, S.O.; Asero, R.; Ballmer-Weber, B.K.; Knol, E.F.; Strobel, S.; Vieths, S.; Kleine-Tebbe, J. EAACI Task Force, Testing for IgG4 against foods is not recommended as a diagnostic tool: EAACI Task Force Report. *Allergy* **2008**, *63*, 793–796. [CrossRef]

Disclaimer/Publisher's Note: The statements, opinions and data contained in all publications are solely those of the individual author(s) and contributor(s) and not of MDPI and/or the editor(s). MDPI and/or the editor(s) disclaim responsibility for any injury to people or property resulting from any ideas, methods, instructions or products referred to in the content.

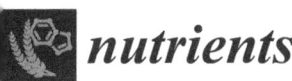

Article

Association of Exclusive Breastfeeding with Asthma Risk among Preschool Children: An Analysis of National Health and Nutrition Examination Survey Data, 1999 to 2014

Chi-Nien Chen [1,2], Yu-Chen Lin [1,3], Shau-Ru Ho [1,3], Chun-Min Fu [1,2,3], An-Kuo Chou [1] and Yao-Hsu Yang [1,2,3,*]

1 Department of Pediatrics, National Taiwan University Hospital Hsin-Chu Branch, Hsinchu 30059, Taiwan
2 Department of Pediatrics, National Taiwan University College of Medicine, Taipei 10051, Taiwan
3 Department of Pediatrics, National Taiwan University Children's Hospital, Taipei 10041, Taiwan
* Correspondence: yan0126@ms15.hinet.net

Abstract: Breastmilk contains many important nutrients, anti-inflammatory agents, and immunomodulators. It is the preferred nutrition source for infants. However, the association of the duration of exclusive breastmilk feeding (BMF) with asthma development is unclear. Data on children from the United States who participated in the National Health and Nutrition Examination Survey (NHANES) from 1999 to 2014 were obtained. We examined the association between the duration of exclusive BMF and asthma in 6000 children (3 to 6 years old). After calculating the duration of exclusive breastfeeding according to answers to NHANES questionnaires, the estimated duration of exclusive BMF was divided into five categories: never breastfed or BMF for 0 to 2 months after birth; BMF for 2 to 4 months after birth; BMF for 4 to 6 months after birth; and BMF for $\geq$6 months after birth. The overall prevalence of asthma in children aged 3 to 6 years was approximately 13.9%. The risk of asthma was lower in children with an exclusive BMF duration of 4 to 6 months (aOR, 0.69; 95% CI, 0.48–0.98), after adjustment for potentially confounding factors. Subgroup analysis revealed that children of younger ages (3 to 4 years old) benefited most from the protective effects of exclusive BMF for 4 to 6 months (aOR, 0.47; 95% CI, 0.27, 0.8). We found that exclusive BMF, especially BMF for 4 to 6 months, is associated with a decreased risk of asthma in preschool-age children. The protective effect appeared to be diminished in older children. The potential mechanism needs further investigation.

Keywords: breastfeeding; breastmilk; pediatric asthma; allergy; cohort study

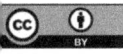

1. Introduction

Asthma is the most common chronic disease in childhood, affecting 8.4% of children in the United States [1]. Most children who suffer from asthma experience their first attack when they are of preschool age, and asthma is a major cause of hospitalization and emergency room visits by preschool children. Asthma prevalence has increased in recent decades [2,3]. It is a chronic airway inflammatory disease, and lung development is a complex process that begins during the intrauterine period and extends through early infancy after birth [4]. Therefore, a beneficial strategy to prevent the development of pediatric asthma is needed, and such a strategy should focus on children's early postnatal period.

Breastfeeding is recognized as having many benefits for short-term and long-term health, including decreasing the risks of upper airway infection, gastrointestinal infection, obesity, and diabetes [5]. From a cost perspective, an increase in the rate of breastfeeding could save billions of dollars and improve maternal and child health [6,7]. The World Health Organization (WHO) and the American Academy of Pediatrics (AAP) recommended that infants should be exclusively breastfed for 6 months, due to the advantages of breastfeeding [8,9]. Breastmilk contains some unique substances that have positive biological effects on the regulation of immune function and the promotion of lung growth. Exclusive breastfeeding for more than 4 months could improve lung growth and lung function in children [10,11]. Accordingly, breastfeeding is considered to have protective effects against the development of asthma.

Some potential mechanisms may explain this association, including microbiome composition, bioactive factors in breastmilk, and the epigenetic effects of breastmilk. Several epidemiologic studies have shown the protective effect of breastfeeding against pediatric asthma [12,13]. Recently, a meta-analysis by Harvey et al. [14] reported a 55% decrease in the risk of wheeze-related outcomes among breastfed children, compared with children who were never breastfed during early childhood. However, some other studies have reported inconsistent results regarding the protective effect of breastfeeding [15,16]. Another meta-analysis study on childhood asthma found that longer durations of breastfeeding and exclusive breastfeeding may only provide a protective effect for pre-school age children [17]. Whether breastfeeding protects against asthma in early childhood and/or for more extended periods is controversial. However, performing a randomized controlled trial of infant feeding practices to clarify this relationship was not practicable.

Therefore, we hypothesized that a longer duration of exclusive breastmilk feeding (BMF) may be associated with a decreased risk of asthma in early childhood. To test this hypothesis, we examined the relationship between BMF and asthma in a nationally representative sample of children in the United States, using data from the National Health and Nutrition Examination Survey (NHANES) from 1999 to 2014.

2. Materials and Methods

The NHANES comprises a series of stratified and multistage surveys designed to investigate the health and nutritional status of adults and children in the United States The survey enrolls a nationally representative sample of approximately 5000 participants each year. A standardized questionnaire is used to collect data on demographic variables, dietary behavior, medical conditions, health insurance, and early childhood conditions for further investigation. The data collection and survey protocols are described elsewhere [18–20]. For the 1999–2000 to 2013–2014 surveys, the overall response rates ranged from 71% to 84%.

Demographic variables included age, sex, and race/ethnicity. Poverty-to-income ratio (PIR) and insurance coverage data were collected from standardized demographic questionnaires. Race/ethnicity was categorized as Hispanic, non-Hispanic White, non-Hispanic Black, and other (including multiracial) (see Table 1). The PIR was categorized as <1.85 or ≥1.85, as described in previous research [21].

Table 1. Clinical characteristics of the study participants and univariate analysis of the risk of asthma.

Characteristics		Total		Ever Asthma			
		N = 6000		Yes (n = 833)		No (n = 5167)	
		n	%	n	%	n	%
Age:	3–4 y	3110	51.8	391	46.9	2719	52.6
	5–6 y	2890	48.2	442	53.1	2448	47.4
Sex:	male	3060	51	502	60.3	2558	49.5
	female	2940	49	331	39.7	2609	50.5
Race:	Mexican-American	1581	26.3	135	16.2	1446	28
	Other-Hispanic	497	8.3	85	10.2	412	8
	Non-Hispanic White	1772	29.5	204	24.5	1568	30.3
	Non-Hispanic Black	1600	26.7	322	38.7	1278	24.7
	Other/Multiracial	550	9.2	87	10.4	463	9
Poverty-to-income ratio:	<1.85	3710	61.8	537	64.5	3173	61.4
	≥1.85	2290	38.2	296	35.5	1994	38.6

Table 1. Cont.

Characteristics		Total		Ever Asthma			
		N = 6000		Yes (n = 833)		No (n = 5167)	
Maternal smoking: yes		768	12.8	134	16.1	634	12.3
no		5232	87.2	699	83.9	4533	87.7
Insurance coverage: yes		5389	89.8	778	93.4	4611	89.2
no		611	10.2	55	6.6	556	10.8
Low birth rate: yes		590	9.8	124	14.9	466	9
no		5410	90.2	709	85.1	4701	91
Maternal age: ≥35 y		1291	21.5	180	21.6	1111	21.5
<35 y		4709	78.5	653	78.4	4056	78.5
Household smoking:		949	15.8	152	18.2	797	15.4
Survey Cycle	1999–2000	593	9.9	96	11.5	497	9.6
	2001–2002	745	12.4	96	11.5	649	12.6
	2003–2004	716	11.9	100	12	616	11.9
	2005–2006	831	13.9	114	13.7	717	13.9
	2007–2008	720	12	103	12.4	617	11.9
	2009–2010	751	12.5	101	12.1	650	12.6
	2011–2012	818	13.6	117	14.1	701	13.6
	2013–2014	826	13.8	106	12.7	720	13.9

Our study was approved by the Institute Review Board (IRB) of National Taiwan University Hospital's Hsin-Chu Branch (IRB No. 107-089-E).

2.1. Breastmilk Exposure Assessment

Exclusive BMF duration was estimated on the basis of dietary and behavioral questionnaires targeting children aged 3 to 6 years. In the NHANES surveys from 1999 to 2000 to 2007 to 2008, the duration of exclusive BMF was assessed by the questions set out below and categorized as follows: "Never"; "<2 months"; ">=2 to <4 months"; ">=4 to <6 months"; and ">=6 months". The categories were determined by calculating the duration of exclusive breastfeeding according to answers provided to the following questions in the questionnaires.

"DBQ010- Was ever breastfed or fed breast milk?"

"DBD030- How old was SP when he/she completely stopped breastfeeding or being fed breast milk?"

"DBD040- How old was (SP) when he/she was first fed formula on a daily basis?"

In the NHANES surveys from 2009–2010 to 2013–2014, the duration of exclusive BMF was assessed by the questions below:

"DBQ010- Was ever breastfed or fed breast milk?"

"DBD030- How old was SP when he/she completely stopped breastfeeding or being fed breast milk?"

"DBD041- How old was (SP) when he/she was first fed formula?"

2.2. Asthma Outcome Assessment

Among preschool-age children, a diagnosis of asthma may be uncertain because conventional pulmonary function tests are not able to confirm the diagnosis. Therefore, the diagnosis of asthma in early childhood is mainly based on clinical judgment. In our study, the diagnosis of asthma was defined by a response of "Yes" to the question: *"Has a doctor or other health professional ever told you/SP that you have asthma?"* We restricted our study to subjects over three years of age, primarily to reduce the overdiagnosis of early childhood asthma. Because a viral infection mainly causes a wheezing illness in children of younger ages, such an infection is often mistaken for asthma due to such early wheezing symptoms.

2.3. Statistical Analysis

Descriptive analyses were performed using the PROC SURVEYMEANS procedure to account for the survey's complex weighting factors. To explore the association of exclusive breastmilk feeding duration with the risk of asthma, we performed logistic regression analyses using the PROC SURVEYLOGISTIC procedure. Multivariable models, including variables such as age, sex, race/ethnicity, family PIR, maternal age at delivery, family smoking exposure, low birth weight, survey cycle, and insurance coverage, were assessed. Participants with missing data for these variables were excluded from complete data analysis. Crude odds ratios (ORs), adjusted ORs, and 95% confidence intervals (CIs) were estimated. All reported p values < 0.05 were considered significant. Statistical analyses were performed using SAS statistical software (version 9.4, SAS Institute Inc., Cary, NC, USA).

3. Results

A total of 82,091 participants were enrolled in the NHANES between 1999 and 2014. Among them, 6768 were children aged 3 to 6 years. After excluding children with missing data, a total of 6000 children aged 3 to 6 years were analyzed in our cohort study (Figure 1). The baseline characteristics of the study participants are listed in Table 1. Trends in exclusive breastfeeding duration and asthma are presented in Table 2.

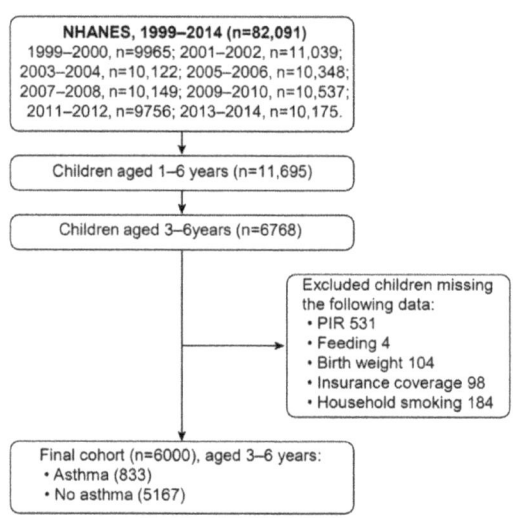

Figure 1. Flow chart of study population.

Table 2. Association of breastmilk feeding duration with risk of asthma.

Duration	Total	Asthma	Prevalence	Crude OR	95% CI	Adjusted OR *	95% CI
Never	2140	358	16.73	1	Ref.	1	Ref.
0–2 m	1692	215	12.71	0.69	0.55–0.86	0.82	0.65–1.04
2–4 m	715	97	13.57	0.78	0.56–1.09	0.93	0.64–1.34
4–6 m	649	66	10.17	0.52	0.37–0.73	0.69	0.48–0.98
≥6 m	804	97	12.06	0.74	0.51–1.07	0.9	0.62–1.3

* Adjusted for age, sex, race, poverty-to-income ratio, maternal age at delivery, maternal smoking during pregnancy, low birth weight, household smoking exposure, insurance coverage, and survey cycle.

Table 2 summarizes the associations between different exclusive breastfeeding durations and asthma, with crude and adjusted ORs and 95% CIs after adjustment for potential confounding factors. The aORs associated with exclusive breastfeeding durations of 4 to 6 months and more than 6 months compared with "Never" were 0.69 (95% CI, 0.48 to 0.98) and 0.9 (95% CI, 0.62 to 1.3), respectively.

Subgroup analysis was performed to determine the effects on different age groups. No statistically significant association was found between BMF duration and asthma development in children aged 5 to 6 years (Table 3). Among children aged 3 to 4 years, the aORs associated with exclusive breastfeeding for 4 to 6 months and more than 6 months compared with "Never" were 0.47 (95% CI, 0.27 to 0.8) and 0.82 (95% CI, 0.49 to 1.36), respectively. However, for children aged 5 to 6 years, the aORs associated with exclusive breastfeeding for 4 to 6 months and more than 6 months, compared with "Never," were 0.94 (95% CI, 0.55 to 1.62) and 0.94 (95% CI, 0.58 to 1.54), respectively. Figure 2 illustrates the relationship between exclusive breastfeeding duration and asthma risk by age. A U-shaped relationship between exclusive breastfeeding duration and the risk of asthma in children aged 3 to 4 (Figure 2A) and a duration of 4 to 6 months was associated with the lowest risk of asthma among them.

Table 3. Association of exclusive breastmilk feeding duration with risk of asthma by age.

	3–4 y					5–6 y				
Duration	N	Asthma	Prevalence	aOR *	95% CI	N	Asthma	Prevalence	aOR *	95% CI
Never	1075	188	17.49	1	Ref.	1065	170	15.96	1	Ref.
0–2 m	934	100	10.71	0.54	0.37–0.79	758	115	15.17	1.16	0.85–1.59
2–4 m	356	33	9.27	0.54	0.3–0.96	359	64	17.83	1.41	0.92–2.16
4–6 m	347	24	6.92	0.47	0.27–0.8	302	42	13.91	0.94	0.55–1.62
≥6 m	398	46	11.56	0.82	0.49–1.36	406	51	12.56	0.94	0.58–1.54

* Adjusted for sex, race, poverty-to-income ratio, maternal age at delivery, maternal smoking during pregnancy, low birth weight, household smoking exposure, insurance coverage and survey cycle.

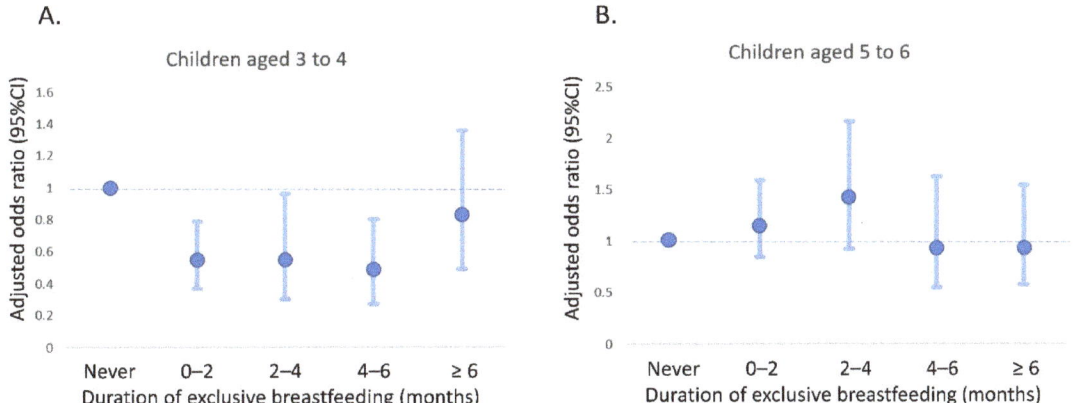

Figure 2. Association of exclusive breastmilk feeding duration with risk of asthma by age. (A) children aged 3 to 4 months; (B) children aged 5 to 6 months.

4. Discussion

We analyzed the data of a nationally representative sample of American children from 1999 to 2014 and found that, for preschool children, exclusive breastfeeding for 4 to 6 months was associated with a lower risk of developing asthma than never breastfeeding. The main findings suggest that the protective effect of breastfeeding is strongest at a young age (3 to 4 years old).

Our study's finding was in line with that of a previous Korean cohort study by Kim et al. [22], who found that exclusive breastfeeding for more than 6 months did not have a statistically significant effect on the development of asthma. This finding contrasts with that of a study from Japan that concluded that exclusive breastfeeding for 6 to 7 months was associated with a lower risk of hospitalization for asthma [23]. In addition, three different systematic reviews and meta-analyses that focused on breastmilk and asthma or childhood wheezing reported the existence of heterogeneity among the studies [24–26]. Possible explanations for the conflicting evidence may be different study designs or inconsistent definitions of breastfeeding and asthma outcomes. Whether breastfeeding can decrease the risk of asthma is controversial. Some studies found that breastfeeding did not have a protective effect against the development of asthma [15,16]. The main reason for the inconsistent findings among previous studies may be variations in study methods and definitions of breastfeeding. Some researchers analyzed exposure to breastfeeding as "ever" or "never", and some analyzed the duration of breastmilk feeding. Different definitions and exposure measurements likely require different outcome assessments to clarify the true effect of BMF on the development of asthma. Therefore, we precisely defined breastmilk exposure as the exclusive duration of breastmilk feeding, to evaluate the relationship between infant feeding practices and subsequent asthma risk. In addition, as it is quite difficult to diagnose asthma in younger children, a clear definition and diagnosis of asthma was needed to allow comparisons between different studies and to reach a consensus standard [27].

An interesting finding of our study was that the protective effect against asthma disappeared with exclusive breastfeeding for more than six months. An explanation may be that maternal or family history of asthma may determine the initiation and duration of BMF, indicating that babies with an increased risk of asthma based on family history may have been more likely to be breastfed longer than those without such a family history. These decisions may neutralize the protective effects of breastfeeding on asthma among children with an increased risk of asthma due to family history [28,29].

4.1. Interpretation of the Subgroup Analysis by Age

Breastfeeding does not seem to be very effective in protecting older children against asthma. Our results demonstrated that exclusive breastfeeding for 4 to 6 months had the most protective effect against asthma development in preschool children aged 3 to 4 years; this effect was not observed in children aged 5 to 6 years. This may be related to the development of asthma caused by environmental factors. Indoor and outdoor air pollutants, biological allergens, and environmental chemicals can cause pre-existing airway inflammation exacerbation, leading to airway hyperresponsiveness and asthma after cumulative exposures during aging [30,31]. Other explanations may be related to the allergic march and the diagnosis of asthma. Early asthmatic wheezing and other minor symptoms may start in early childhood. These symptoms may persist or deteriorate throughout school age and adolescence [32]. The diagnosis of asthma using lung function tests cannot be performed in young children, due to the limited cooperation by young children and suboptimal forced exhalation maneuvers [33]. The diagnosis of asthma is more accurate in older children. Therefore, we restricted the primary analysis group to children over three years of age to reduce the impact of the difficulty in diagnosing asthma in children at younger ages.

4.2. Mechanisms Driving the Protective Effect of BMF against Asthma

Breastfeeding may influence epigenetic processes through global DNA methylation patterns [34,35]. Although many epigenetic mechanisms for breastfeeding and epigenetic processes have been postulated, further well-designed studies should be performed to eliminate confounding effects. Possible confounding factors may include maternal prepregnancy factors (such as maternal age, parity, body mass index, and pre-existing conditions), gestational factors (drug exposure, tobacco use, and delivery mode), and socioeconomic factors (educational attainment, occupation, and family income) [36].

Immunomodulatory constituents and anti-inflammatory agents in breastmilk are important for the prevention of childhood asthma. Breastfeeding plays a key role in the development of oral and intestinal microbiota in infants. Breastmilk provides pioneering species and aids in the establishment of the final intestinal microbiota composition. Human milk oligosaccharides (HMOs) also have the ability to influence the development of the immune system [37]. Most HMOs are indigestible in newborn children and have a prebiotic effect. In the lower intestinal tract, HMOs provide substrates for gut bacteria and are especially utilized by Bacteroides and Bifidobacteria [38]. A predominance of these intestinal bacteria might prevent the proliferation of pathogenic bacteria, improve gut barrier function, and mitigate the risks of severe intestinal infections. It has been proposed that gut microbiota alterations in early childhood can change immunological tolerance and predispose individuals to allergic disorders, including asthma [39].

Some studies have proven that specific HMOs can regulate the immune response directly via viral pathogen mitigation and regulation of host immune cells. In addition, there is another possible mechanism by which HMOs protect against asthma. Approximately 1% of HMOs are absorbed into the blood circulation and finally reach end organs, such as the lungs [40]. HMOs can affect the turnover of airway epithelial cells and the formation of glycocalyx mucus, and interact with immune cells and pathogens to protect against asthma [41].

4.3. Strengths and Limitations

This study had several strengths. First, we used data from a large nationally representative cohort for analysis, and the results summarize the trends of BMF practices and their effects on asthma outcomes over the course of 16 years. We assessed the protective effect of BMF while controlling for multiple confounding factors. Performing a randomized controlled trial of infant feeding practices would not have been practicable; therefore, we provided beneficial evidence of the association by assessing the dose-response effects of BMF stratified by exclusive BMF duration.

This study had some limitations. First, this was a cross-sectional study, and the study design could not fully eliminate the possibility of reverse causation. Participants with a longer duration of exclusive BMF may have had early allergic or wheezing symptoms and signs, and mothers may have intentionally prolonged the duration of breastfeeding. Some of the mothers may have practiced exclusive BMF to promote better offspring outcomes. There were no specific questionnaire questions regarding an association between the timing of wheezing or allergic symptoms and the age of asthma onset. Without a time-sequence evaluation, it was difficult to identify this association clearly. Second, because of the study design, this study could not differentiate between the effects of direct breastfeeding and feeding with expressed breastmilk. Direct breastfeeding may have better protective effects than other modes of BMF [12]. There have been various definitions of breastmilk exposure among different studies, which may have influenced the outcomes, resulting in the uncertain benefit of BMF. Third, recall bias regarding BMF duration should be considered [42]. Inaccuracies in the recall of BMF may have led to the reporting of shorter or longer BMF durations, especially for those children of older ages. We used the NHANES database questions to estimate the duration of exclusive breastfeeding. There may be other diets that could not be fully captured by the database questions, potentially leading to biased estimates of the duration of exclusive breastfeeding. Accordingly, the results should be interpreted carefully. Fortunately, the impact of recall bias may be less than expected, because overall BMF durations were similar in other surveys [43]. Fourth, family medical history and environmental factors may increase children's asthma risk. For example, a family history of allergic diseases, pets in the family home, and/or living in an urban or rural area are all potential influencing factors [44–46]. Researchers should consider such factors in future analysis. Unfortunately, in the NHANES database, such variables were not completely accounted for or were not available for a public study. Future research needs to investigate whether such factors, other than breastmilk itself, have substantial effects on children's asthma.

In the future, a prospective cohort study is needed to clarify the temporal issues associated with potential reverse causation and more comprehensive data, such as data on the duration and types of breastfeeding, are needed to develop strategies to protect against asthma development.

5. Conclusions

In conclusion, we demonstrated a U-shaped relationship between exclusive breastfeeding duration and the risk of asthma in children aged 3 to 4 years, and a duration of 4 to 6 months was associated with a lower risk of asthma in preschool children, especially younger children, based on data from the National Health and Nutrition Examination Survey (NHANES) from 1999 to 2014. Public health policies to promote exclusive breastmilk feeding (BMF) may help to prevent the development of asthma in early childhood. Future studies are needed to investigate reverse causation and to elucidate the mechanism and interactions with potential confounding factors.

Author Contributions: Conceptualization, C.-N.C. and Y.-H.Y.; methodology, C.-N.C. and Y.-H.Y.; software, C.-N.C.; formal analysis, C.-N.C., Y.-C.L., S.-R.H. and Y.-H.Y.; investigation, C.-N.C., Y.-C.L., S.-R.H., C.-M.F. and A.-K.C.; resources, C.-N.C., C.-M.F. and Y.-H.Y.; data curation, C.-N.C. and Y.-H.Y.; writing—original draft preparation, C.-N.C., Y.-C.L. and S.-R.H.; writing—review and editing, C.-M.F., A.-K.C. and Y.-H.Y.; supervision, Y.-H.Y.; project administration, C.-N.C. and Y.-H.Y.; funding acquisition, C.-N.C. All authors have read and agreed to the published version of the manuscript.

Funding: This work was supported by funding from the National Taiwan University Hospital Hsin-Chu Branch (grant number 111-HCH024).

Institutional Review Board Statement: The study was conducted according to the guidelines of the Declaration of Helsinki and approved by the National Taiwan University Hospital Hsin-Chu branch Institutional Review Board. (No. 107-089-E) (date of approval: 24 October 2018).

Informed Consent Statement: The ethics committee agreed that informed consent was waived due to the retrospective and de-identified analysis applied in this study.

Data Availability Statement: All information is available on the NHANES website.

Conflicts of Interest: The authors declare no conflict of interest.

References

1. Stern, J.; Pier, J.; Litonjua, A.A. Asthma epidemiology and risk factors. *Semin. Immunopathol.* **2020**, *42*, 5–15. [CrossRef] [PubMed]
2. Asher, M.I.; Montefort, S.; Björkstén, B.; Lai, C.K.; Strachan, D.P.; Weiland, S.K.; Williams, H. Worldwide time trends in the prevalence of symptoms of asthma, allergic rhinoconjunctivitis, and eczema in childhood: ISAAC phases one and three repeat multicountry cross-sectional surveys. *Lancet* **2006**, *368*, 733–743. [CrossRef]
3. Akinbami, L.J.; Simon, A.E.; Rossen, L.M. Changing trends in asthma prevalence among children. *Pediatrics* **2016**, *137*, 1–7. [CrossRef] [PubMed]
4. Burri, P.H. Structural aspects of postnatal lung development—Alveolar formation and growth. *Biol. Neonate* **2006**, *89*, 313–322. [CrossRef] [PubMed]
5. Louis-Jacques, A.F.; Stuebe, A.M. Enabling breastfeeding to support lifelong health for mother and child. *Obstet. Gynecol. Clin. N. Am.* **2020**, *47*, 363–381. [CrossRef] [PubMed]
6. Bartick, M.; Reinhold, A. The burden of suboptimal breastfeeding in the United States: A pediatric cost analysis. *Pediatrics* **2010**, *125*, e1048–e1056. [CrossRef] [PubMed]
7. Bartick, M.C.; Jegier, B.J.; Green, B.D.; Schwarz, E.B.; Reinhold, A.G.; Stuebe, A.M. Disparities in breastfeeding: Impact on maternal and child health outcomes and costs. *J. Pediatr.* **2017**, *181*, 49–55.e6. [CrossRef] [PubMed]
8. Meek, J.Y.; Noble, L. Policy statement: Breastfeeding and the use of human milk. *Pediatrics* **2022**, *150*, e2022057988. [CrossRef] [PubMed]
9. World Health Organization. *International Code of Marketing of Breast-Milk Substitutes*; World Health Organization: Geneva, Switzerland, 1981.
10. Guilbert, T.W.; Stern, D.A.; Morgan, W.J.; Martinez, F.D.; Wright, A.L. Effect of breastfeeding on lung function in childhood and modulation by maternal asthma and atopy. *Am. J. Respir. Crit. Care Med.* **2007**, *176*, 843–848. [CrossRef] [PubMed]
11. Ogbuanu, I.U.; Karmaus, W.; Arshad, S.H.; Kurukulaaratchy, R.J.; Ewart, S. Effect of breastfeeding duration on lung function at age 10 years: A prospective birth cohort study. *Thorax* **2009**, *64*, 62–66. [CrossRef]
12. Klopp, A.; Vehling, L.; Becker, A.B.; Subbarao, P.; Mandhane, P.J.; Turvey, S.E.; Lefebvre, D.L.; Sears, M.R.; Azad, M.B. Modes of infant feeding and the risk of childhood asthma: A prospective birth cohort study. *J. Pediatr.* **2017**, *190*, 192–199.e2. [CrossRef] [PubMed]
13. Fredriksson, P.; Jaakkola, N.; Jaakkola, J.J. Breastfeeding and childhood asthma: A six-year population-based cohort study. *BMC Pediatr.* **2007**, *7*, 39. [CrossRef] [PubMed]

14. Harvey, S.M.; Murphy, V.E.; Whalen, O.M.; Gibson, P.G.; Jensen, M.E. Breastfeeding and wheeze-related outcomes in high-risk infants: A systematic review and meta-analysis. *Am. J. Clin. Nutr.* **2021**, *113*, 1609–1618. [CrossRef]
15. Bion, V.; Lockett, G.A.; Soto-Ramírez, N.; Zhang, H.; Venter, C.; Karmaus, W.; Holloway, J.W.; Arshad, S.H. Evaluating the efficacy of breastfeeding guidelines on long-term outcomes for allergic disease. *Allergy* **2016**, *71*, 661–670. [CrossRef]
16. Chiu, C.Y.; Liao, S.L.; Su, K.W.; Tsai, M.H.; Hua, M.C.; Lai, S.H.; Chen, L.C.; Yao, T.C.; Yeh, K.W.; Huang, J.L. Exclusive or Partial Breastfeeding for 6 Months Is Associated with Reduced Milk Sensitization and Risk of Eczema in Early Childhood: The PATCH Birth Cohort Study. *Medicine* **2016**, *95*, e3391. [CrossRef]
17. Xue, M.; Dehaas, E.; Chaudhary, N.; O'Byrne, P.; Satia, I.; Kurmi, O.P. Breastfeeding and risk of childhood asthma: A systematic review and meta-analysis. *ERJ Open Res.* **2021**, *7*, 00504–02021. [CrossRef]
18. Orozco, J.; Echeverria, S.E.; Armah, S.M.; Dharod, J.M. Household food insecurity, breastfeeding, and related feeding practices in US infants and toddlers: Results from NHANES 2009–2014. *J. Nutr. Educ. Behav.* **2020**, *52*, 588–594. [CrossRef]
19. Ahluwalia, N.; Dwyer, J.; Terry, A.; Moshfegh, A.; Johnson, C. Update on NHANES dietary data: Focus on collection, release, analytical considerations, and uses to inform public policy. *Adv. Nutr.* **2016**, *7*, 121–134. [CrossRef]
20. Jackson-Browne, M.S.; Eliot, M.; Patti, M.; Spanier, A.J.; Braun, J.M. PFAS (per- and polyfluoroalkyl substances) and asthma in young children: NHANES 2013–2014. *Int. J. Hyg. Environ. Health* **2020**, *229*, 113565. [CrossRef]
21. Rai, D.; Bird, J.K.; McBurney, M.I.; Chapman-Novakofski, K.M. Nutritional status as assessed by nutrient intakes and biomarkers among women of childbearing age–is the burden of nutrient inadequacies growing in America? *Public Health Nutr.* **2015**, *18*, 1658–1669. [CrossRef]
22. Kim, J.H.; Lee, S.W.; Lee, J.E.; Ha, E.K.; Han, M.Y.; Lee, E. Breastmilk feeding during the first 4 to 6 months of age and childhood disease burden until 10 years of age. *Nutrients* **2021**, *13*, 2825. [CrossRef]
23. Yamakawa, M.; Yorifuji, T.; Kato, T.; Yamauchi, Y.; Doi, H. Breast-feeding and hospitalization for asthma in early childhood: A nationwide longitudinal survey in Japan. *Public Health Nutr.* **2015**, *18*, 1756–1761. [CrossRef] [PubMed]
24. Gdalevich, M.; Mimouni, D.; Mimouni, M. Breast-feeding and the risk of bronchial asthma in childhood: A systematic review with meta-analysis of prospective studies. *J. Pediatr.* **2001**, *139*, 261–266. [CrossRef] [PubMed]
25. Dogaru, C.M.; Nyffenegger, D.; Pescatore, A.M.; Spycher, B.D.; Kuehni, C.E. Breastfeeding and childhood asthma: Systematic review and meta-analysis. *Am. J. Epidemiol.* **2014**, *179*, 1153–1167. [CrossRef]
26. Lodge, C.J.; Tan, D.J.; Lau, M.X.; Dai, X.; Tham, R.; Lowe, A.J.; Bowatte, G.; Allen, K.J.; Dharmage, S.C. Breastfeeding and asthma and allergies: A systematic review and meta-analysis. *Acta Paediatr.* **2015**, *104*, 38–53. [CrossRef]
27. Papadopoulos, N.G.; Čustović, A.; Cabana, M.D.; Dell, S.D.; Deschildre, A.; Hedlin, G.; Hossny, E.; Le Souëf, P.; Matricardi, P.M.; Nieto, A.; et al. Pediatric asthma: An unmet need for more effective, focused treatments. *Pediatr. Allergy Immunol.* **2019**, *30*, 7–16. [CrossRef]
28. Azad, M.B.; Vehling, L.; Lu, Z.; Dai, D.; Subbarao, P.; Becker, A.B.; Mandhane, P.J.; Turvey, S.E.; Lefebvre, D.L.; Sears, M.R. Breastfeeding, maternal asthma and wheezing in the first year of life: A longitudinal birth cohort study. *Eur. Respir. J.* **2017**, *49*, 1602019. [CrossRef]
29. Peters, R.L.; Kay, T.; McWilliam, V.L.; Lodge, C.J.; Ponsonby, A.L.; Dharmage, S.C.; Lowe, A.J.; Koplin, J.J. The interplay between eczema and breastfeeding practices may hide breastfeeding's protective effect on childhood asthma. *J. Allergy Clin. Immunol.* **2021**, *9*, 862–871.e5. [CrossRef] [PubMed]
30. Guarnieri, M.; Balmes, J.R. Outdoor air pollution and asthma. *Lancet* **2014**, *383*, 1581–1592. [CrossRef]
31. Vincent, M.J.; Bernstein, J.A.; Basketter, D.; LaKind, J.S.; Dotson, G.S.; Maier, A. Chemical-induced asthma and the role of clinical, toxicological, exposure and epidemiological research in regulatory and hazard characterization approaches. *Regul. Toxicol. Pharmacol.* **2017**, *90*, 126–132. [CrossRef]
32. Bantz, S.K.; Zhu, Z.; Zheng, T. The atopic march: Progression from atopic dermatitis to allergic rhinitis and asthma. *J. Clin. Cell. Immunol.* **2014**, *5*, 202. [CrossRef]
33. Beydon, N.; Davis, S.D.; Lombardi, E.; Allen, J.L.; Arets, H.G.; Aurora, P.; Bisgaard, H.; Davis, G.M.; Ducharme, F.M.; Eigen, H.; et al. An official American thoracic society/European respiratory society statement: Pulmonary function testing in preschool children. *Am. J. Respir. Crit. Care Med.* **2007**, *175*, 1304–1345. [CrossRef]
34. Oddy, W.H. Breastfeeding, childhood asthma, and allergic disease. *Ann. Nutr. Metab.* **2017**, *70* (Suppl. S2), 26–36. [CrossRef] [PubMed]
35. Hartwig, F.P.; De Mola, C.L.; Davies, N.M.; Victora, C.G.; Relton, C.L. Breastfeeding effects on DNA methylation in the offspring: A systematic literature review. *PLoS ONE* **2017**, *12*, e0173070. [CrossRef]
36. Miliku, K.; Azad, M.B. Breastfeeding and the developmental origins of asthma: Current evidence, possible mechanisms, and future research priorities. *Nutrients* **2018**, *10*, 995. [CrossRef]
37. Corpeleijn, W.E.; Vermeulen, M.J.; van Vliet, I.; Kruger, C.; Van Goudoever, J.B. Human milk banking-facts and issues to resolve. *Nutrients* **2010**, *2*, 762–769. [CrossRef]
38. Marcobal, A.; Sonnenburg, J.L. Human milk oligosaccharide consumption by intestinal microbiota. *Clin. Microbiol. Infect.* **2012**, *18* (Suppl. S4), 12–15. [CrossRef]
39. Moossavi, S.; Miliku, K.; Sepehri, S.; Khafipour, E.; Azad, M.B. The prebiotic and probiotic properties of human milk: Implications for infant immune development and pediatric asthma. *Front. Pediatr.* **2018**, *6*, 197. [CrossRef]
40. Bode, L. The functional biology of human milk oligosaccharides. *Early Hum. Dev.* **2015**, *91*, 619–622. [CrossRef]

41. Orczyk-Pawiłowicz, M.; Lis-Kuberka, J. The impact of dietary fucosylated oligosaccharides and glycoproteins of human milk on infant well-being. *Nutrients* **2020**, *12*, 1105. [CrossRef]
42. Van Zyl, Z.; Maslin, K.; Dean, T.; Blaauw, R.; Venter, C. The accuracy of dietary recall of infant feeding and food allergen data. *J. Hum. Nutr. Diet.* **2016**, *29*, 777–785. [CrossRef] [PubMed]
43. Li, R.; Perrine, C.G.; Anstey, E.H.; Chen, J.; MacGowan, C.A.; Elam-Evans, L.D. Breastfeeding trends by race/ethnicity among US children born from 2009 to 2015. *JAMA Pediatr.* **2019**, *173*, e193319. [CrossRef]
44. Ren, J.; Xu, J.; Zhang, P.; Bao, Y. Prevalence and Risk Factors of Asthma in Preschool Children in Shanghai, China: A Cross-Sectional Study. *Front. Pediatr.* **2021**, *9*, 793452. [CrossRef] [PubMed]
45. Luo, S.; Sun, Y.; Hou, J.; Kong, X.; Wang, P.; Zhang, Q.; Sundell, J. Pet keeping in childhood and asthma and allergy among children in Tianjin area, China. *PLoS ONE* **2018**, *13*, e0197274. [CrossRef] [PubMed]
46. Grant, T.L.; Wood, R.A. The influence of urban exposures and residence on childhood asthma. *Pediatr. Allergy Immunol.* **2022**, *33*, e13784. [CrossRef]

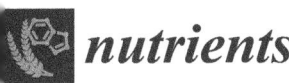

Article

House Dust Mite Exposure through Human Milk and Dust: What Matters for Child Allergy Risk?

Patricia Macchiaverni [1,2,*], Ulrike Gehring [3], Akila Rekima [1,2], Alet H. Wijga [4] and Valerie Verhasselt [1,2]

1. Centre of Research for Immunology and Breastfeeding (CIBF), Medical School and School of Biomedical Science, University of Western Australia, Perth, WA 6009, Australia; akila.rekima@uwa.edu.au (A.R.); valerie.verhasselt@uwa.edu.au (V.V.)
2. Immunology and Breastfeeding Group, Neonatal and Life Course Health Program, Telethon Kids Institute, Perth, WA 6009, Australia
3. Institute for Risk Assessment Sciences, Utrecht University, 3508 TC Utrecht, The Netherlands; U.Gehring@uu.nl
4. Centre for Prevention and Health Services Research, National Institute for Public Health and the Environment, 3720 BA Bilthoven, The Netherlands; alet.wijga@rivm.nl
* Correspondence: patricia.macchiaverni@telethonkids.org.au or patricia.macchiaverni@uwa.edu.au

Abstract: Allergies are major noncommunicable diseases associated with significant morbidity, reduced quality of life, and high healthcare costs. Despite decades of research, it is still unknown if early-life exposure to indoor allergens plays a role in the development of IgE-mediated allergy and asthma. The objective of this study is to contribute to the identification of early-life risk factors for developing allergy. We addressed whether two different sources of house dust mite *Der p* 1 allergen exposure during early life, i.e., human milk and dust, have different relationships with IgE levels and asthma outcomes in children. We performed longitudinal analyses in 249 mother–child pairs using data from the PIAMA birth cohort. Asthma symptoms and serum total and specific IgE levels in children were available for the first 16 years of life. *Der p* 1 levels were measured in human milk and dust samples from infant mattresses. We observed that infant exposure to *Der p* 1 through human milk was associated with an increased risk of having high levels of serum IgE (top tertile > 150 kU/mL) in childhood as compared to infants exposed to human milk with undetectable *Der p* 1 [adjusted OR (95% CI) 1.83 (1.05–3.20) p = 0.0294]. The *Der p* 1 content in infant mattress dust was not associated with increased IgE levels in childhood. The risk of asthma and *Der p* 1 sensitization was neither associated with *Der p* 1 in human milk nor with *Der p* 1 in dust. In conclusion, high levels of IgE in childhood were associated with *Der p* 1 exposure through human milk but not exposure from mattress dust. This observation suggests that human milk is a source of *Der p* 1 exposure that is relevant to allergy development and fosters the need for research on the determinants of *Der p* 1 levels in human milk.

Keywords: breastmilk; house dust mite; *Der p* 1; Asthma; total IgE

Citation: Macchiaverni, P.; Gehring, U.; Rekima, A.; Wijga, A.H.; Verhasselt, V. House Dust Mite Exposure through Human Milk and Dust: What Matters for Child Allergy Risk? *Nutrients* 2022, 14, 2095. https://doi.org/10.3390/nu14102095

Academic Editor: Hiam Abdala-Valencia

Received: 1 April 2022
Accepted: 12 May 2022
Published: 17 May 2022

Publisher's Note: MDPI stays neutral with regard to jurisdictional claims in published maps and institutional affiliations.

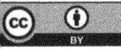

Copyright: © 2022 by the authors. Licensee MDPI, Basel, Switzerland. This article is an open access article distributed under the terms and conditions of the Creative Commons Attribution (CC BY) license (https://creativecommons.org/licenses/by/4.0/).

1. Introduction

Allergy is an abnormal immune response directed against harmless molecules called allergens. In allergic disorders, such as allergic asthma, the immune response is associated with B cells differentiation that undergo immunoglobulin class-switch recombination to produce IgE antibodies. IgE antibodies are the hallmark of allergic responses and are responsible for acute allergic symptoms upon their cross-linking on mast cells by allergens [1]. Increased levels of IgE can also drive amplification mechanisms in allergic disorders even in the absence of ongoing exposure to specific antigens [1].

Many factors affect the induction of IgE antibodies, including the host genotype, nature of allergen, allergen concentration in the environment and the route of exposure [1]. Recent studies demonstrated that food allergens induce allergic sensitization when in contact with an impaired skin barrier [2], whereas the oral route is thought to favour oral tolerance and allergy protection [3–5]. On the other hand, skin [6], respiratory [7] and oral exposure to house dust mite (HDM) allergen, were associated with increased risks of allergic sensitisation, respiratory problems [8] and food allergies in infants [9].

Dermatophagoides pteronyssinus is the most widely distributed HDM, and the role of *Der p* 1 allergen in allergic sensitization and disease is largely recognized [7]. Allergic inflammation induced by *Der p* 1 also stimulates allergic responses to bystander allergens [10], thereby contributing to the progression of the atopic march. Although it is usually found in high concentrations in indoor environments [7], the dust is not the only matrix where HDM allergens are found. *Der p* 1 was detected in up to 78% of human milk samples from Australia, France, Brazil and the Netherlands [8,11–13]. This observation reinforces that exposure to *Der p* 1 occurs in the first months of life by both respiratory and oral routes.

The design of successful strategies for allergy prevention requires the identification of risk factors in early life; a period that is considered to be a window of susceptibility for the long-term risk of disease [14]. The present work used data from the Prevention and Incidence of Asthma and Mite Allergy (PIAMA) birth cohort to investigate whether the source of *Der p* 1 exposure in early childhood, i.e., human milk versus exposure from mattress dust, influences IgE levels and asthma prevalence throughout the first 16 years of life.

Here, we demonstrated that *Der p*1 in human milk, but not dust, was associated with an increased risk of having high levels of IgE in childhood. This highlights the need to conduct research on *Der p*1 exposure through milk to investigate strategies for allergy prevention.

2. Materials and Methods

2.1. Study Design and Population

The study population consisted of mother–child pairs from the Prevention and Incidence of Asthma and Mite Allergy (PIAMA) birth cohort, detailed in [15]. In brief, all participants had been followed up since birth by repeated questionnaires at ages 3 months, 1 year, and then annually until age 8, and at ages 11, 14 and 17 years. Medical examinations, including the collection of blood samples for measurements of allergen-specific and total IgE were performed in (different) sub-populations at ages 1, 4, 8, 12 and 16 years. Human milk and dust samples were collected in a sub-group of the population around the infant's age of 3 months. A total of 249 mother–child pairs with measurements of *Der p* 1 in human milk samples and information on at least one infant health outcome (asthma and/or total IgE) for at least one time point between 4 and 16 years were included. Details on this cohort study were published elsewhere [15].

2.2. Samples Collection and Der p 1 Quantification in Human Milk and Mattress Dust

Human milk samples were collected as previously described [16]. *Der p* 1 levels were determined in the aqueous fraction of human milk using an adapted protocol for a high specificity and sensitivity detection, as previously described [8,11,17]. The lower limit of detection (LOD) was 60 pg/mL for twice-diluted human milk samples. Dust samples were collected from infant mattresses according to a standardized protocol, as previously described [18]. Dust extracts were analysed for *Der p* 1 using sandwich enzyme immunoassay (Indoor Biotechnologies, Cardiff, UK). Levels of *Der p* 1 were expressed per gram of dust for samples with detectable amounts of dust ($\geq$11 mg dust). The LOD was 8 ng/mL for 5-fold diluted dust samples. Samples with non-detectable amounts of allergen were assigned a value of two-thirds the detection limit. *Der p* 1 levels in infant mattress dust were available for 198 of the 249 participants.

2.3. Health Outcomes: IgE Levels and Asthma

Total and specific IgE levels for *Dermatophagoides pteronyssinus* (*Der p*) were measured by a radioallergosorbent-test-like method (Sanquin Laboratories. Amsterdam, The

Netherlands) at ages of 4, 8, 12, and 16 years in children of both allergic and non-allergic mothers [19]. Allergic sensitization was defined as Der p-specific IgE ≥ 0.35 kU/L. Parents completed questionnaires for asthma annually until the age of 8 years and then at ages 11, 14, and 16 years. Asthma was defined from age 3 onwards as at least two positive answers to the following three questions: (1) Has a doctor ever diagnosed asthma in your child? (2) Has your child had wheezing or whistling in the chest in the last 12 months? (3) Has your child been prescribed asthma medication during the last 12 months. This definition was developed by a panel of experts within the MeDALL consortium [20].

2.4. Statistical Analysis

For all analyses, Der p 1 levels in human milk and dust were dichotomized into two categorical variables using the LOD as cut-off values. Total IgE levels were dichotomized into two categorical variables using the top tertile level (>150 kU/L) as cut-off value for "high IgE". Longitudinal associations of human milk Der p 1 levels with high IgE, allergic sensitization, and asthma were assessed by generalized estimation equations with a logit link and compound symmetry within a participant correlation structure. Analyses were performed with and without adjustment for the same covariates as in earlier analyses within the same cohort [19] (child's age at the time of outcome assessment, maternal asthma and maternal allergy to house dust mites, sex, and pets in the child's home during the first year of life). Associations of Der p 1 levels with allergic outcomes are presented as odd ratios with 95% confidence intervals (CI). Statistical significance was defined by a two-sided a-level of 5%. Calculations were performed using the Statistical Analysis System (SAS 9.4, Cary, NC, USA).

3. Results

3.1. Characteristics of the Study Population

Characteristics of the study population, such as season of birth, gestational age and duration of breastfeeding are summarized in Table 1. By design, households of mothers with asthma or allergies were over-represented in the study participants when compared with the full PIAMA cohort [15].

Table 1. Characteristics of the study population.

	Study Participants
Infant male sex	126/249 (51%)
Maternal asthma, n/N (%)	40/249 (16%)
Maternal allergy to house dust (mites), n/N (%)	95/244 (39%)
Season of birth, n/N (%)	
Winter	85/249 (34%)
Spring	80/249 (32%)
Summer	49/249 (20%)
Autumn	35/249 (14%)
Maternal age at birth, mean (SD)	31.1 (3.8), n = 244
Gestational age at birth, mean (SD)	40.1 (1.4), n = 249
Infant birth weight (grams), mean (SD)	3532 (492), n = 249
Caesarian section, n/N (%)	20/248 (8%)
Infant age at human milk collection (days), mean (SD)	108 (29), n = 245
Duration of breastfeeding (weeks), mean (SD)	30 (13), n = 249
Pets in the child's home during 1st year, n/N (%)	104/248 (42%)

Maternal history of allergies and/or asthma was defined from a validated self-reported questionnaire [15,21].

3.2. Presence of Der p 1 Allergen in Human Milk and Infant Mattress Dust

Der p 1 was detected in more than one-third of human milk samples, and the median concentration among these samples was 174 pg/mL (range ≤ LOD-1238 pg/mL, Table 2). We found Der p 1 in 41% of dust samples from the infants' mattresses, and the median concentration among these samples was 1165 ng/g of dust (range ≤ LOD-20,502 ng/g of dust, Table 2).

Table 2. Distribution of Der p 1 levels in human milk and dust samples collected from child's mattress.

Der p 1 Detection	Human Milk (pg/mL)	Dust from Infant's Mattress (ng/g)
Number of samples	218	198
Samples with detected Der p 1 (%)	79 (36)	81 (41)
Median * (concentration range)	174 [<LOD-1238]	1165 [<LOD-20,502]

* For ≥ LOD samples. Detection limit 60 pg/mL and 8 ng/mL for human milk and dust, respectively.

3.3. Associations of Der p 1 Allergen in Human Milk with Child IgE Levels and Asthma

We first analysed levels of total IgE in children breastfed by mothers with detectable versus non-detectable Der p 1 in breastmilk. The estimating equation (GEE) analysis of IgE levels at all ages demonstrated that there was a difference of 90.8 kU/mL in IgE levels when comparing children breastfed by mothers with detectable and non-detectable Der p 1 in human milk at all ages [95% CI (−6.6; 188.2)], $p = 0.06$. The odds ratio of having high levels of IgE (>150 kU/L) was higher in children exposed to Der p 1 in human milk (Figure 1 and Supplementary Table S1). Age-specific associations of high IgE levels in serum with the presence of Der p 1 in human milk were statistically significant at 12 and 16 years of age (Figure 1 and Supplementary Table S1). Overall and age-specific associations persisted after adjustment for confounders (Supplementary Table S1). We further assessed whether the prevalence of Der p sensitization (Der p spec IgE ≥ 0.35 kU/L) at 4–16 years of age was associated with the presence of Der p 1 in human milk. No significant difference was observed when comparing children breastfed by mothers with detectable versus non-detectable Der p 1 in human milk (Supplementary Figure S1). Finally, we analysed whether the presence of Der p 1 in human milk was associated with asthma symptoms in the first 16 years of life. A total of 243 children with 1875 observations were included in models with confounder adjustments. The prevalence (Figure 2A) and odds ratios of asthma symptoms tended to increase in children breastfed by mothers with Der p 1 in human milk as compared to unexposed children, but associations were not statistically significant [OR (95% CI) 1.38 (0.63–3.04) and 1.47 (0.66–3.27)] for crude and adjusted associations, respectively. The number of asthma cases was small to assess age-specific associations.

3.4. Associations of Der p 1 Allergen in Mattress Dust with Child IgE Levels and Asthma

We analysed levels of total IgE in children with detectable versus non-detectable Der p 1 in mattress dust collected during the same period of time as breastmilk. When comparing both groups, the mean difference (95% CI) in total IgE levels was −33.7 kU/mL (−146.9; 79.5), $p = 0.55$. The odd ratios of having high levels of IgE (>150 kU/L) were similar in children from both groups (Figure 1 and Supplementary Table S1). We then analysed whether the presence of Der p 1 in mattress dust was associated with asthma symptoms from 3 to 17 years of life. Although the prevalence (Figure 2B) and odds ratios for asthma symptoms tended to be lower in children with detectable Der p 1 in mattress dust compared to those with non-detectable Der p 1 in mattress dust [OR (95% CI) 0.79 (0.32–1.95) and 0.63 (0.26–1.52)] for crude and adjusted associations, respectively, no significant association was found. The number of asthma cases was small when assessing age-specific associations.

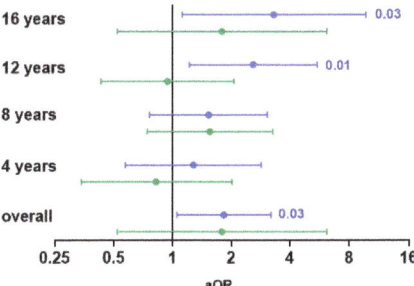

Figure 1. Adjusted associations of high IgE levels in children with *Der p* 1 levels in human milk and infant's mattress dust. Adjusted odds ratios (aORs) for high levels of IgE (top tertile, > 150 kU/L) at 4–16 years of age in children exposed to detectable versus non-detectable *Der p* 1 in human milk (blue circles) and in infant's mattress dust (green circles). ORs were adjusted for child's age at the time of reporting asthma and maternal asthma, as well as for maternal allergy to house dust mites, sex, and pets in the child's home during the first year of life.

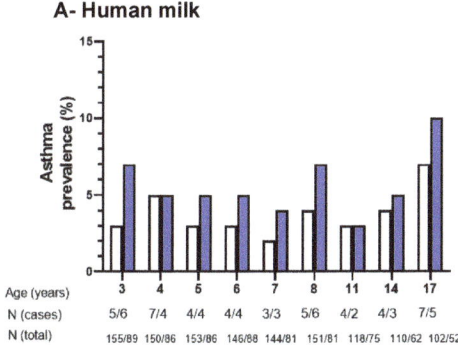

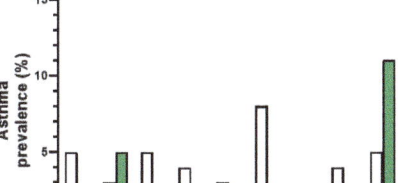

Figure 2. Prevalence of asthma according to the presence of *Der p* 1 in human milk and infant's mattress. Prevalence of asthma in the past 12 months in 3–17-year-old children exposed to non-detectable (empty columns) and detectable (filled column) *Der p* 1 in human milk (**A**) and mattress dust (**B**). N represents the number of children with asthma symptom (cases) and the total population (total). Fisher's exact test was used to compare the prevalence of asthma between groups.

4. Discussion

The lack of knowledge about the sources of allergen exposure in early life hampers the design of successful strategies for the primary prevention of allergies. Here, we confirm previous findings showing that infant mattress and human milk are sources of HDM allergen (*Der p* 1) exposure in early in life [8,9,11–13,22]. Importantly, our data suggest an increased risk of having high levels of IgE and a trend of increased asthma risk in children breastfed by mothers with detectable *Der p* 1 in human milk, while such an association was not found for *Der p* 1 in infant mattresses. This observation is consistent with previous findings from the French EDEN birth cohort, where a significantly increased risk of allergic sensitization and respiratory allergies was found in children exposed to *Der p* 1 through human milk [8] but was not related to the proxy of infant exposure to *Der p* 1. The lack of association between *Der p* 1 in dust and infant asthma outcomes is also consistent with previous observations within a larger group of PIAMA participants [19] and other cohorts [23]. This provides evidence that *Der p* 1 exposure though human milk may represent an independent factor that influences infant IgE levels and may set infants on a trajectory towards allergy-prone immunity. The causal relation between *Der p* 1 in breastmilk and increased susceptibility to both respiratory and food allergies was previously confirmed in a mouse pre-clinical study [8,11]. By virtue of their proteolytic activity and capacity to activate pattern recognition receptors, *Der p* 1 allergens induced T helper 2 (Th2) immune responses and triggered allergies to both Der p and bystander allergens. [24]. This may explain why we mainly found an increase in total IgE but not *Der p*-specific IgE.

Interestingly, the odds ratio for having high levels of serum IgE in relation to *Der p* 1 levels in human milk increased with age. Previous studies showed that breastfeeding may convey some protection from asthma during the first years of life, while the benefit would disappear later on [25]. Sears et al. investigated the long-term outcomes of asthma and atopy in breastfed and non-breastfed infants and demonstrated that breastfeeding increased the risk of allergic sensitization to common respiratory allergens from 13 to 21 years and doubled the risk of asthma from 9 years until adulthood [26]. Another study that investigated the long-term effects of exclusive breastfeeding on allergic outcomes in a cohort of 8583 children showed that breastfeeding was protective against asthma at 7 years of age, but this risk was reversed by the age of 14 years, becoming a consistent risk factor until 44 years in infants from atopic mothers [27]. The mechanisms underlying such a long-term association of breastfeeding with developing allergies are currently unknown. We can speculate that *Der p* 1 in human milk may set infants on a trajectory where subsequent gene–environment interactions will lead to the development of allergies.

Even though the total level of IgE was shown to be an important predictor of asthma in population-based studies [28,29] a limitation of our study is the relatively small sample size and consequently the small number of children with asthma outcomes. Moreover, because of the small sample size, we could account for a limited set of potential confounders only (the same as in previous analyses for consistency) [19]. We therefore cannot rule out residual confounding. This prevents us from drawing a firm conclusion for the relevant sources of *Der p* 1 exposure regarding asthma risk, and this stresses the need for larger prospective studies to replicate our findings.

In conclusion, *Der p* 1 exposure through human milk was associated with high levels of IgE in children, while exposure through mattress dust was not. This observation may explain the current lack of consensus on the role of early-life mite allergen exposure in infant allergic symptoms and markers [23]. Since earlier findings suggest that *Der p* 1 content in the indoor environment is not related to the presence of *Der p* 1 in human milk [22], human milk should be included as an independent source of early-life *Der p* 1 exposure in research investigating strategies for allergy prevention.

While there is no doubt that breastfeeding is the most powerful way to prevent infectious diseases and reduce child mortality [30], its effects on allergy prevention are controversial [30–32]. By identifying which factors in breastmilk are protective for allergy and learning how to modulate them, we will make breastmilk more able to prevent allergic diseases.

Supplementary Materials: The following supporting information can be downloaded at: https://www.mdpi.com/article/10.3390/nu14102095/s1, Table S1: Associations between having a high level of IgE and the presence of Der p 1 in human milk and infant's mattress dust. Figure S1: Prevalence of *Der p* sensitization in children according to the presence of *Der p* 1 in human milk.

Author Contributions: P.M. contributed to *Der p* 1 quantification in human milk, performed the analysis and interpretation of data, and wrote the manuscript with V.V., U.G. and A.H.W., who were the principal investigators of the PIAMA study and contributed to the design, follow-up and data collection of the PIAMA study. A.H.W. initiated and coordinated the collection of the human milk samples. U.G. carried out the statistical analyses for this study and contributed to the data interpretation. A.R. performed *Der p* 1 quantification in human milk and contributed to data analysis and interpretation. V.V. proposed and conceived this study, contributed to data analysis and supervised the project realization. All authors approved the final manuscript as submitted and agreed to be accountable for all aspects of the work. All authors have read and agreed to the published version of the manuscript.

Funding: The PIAMA study received funding from the Netherlands Organization for Health Research and Development; the Netherlands Organization for Scientific Research, the Netherlands Asthma Fund; the Netherlands Ministry of Spatial Planning, Housing, and the Environment; and the Netherlands Ministry of Health, Welfare, and Sport. This work was supported by the Institut National de la Santé et Recherche Médicale (INSERM), the Université de Nice Sophia-Antipolis (UNS), and the University of Western Australia.

Institutional Review Board Statement: The study was conducted in accordance with the Declaration of Helsinki and approved by the Institutional Review Boards: Start of project—Ethic Committee Name: Rotterdam, MEC (Medisch Ethische Commisie Erasmus Universiteit Rotterdam/Academische Ziekenhuizen Rotterdam), Approval Code: 132.636/1994/39, Approval Date: 13 June 1994; Ethic Committee Name: Rotterdam, MEC (Medisch Ethische Commisie Erasmus Universiteit Rotterdam/Academische Ziekenhuizen Rotterdam), Approval Code: 137.326/1994/130, Approval Date: 16 February 1995; Ethic Committee Name: Groningen, MEC (Medisch Ethische Commisie Academisch ziekenhuis Groningen), Approval Code: 94/08/92, Approval Date: 26 August 1994; Ethic Committee Name: Utrecht/Bilthoven, MEC-TNO (Medisch Ethische Commisie -Toegepast Natuurwetenschappelijk Onderzoek), Approval Code: 95/50, Approval Date: 28 February 1996. Aged 4 years—Ethic Committee Name: Utrecht, CCMO (Centrale Commissie Mensgebonden Onderzoek), Approval Code: P000777C, Approval Date: 25 September 2000. Age 8 years: Ethic Committee Name: Utrecht, CCMO (Centrale Commissie Mensgebonden Onderzoek), Approval Code: P04.0071C, Approval Date: 5 August 2004; Ethic Committee Name: Utrecht, METC (Medisch Ethische Toetsings Commissie), Approval Code: 04-101 / K, Approval Date: 27 July 2004; Ethic Committee Name: Rotterdam, MEC (Medisch Ethische Commisie Erasmus Universiteit Rotterdam), Approval Code: P04.0071C/MEC 2004-152, Approval Date: 1 July 2004; Ethic Committee Name: Groningen, MEC (Medisch Ethische Commisie Academisch ziekenhuis Groningen), Approval Code: P04.0071C/ M 4.019912, Approval Date: 28 June 2004. Aged 12 years—Ethic Committee Name: Utrecht, METC (Medisch Ethische Toetsings Commissie), Approval Code: 07-337/K, Approval Date: 20 May 2008. Aged 16 years—Ethic Committee Name: Utrecht, METC (Medisch Ethische Toetsings Commissie), Approval Code: 12-019/K, Approval Date: 25 May 2012 (Amendement 1, 12 July 2012/Amendement 2, 20 September 2012); Ethic Committee Name: Groningen, METC (Medisch Ethische Toetsings Commissie), Approval Code: 12-019/K, Approval Date: Amendement, 16 August 2012.

Informed Consent Statement: Informed consent was obtained from parents or legal guardians of all subjects involved in the study.

Data Availability Statement: Not applicable.

Acknowledgments: The authors would like to thank the PIAMA participants who contributed to the study. They would also like to thank Marieke Oldenwening, Ada Wolse and Marjan Tewis for their contributions to the data collection and data management. We thank Lieke van den Elsen for the critical reading of the manuscript.

Conflicts of Interest: Patricia Macchiaverni, Ulrike Gehring, Akila Rekima, Alet. H. Wijga and Valerie Verhasselt declare no conflicts of interest. The funders had no role in the design of the study; in the collection, analyses, or interpretation of data; in the writing of the manuscript, or in the decision to publish the results.

References

1. Galli, S.J.; Tsai, M.; Piliponsky, A.M. The development of allergic inflammation. *Nature* **2008**, *454*, 445–454. [CrossRef] [PubMed]
2. Lack, G.; Fox, D.; Northstone, K.; Golding, J. Avon Longitudinal Study of Parents and Children Study Team Factors associated with the development of peanut allergy in childhood. *N. Engl. J. Med.* **2003**, *348*, 977–985. [CrossRef] [PubMed]
3. Du Toit, G.; Sampson, H.A.; Plaut, M.; Burks, A.W.; Akdis, C.A.; Lack, G. Food allergy: Update on prevention and tolerance. *J. Allergy Clin. Immunol.* **2018**, *141*, 30–40. [CrossRef] [PubMed]
4. Verhasselt, V.; Genuneit, J.; Metcalfe, J.R.; Tulic, M.K.; Rekima, A.; Palmer, D.J.; Prescott, S.L. Ovalbumin in breastmilk is associated with a decreased risk of IgE-mediated egg allergy in children. *Allergy* **2020**, *75*, 1463–1466. [CrossRef]
5. Verhasselt, V.; Milcent, V.; Cazareth, J.; Kanda, A.; Fleury, S.; Dombrowicz, D.; Glaichenhaus, N.; Julia, V. Breast milk-mediated transfer of an antigen induces tolerance and protection from allergic asthma. *Nat. Med.* **2008**, *14*, 170–175. [CrossRef]
6. Serhan, N.; Basso, L.; Sibilano, R.; Petitfils, C.; Meixiong, J.; Bonnart, C.; Reber, L.L.; Marichal, T.; Starkl, P.; Cenac, N.; et al. House dust mites activate nociceptor-mast cell clusters to drive type 2 skin inflammation. *Nat. Immunol.* **2019**, *20*, 1435–1443. [CrossRef]
7. Miller, J.D. The Role of Dust Mites in Allergy. *Clin. Rev. Allergy Immunol.* **2019**, *57*, 312–329. [CrossRef]
8. Baiz, N.; Macchiaverni, P.; Tulic, M.K.; Rekima, A.; Annesi-Maesano, I.; Verhasselt, V.; Group, E.M.-C.C.S. Early oral exposure to house dust mite allergen through breast milk: A potential risk factor for allergic sensitization and respiratory allergies in children. *J. Allergy Clin. Immunol.* **2017**, *139*, 369–372.e310. [CrossRef]
9. Rekima, A.; Bonnart, C.; Macchiaverni, P.; Metcalfe, J.; Tulic, M.K.; Halloin, N.; Rekima, S.; Genuneit, J.; Zanelli, S.; Medeiros, S.; et al. A role for early oral exposure to house dust mite allergens through breastmilk in IgE-mediated food allergy susceptibility. *J. Allergy Clin. Immunol.* **2020**, *145*, 1416–1429. [CrossRef]
10. Gough, L.; Sewell, H.F.; Shakib, F. The proteolytic activity of the major dust mite allergen Der p 1 enhances the IgE antibody response to a bystander antigen. *Clin. Exp. Allergy* **2001**, *31*, 1594–1598. [CrossRef]
11. Macchiaverni, P.; Rekima, A.; Turfkruyer, M.; Mascarell, L.; Airouche, S.; Moingeon, P.; Adel-Patient, K.; Condino-Neto, A.; Annesi-Maesano, I.; Prescott, S.L.; et al. Respiratory allergen from house dust mite is present in human milk and primes for allergic sensitization in a mouse model of asthma. *Allergy* **2014**, *69*, 395–398. [CrossRef]
12. Macchiaverni, P.; Ynoue, L.H.; Arslanian, C.; Verhasselt, V.; Condino-Neto, A. Early Exposure to Respiratory Allergens by Placental Transfer and Breastfeeding. *PLoS ONE* **2015**, *10*, e0139064. [CrossRef] [PubMed]
13. Macchiaverni, P.; Rekima, A.; van den Elsen, L.; Renz, H.; Verhasselt, V. Allergen shedding in human milk: Could it be key for immune system education and allergy prevention? *J. Allergy Clin. Immunol.* **2021**, *148*, 679–688. [CrossRef]
14. Renz, H.; Adkins, B.D.; Bartfeld, S.; Blumberg, R.S.; Farber, D.L.; Garssen, J.; Ghazal, P.; Hackam, D.J.; Marsland, B.J.; McCoy, K.D.; et al. The neonatal window of opportunity-early priming for life. *J. Allergy Clin. Immunol.* **2018**, *141*, 1212–1214. [CrossRef] [PubMed]
15. Brunekreef, B.; Smit, J.; de Jongste, J.; Neijens, H.; Gerritsen, J.; Postma, D.; Aalberse, R.; Koopman, L.; Kerkhof, M.; Wilga, A.; et al. The prevention and incidence of asthma and mite allergy (PIAMA) birth cohort study: Design and first results. *Pediatr. Allergy Immunol.* **2002**, *13*, 55–60. [CrossRef] [PubMed]
16. Wijga, A.; Houwelingen, A.C.; Smit, H.A.; Kerkhof, M.; Vos, A.P.; Neijens, H.J.; Brunekreef, B.; Study, P.B.C. Fatty acids in breast milk of allergic and non-allergic mothers: The PIAMA birth cohort study. *Pediatr. Allergy Immunol.* **2003**, *14*, 156–162. [CrossRef]
17. Tulic, M.K.; Vivinus-Nebot, M.; Rekima, A.; Rabelo Medeiros, S.; Bonnart, C.; Shi, H.; Walker, A.; Dainese, R.; Boyer, J.; Vergnolle, N.; et al. Presence of commensal house dust mite allergen in human gastrointestinal tract: A potential contributor to intestinal barrier dysfunction. *Gut* **2016**, *65*, 757–766. [CrossRef]
18. Van Strien, R.T.; Koopman, L.P.; Kerkhof, M.; Spithoven, J.; de Jongste, J.C.; Gerritsen, J.; Neijens, H.J.; Aalberse, R.C.; Smit, H.A.; Brunekreef, B. Mite and pet allergen levels in homes of children born to allergic and nonallergic parents: The PIAMA study. *Environ. Health Perspect.* **2002**, *110*, A693–A698. [CrossRef]
19. Gehring, U.; de Jongste, J.C.; Kerkhof, M.; Oldewening, M.; Postma, D.; van Strien, R.T.; Wijga, A.H.; Willers, S.M.; Wolse, A.; Gerritsen, J.; et al. The 8-year follow-up of the PIAMA intervention study assessing the effect of mite-impermeable mattress covers. *Allergy* **2012**, *67*, 248–256. [CrossRef]
20. Pinart, M.; Benet, M.; Annesi-Maesano, I.; von Berg, A.; Berdel, D.; Carlsen, K.C.; Carlsen, K.H.; Bindslev-Jensen, C.; Eller, E.; Fantini, M.P.; et al. Comorbidity of eczema, rhinitis, and asthma in IgE-sensitised and non-IgE-sensitised children in MeDALL: A population-based cohort study. *Lancet Respir. Med.* **2014**, *2*, 131–140. [CrossRef]
21. Wijga, A.H.; Kerkhof, M.; Gehring, U.; de Jongste, J.C.; Postma, D.S.; Aalberse, R.C.; Wolse, A.P.; Koppelman, G.H.; van Rossem, L.; Oldewening, M.; et al. Cohort profile: The prevention and incidence of asthma and mite allergy (PIAMA) birth cohort. *Int. J. Epidemiol.* **2014**, *43*, 527–535. [CrossRef] [PubMed]
22. Macchiaverni, P.; Gehring, U.; Rekima, A.; Wijga, A.; Verhasselt, V. House dust mites: Does a clean mattress mean Der p 1-free breastmilk? *Pediatr. Allergy Immunol.* **2020**, *31*, 990–993. [CrossRef]

23. Custovic, A.; Murray, C.S.; Simpson, A. Dust-mite inducing asthma: What advice can be given to patients? *Expert Rev. Respir. Med.* **2019**, *13*, 929–936. [CrossRef] [PubMed]
24. Jacquet, A.; Robinson, C. Proteolytic, lipidergic and polysaccharide molecular recognition shape innate responses to house dust mite allergens. *Allergy* **2020**, *75*, 33–53. [CrossRef]
25. Dogaru, C.M.; Nyffenegger, D.; Pescatore, A.M.; Spycher, B.D.; Kuehni, C.E. Breastfeeding and childhood asthma: Systematic review and meta-analysis. *Am. J. Epidemiol.* **2014**, *179*, 1153–1167. [CrossRef]
26. Sears, M.R.; Greene, J.M.; Willan, A.R.; Taylor, D.R.; Flannery, E.M.; Cowan, J.O.; Herbison, G.P.; Poulton, R. Long-term relation between breastfeeding and development of atopy and asthma in children and young adults: A longitudinal study. *Lancet* **2002**, *360*, 901–907. [CrossRef]
27. Matheson, M.C.; Erbas, B.; Balasuriya, A.; Jenkins, M.A.; Wharton, C.L.; Tang, M.L.; Abramson, M.J.; Walters, E.H.; Hopper, J.L.; Dharmage, S.C. Breast-feeding and atopic disease: A cohort study from childhood to middle age. *J. Allergy Clin. Immunol.* **2007**, *120*, 1051–1057. [CrossRef]
28. Sunyer, J.; Anto, J.M.; Castellsague, J.; Soriano, J.B.; Roca, J. Total serum IgE is associated with asthma independently of specific IgE levels. The Spanish Group of the European Study of Asthma. *Eur. Respir. J.* **1996**, *9*, 1880–1884. [CrossRef]
29. Sonntag, H.J.; Filippi, S.; Pipis, S.; Custovic, A. Blood Biomarkers of Sensitization and Asthma. *Front. Pediatr.* **2019**, *7*, 251. [CrossRef]
30. Victora, C.G.; Bahl, R.; Barros, A.J.; Franca, G.V.; Horton, S.; Krasevec, J.; Murch, S.; Sankar, M.J.; Walker, N.; Rollins, N.C.; et al. Breastfeeding in the 21st century: Epidemiology, mechanisms, and lifelong effect. *Lancet* **2016**, *387*, 475–490. [CrossRef]
31. de Silva, D.; Halken, S.; Singh, C.; Muraro, A.; Angier, E.; Arasi, S.; Arshad, H.; Beyer, K.; Boyle, R.; du Toit, G.; et al. Preventing food allergy in infancy and childhood: Systematic review of randomised controlled trials. *Pediatr. Allergy Immunol.* **2020**, *31*, 813–826. [CrossRef] [PubMed]
32. Gungor, D.; Nadaud, P.; LaPergola, C.C.; Dreibelbis, C.; Wong, Y.P.; Terry, N.; Abrams, S.A.; Beker, L.; Jacobovits, T.; Jarvinen, K.M.; et al. Infant milk-feeding practices and food allergies, allergic rhinitis, atopic dermatitis, and asthma throughout the life span: A systematic review. *Am. J. Clin. Nutr.* **2019**, *109*, 772S–799S. [CrossRef] [PubMed]

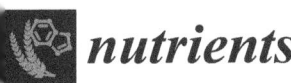

Article

Direct Binding of Bovine IgG-Containing Immune Complexes to Human Monocytes and Their Putative Role in Innate Immune Training

Mojtaba Porbahaie [1], Huub F. J. Savelkoul [1], Cornelis A. M. de Haan [2], Malgorzata Teodorowicz [1] and R. J. Joost van Neerven [1,3,*]

[1] Cell Biology and Immunology, Wageningen University & Research, 6708 WD Wageningen, The Netherlands
[2] Virology Division, Infectious Diseases and Immunology, Utrecht University, 3584 CS Utrecht, The Netherlands
[3] FrieslandCampina, 3818 LE Amersfoort, The Netherlands
* Correspondence: joost.vanneerven@wur.nl

Citation: Porbahaie, M.; Savelkoul, H.F.J.; de Haan, C.A.M.; Teodorowicz, M.; van Neerven, R.J.J. Direct Binding of Bovine IgG-Containing Immune Complexes to Human Monocytes and Their Putative Role in Innate Immune Training. *Nutrients* 2022, 14, 4452. https://doi.org/10.3390/nu14214452

Academic Editor: Rosa Casas

Received: 19 August 2022
Accepted: 20 October 2022
Published: 22 October 2022

Publisher's Note: MDPI stays neutral with regard to jurisdictional claims in published maps and institutional affiliations.

Copyright: © 2022 by the authors. Licensee MDPI, Basel, Switzerland. This article is an open access article distributed under the terms and conditions of the Creative Commons Attribution (CC BY) license (https://creativecommons.org/licenses/by/4.0/).

Abstract: Bovine milk IgG (bIgG) was shown to bind to and neutralize the human respiratory synovial virus (RSV). In animal models, adding bIgG prevented experimental RSV infection and increased the number of activated T cells. This enhanced activation of RSV-specific T cells may be explained by receptor-mediated uptake and antigen presentation after binding of bIgG-RSV immune complexes (ICs) with FcγRs (primarily CD32) on human immune cells. This indirect effect of bIgG ICs on activation of RSV-specific T cells was confirmed previously in human T cell cultures. However, the direct binding of ICs to antigen-presenting cells has not been addressed. As bovine IgG can induce innate immune training, we hypothesized that this effect could be caused more efficiently by ICs. Therefore, we characterized the expression of CD16, CD32, and CD64 on (peripheral blood mononuclear cells (PBMCs), determined the optimal conditions to form ICs of bIgG with the RSV preF protein, and demonstrated the direct binding of these ICs to human CD14$^+$ monocytes. Similarly, bIgG complexed with a murine anti-bIgG mAb also bound efficiently to the monocytes. To evaluate whether the ICs could induce innate immune training more efficiently than bIgG itself, the resulted ICs, as well as bIgG, were used in an in vitro innate immune training model. Training with the ICs containing bIgG and RSV preF protein—but not the bIgG alone—induced significantly higher TNF-α production upon LPS and R848 stimulation. However, the preF protein itself nonsignificantly increased cytokine production as well. This may be explained by its tropism to the insulin-like growth factor receptor 1 (IGFR1), as IGF has been reported to induce innate immune training. Even so, these data suggest a role for IgG-containing ICs in inducing innate immune training after re-exposure to pathogens. However, as ICs of bIgG with a mouse anti-bIgG mAb did not induce this effect, further research is needed to confirm the putative role of bIgG ICs in enhancing innate immune responses in vivo.

Keywords: immune complex; trained immunity; RSV; bovine IgG; preF protein

1. Introduction

Consumption of raw cow's milk has been shown to be associated with a lower prevalence of asthma and hay fever and even reduced respiratory tract infections in a single study [1,2]. On the other hand, cow's milk is a major cause of food allergy in approximately 1–4% of very young children [3]. Cow's milk contains several immunomodulatory proteins that can support the immune system of humans [4–7]. Bovine IgG or bIgG is one of the major bovine milk proteins that is thought to contribute to the inverse association of raw milk consumption with respiratory tract infections and allergies [8–10]. In the gastrointestinal tract or the tonsillar crypts in Waldeyer's ring, dietary components may come into direct contact with respiratory pathogens from the nasal cavity after swallowing [11,12]. This implies that bIgG can directly encounter bacteria and viruses and form immune complexes

(IC). After uptake into the mucosal tissue, these ICs can interact with receptors on immune cells such as neutrophils and macrophages, which phagocytose and eliminate the pathogen. Moreover, upon internalization of ICs, monocytes and dendritic cells (DCs) can process and present antigenic pathogen-derived peptides to T lymphocytes [7,13].

IgG is known to interact with a conserved family of transmembrane glycoproteins known as Fc gamma receptors (FcγRs) [14,15]. On human immune and non-immune cells, three classes of FcγRs are expressed with different affinities for IgG subclasses: high-affinity (10^{-9} M Kd) FcγRI (CD64), and low-affinity (10^{-6} M Kd) FcγRII (CD32) and FcγRIII (CD16) [16,17]. The high-affinity CD64 is predominantly occupied by endogenous serum IgG monomers in vivo [17] and plays a critical role in antibody-dependent cellular phagocytosis (ADCP) in myeloid phagocytes [18]. IgG monomers do not bind to CD32, and only ICs comprising several IgGs bound to antigens can bind to and interact with these low-affinity receptors [19,20]. Along with CD64, CD32 is essential for ADCP by neutrophils and macrophages and also in the process of antigen presentation to the naive T cells by DCs [21–23]. The lower affinity of CD32 for IgG monomers ensures that the antibodies' effector function is only initiated in the presence of a pathogen-derived antigen, preventing an aberrant immune response in the presence of normal levels of antibodies in vivo. CD16, another low-affinity FcγR, is primarily involved in eliminating infected cells via antibody-dependent cellular cytotoxicity (ADCC), mainly mediated by natural killer (NK) cells [21]. Apart from these classical FcγRs, it is known that the neonatal Fc receptor (FcRn) can interact with IgG. FcRn enables the transfer of maternal IgG to the fetus via the placenta, conferring passive immunity to the offspring [24]. FcRn also mediates the salvaging of internalized IgG from degradation through a pH-dependent cellular recycling mechanism [25]. In addition, it was demonstrated that FcRn is important for the internalization of IgG ICs—but not monomers—and the process of antigen presentation by antigen presenting cells (APCs) [26,27].

It has been established that bIgG binds to several human pathogens, including respiratory syncytial virus (RSV) [7,13,28]. Although neutralization of RSV was noted in in vitro studies, the effect of bovine IgG on actual RSV infection that occurs in the nasal cavity cannot be expected; rather, an increased immune response upon re-infection with RSV is anticipated. RSV is one of the most common causes of respiratory tract infections (RTIs) in newborns, which also increases the risk of later-life health complications such as asthma [29,30]. The F protein of RSV is crucial in binding to and infecting human cells, and breast milk preF protein-specific antibodies are a correlate of protection in infants [31]. In addition to binding to and neutralizing human RSV, bIgG facilitates FcγRII-mediated internalization of bIgG-coated pathogens by human neutrophils, monocytes, and DCs [13]. Nederend et al. recently demonstrated that bIgG could neutralize RSV in an in vitro cellular infection model, as did human intravenous immunoglobulin (IVIg) and the prophylactic RSV-specific monoclonal antibody, palivizumab [28]. The latter was more than 100-fold more effective compared to human IV-Ig, and even more compared to bovine IgG, as was expected for a monoclonal antibody. However, as palivizumab is an injection treatment, the clinical efficacy of bIgG cannot be inferred from these findings. Interestingly, the authors showed that activation of RSV preF protein (preF)-specific CD4$^+$ and CD8$^+$ T cells was strongly enhanced in the presence of bovine IgG [28]. They concluded that the interaction between ICs and (activating) FcγRII on autologous monocytes resulted in higher antigen presentation and T cell activation. Moreover, bIgG was found to be protective against experimental RSV infection in mice [28]. Likewise, dietary supplementation of mice with bovine colostrum, a preparation very rich in bIgG, was shown to decrease RSV infection rates and increase the number of CD69$^+$, IFN-γ producing CD8$^+$ T cells [32].

Interestingly, bIgG may also contribute to the resistance against (viral) infections by inducing trained innate immunity in FcγR bearing monocytes [33,34]. This mechanism leads to enhanced cytokine production of innate immune cells after stimulation with Toll-like receptor (TLR) ligands [35,36]. In this concept, primary exposure to the training agent leads to a more robust secondary response to the same and related TLR stimulation. The underlying training mechanism for β-glucans—a compound with established training potential—was shown to be via the engagement of the Dectin-1 receptor and downstream signaling events, including the Raf-1 pathway [37,38]. Following activation of the Dectin-1 receptor, epigenetic alterations in the cells occur by trimethylation of the H3K4 histone protein, a shift in cell metabolism from oxidative phosphorylation to aerobic glycolysis, and consequently, a change in the responsiveness of the cells [39,40]. bIgG has been demonstrated to induce innate immune training resulting in increased production of IL-6 and TNF-α in human monocytes in vitro upon TLR stimulation [33,34].

As monomeric IgG does not interact with low-affinity IgG receptors, we hypothesized that the training effects of bIgG might be induced more efficiently by multimeric IgG immune complexes. To address this question, we studied the direct binding of bovine IgG to human monocytes in the presence or absence of the RSV preF protein or anti-bIgG (α-bIgG) antibodies. We established optimal rations between bIgG and the RSV preF and α-bIgG for efficient binding and tested whether these immune complexes could induce innate immune training.

2. Materials and Methods

2.1. PBMC Isolation

PBMCs were isolated from buffy coats (Sanquin blood bank, Nijmegen) or the fresh blood of donors collected at the Wageningen University blood collection center after obtaining written consent. Gradient centrifugation on Ficoll Paque Plus (GE Healthcare, 17-1440-02, Chicago, IL, USA) was used to isolate PBMCs. Ficoll (15 mL/tube) was transferred to Leucosep tubes (Greiner Bio-One, #227290, Monroe, NC, USA), and the tubes were spun down briefly. Blood samples were added to the tubes after being diluted 1:1 with warm (37 °C) phosphate-buffered saline (PBS) (Gibco, #20012027, Cincinnati, OH, USA). After centrifugation, the PBMCs fraction on top of the porous barrier was transferred to new 50 mL Falcon tubes (Corning, #352070, Corning, NY, USA). Warm PBS was added to wash the cells, and the tubes were spun down. The diluted plasma was discarded, and the cell pellet was resuspended after centrifugation. Following the third wash, the cells were resuspended in RPMI 1640 (Gibco, #61870010, Cincinnati, OH, USA).

2.2. Reagents

Bovine Immunoglobulin G (bIgG) was isolated from bovine colostrum and provided by FrieslandCampina. Expression and purification of a DSCav1-like [41] prefusion-stabilized recombinant soluble RSV F protein (preF) were described previously [42]. Monoclonal anti-bovine IgG antibody (α-bIgG) (Sigma-Aldrich, #B6901, St. Louis, MO, USA) was used for bIgG IC formation. For bIgG detection by flow cytometry, AlexaFlour 647 conjugated goat anti-bovine IgG (Jackson ImmunoResearch, #101-605-165, Ely, Cambridgeshire, UK) was applied.

2.3. FcγR Expression

The expression of various FcγRs was characterized on different immune cells within the PBMC fraction. PBMCs were stained with fluorochrome-conjugated antibodies (Table 1) for immune cell phenotyping. T- and B-cells, monocytes, mDCs, and pDCs were identified, and the FcγRI (CD64), FcγRII (CD32), and FcγRIII (CD16) expression levels were measured. In brief, 1×10^6 cells were plated in a NUNC plate (ThermoFisher, #267245, Cincinnati, OH, USA) and washed with cold (4 °C) FACS buffer (PBS supplemented with 2.5 mM ethylenediaminetetraacetic acid (EDTA) and 0.05% sodium azide). The cells were then stained with the antibody mixture, and the plate was incubated for 30 min at 4 °C in the dark. Then, the cells were washed with two changes of cold FACS buffer, spinning and discarding the supernatant after each wash. After resuspending the cells in FACS buffer, they were measured on CytoFLEX LX (Beckman Coulter, #C11186, Indianapolis, IN, USA), and the generated data were analyzed using FlowJo (FlowJo LLC, v9, Ashland, OR, USA).

The gating strategy for selecting different cell subsets and assessing FcγR expression is described in the supplementary data (Figure S1).

Table 1. Antibody panel used for peripheral blood mononuclear cell (PBMC) phenotyping and assessing the expression of FcγRs.

Antibody	Fluorochrome	Host/Isotype	Clone	Company	Catalog Number
α-CD3	PE-Cy5	Mouse/IgG1	UCHT1	BD	555,334
α-CD11c	BV421	Mouse/IgG1	3.9	Biolegend	301,628
α-CD14	APC-H7	mouse/IgG2b	MφP9	BD	560,180
α-CD19	FITC	Mouse/IgG1	HIB19	BD	555,412
α-CD123	BV605	mouse/IgG2a	7G3	BD	564,197
α-HLA-DR	BV510	mouse/IgG2a	L243	Biolegend	307,646
α-CD64	APC	mouse/IgG1	10.1	Biolegend	305,014
α-CD32	PerCp-Cy5.5	mouse/IgG2b	FUN-2	Biolegend	303,216
α-CD16	PE	mouse/IgG1	B73.1	BD	332,779

Detection of bIgG and bIgG-immune complexes bound to monocytes.

Freshly isolated PBMCs were subjected to various concentrations of bIgG to confirm the binding of bIgG to the monocytes. PBMCs were incubated at 4 °C for 20 min with bIgG (500, 50, 5, and 0 µg/mL) and then were stained with goat AlexaFlour 647 conjugated anti-bovine IgG (Jackson ImmunoResearch, #101-605-165, Ely, Cambridgeshire, UK) and anti-CD14 (Biolegend, #301830, San Diego, CA, USA) for 30 min at 4 °C in the dark. Next, the cells were washed twice with cold FACS buffer. FACS buffer was added, the plate was spun down, and the supernatant was discarded after each centrifugation. The cells were then resuspended in FACS buffer before being analyzed on a CytoFLEX LX flow cytometer. The data were analyzed using FlowJo, and the median fluorescence intensity (MFI) of the bIgG signal was determined on the CD14$^+$ cells (Figure S2 for gating strategy).

To determine the optimal antibody: antigen ratio for the formation of large immune complexes (ICs), bIgG was titrated while keeping the concentration of the antigen constant. Increasing concentrations of bIgG were incubated with respiratory syncytial virus (RSV) preF. As the first step and to dispose of antibody aggregates and obtain monomeric forms, the bIgG stock was spun down (17× g, RT, 15 min), and the supernatant was used for downstream experiments. bIgG at concentrations of 100, 30, 10, 3, 1, 0.3, 0.1, and 0 µg/mL were made using the serial dilution method and combined 1:1 with PreF protein (50 µg/mL) on a sterile NUNC plate. The plate was wrapped in plastic foil and was pre-incubated at 37 °C for 60 min to allow IC formation. After incubation, the plate was cooled down, and the mixture was exposed to freshly isolated PBMCs (3×10^5/well). The plate was wrapped in foil and was incubated in the fridge (4 °C) for 60 min to allow the binding of ICs to the cells. The cells were washed with cold FACS buffer to remove the unbound antibody/antigen residuals following the incubation. The cells were then stained with anti-bIgG (Jackson ImmunoResearch, #101-605-165, Ely, Cambridgeshire, UK) and also anti-CD14 antibody (Biolegend, #325606, San Diego, CA, USA) for monocyte identification. The same bIgG concentrations but without preF protein (bIgG only) and preF protein alone were included as the experiment controls and background values. Cells were subsequently measured using a CytoFLEX LX flow cytometer, the data were processed using FlowJo, and graphs from the bIgG detection MFI were created using MS Excel (MS Office 365). The experiments were performed with two replicates of the same condition and were repeated with the blood of at least three different donors.

A similar approach was applied to identify the optimal ratio between bIgG and mouse anti-bovine IgG monoclonal antibody (α-bIgG) (Sigma-Aldrich, #B6901, St. Louis, MO, USA). The aim was to use a monoclonal antibody with a higher specificity against bIgG.

Various bIgG concentrations (100, 30, 10, 3, 1, 0.3, 0.1, and 0 μg/mL) were incubated with two concentrations of α-bIgG (5 and 1 μg/mL) and the data were handled the same as RSV PreF protein, as described above. The blood samples from at least three donors were used for the titration assays of bIgG and α-bIgG. The optimal antibody: antigen ratio determined in these assays was then utilized in subsequent innate immune training experiments.

2.4. Innate Immune Training

The ability of generated ICs to enhance monocyte responses was evaluated in an in vitro innate immune training model [43]. PBMCs were isolated, and CD14$^+$ monocytes were negatively selected and trained as described elsewhere [33,34]. RPMI 1640 medium (Gibco, #A1049101, Cincinnati, OH, USA) and 100 μg/mL of whole glucan particle (WGP) (InvivoGen, #tlrl-wgp, San Diego, CA, USA) were applied as the experiment negative and positive controls, respectively. The training was done with preF protein only (50 μg/mL), bIgG only (10 μg/mL), and their corresponding immune complexes (ICs) comprised of bIgG: preF as described earlier. In addition, α-bIgG only (5 μg/mL), bIgG only (3 μg/mL), and bIgG: α-bIgG immune complexes (ICs) were also used separately as the training compounds. After training and resting, the cells were stimulated with either 10 pg/mL of LPS (TLR4 ligand) (Sigma-Aldrich, #L2880, St. Louis, MO, USA) or 5 ng/mL of R848 (TLR7/8 ligand) (InvivoGen, #tlrl-r848, San Diego, CA, USA). Cytometric bead array (CBA) and individual cytokines Flex Sets were used for measuring IL-6 (BD, #558276, Franklin Lakes, NJ, USA) and TNF-α (BD, #558273, Franklin Lakes, NJ, USA) in the culture supernatant of the cells (supplementary Figure S3). The experiments were performed with the PBMCs isolated from 7–10 donors.

2.5. Statistical Analysis

CBA data were analyzed by FCAP Array (BD Biosciences, v3.0, Franklin Lakes, NJ, USA) and then were transferred to GraphPad Prism (GraphPad Software, v9, San Diego, CA, USA) for statistical analysis and preparing the figures. The data were normalized and are expressed as fold changes relative to the untrained monocytes (control group- RPMI 1640). The Wilcoxon matched-pairs signed-ranks test was used for head-to-head comparisons, and for multiple comparisons, the Friedman test was utilized to compare different groups with the control. The differences were considered significant when the p-value was <0.05 (*), or <0.01 (**), as indicated in the graphs.

3. Results

3.1. FcγR Expression

To study the relative expression of FcγRs on immune cells, we determined the expression levels of the CD16, CD32, and CD64 on the surface of monocytes, mDC, pDC, and B- and T lymphocytes (Summarized in Table 2). FcγRIII (CD16) was highly expressed on a subset of mDCs (Figure S4A), whereas it was only present on a small percentage (less than 5%) of monocytes, and CD16 was not detected on T- and B cells and on pDCs (Figure S4A). While FcγRII (CD32) expression was high on monocytes and B lymphocytes, this receptor was not present on T cells and pDCs (Figure S4B). CD32 was also present on mDCs; however, the expression levels varied within the mDC subsets (Figure S4B). Monocytes highly expressed FcγRI (CD64); however, in contrast, this receptor was absent on T- and B cells and pDCs (Figure S4C). The expression levels of CD64 on mDCs varied considerably (Figure S4C).

Although indirect immunological effects of bIgG on monocytes and other cell types was described previously [14], the direct binding of bIgG to monocytes has not formally been demonstrated. To demonstrate the binding of bovine IgG to human monocytes, a range of bIgG concentrations was allowed to bind to human PBMCs, washed to remove non-bound bIgG, and binding to monocytes was detected by flow cytometry using AlexaFlour 647-conjugated anti-bovine IgG antibody. Monocytes were selected since they highly express CD32, the same FcγR that bIgG was shown to bind [13]. Bovine IgG showed a dose-dependent binding to human monocytes, especially at high bIgG concentrations (Figure 1A,B). As we had previously noted the presence of some aggregated bIgG on native-PAGE, this binding at high bIgG concentrations might be related to the aggregated bIgG. The presence of bIgG aggregates before centrifugation and their removal by centrifugation is shown in Figure S5. In this figure, the apparent aggregates of IgG are clearly visible in the starting material as in the pellet, but not in the supernatant after centrifugation. Although these data are not quantitative, the difference between the supernatant and pellet fraction indicate the presence of aggregates, as well as the fact that they are (at least partially) depleted by centrifugation prior to use.

Table 2. Direct binding of bIgG and bIgG-immune complexes to monocytes.

Cell Type	FcγRIII (CD16)	FcγRII (CD32)	FcγRI (CD64)
T cells	−	−	−
B cells	−	+	−
Monocytes	+/−	+	+
mDCs	+/−	+	(+)
pDCs	−	−	−

+, the receptor is expressed on the cell; −, the receptor is not expressed on the cell; +/−, the receptor is expressed on a subset of the cell; (+), different levels of receptor expression.

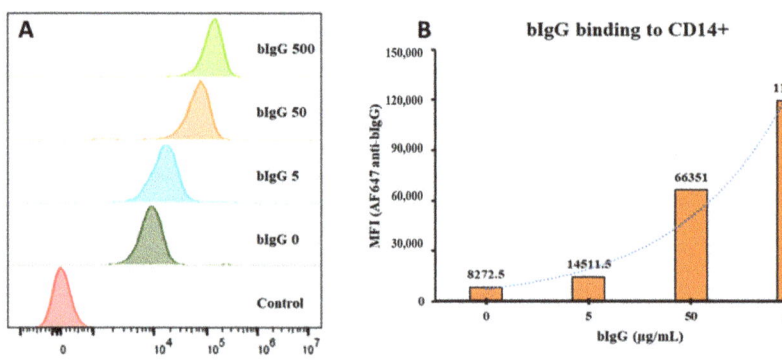

Figure 1. Histogram comparing the mean fluorescence intensity (MFI) of the bovine IgG (bIgG) signal on CD14$^+$ monocytes: Peripheral blood mononuclear cells (PBMCs) were incubated with bIgG (500, 50, 5, or 0 µg/mL) for 20 min (**A**). A dose-dependent increase in the bIgG signal on the CD14$^+$ monocytes was detected with an increase in the concentration of bIgG used (**B**).

To study if the binding to FcγRs on monocytes is increased by immune complexes, various concentrations of bIgG were preincubated with the RSV preF protein or with a monoclonal anti-bIgG to allow the formation of ICs before exposing them to the PBMCs. As shown in Figure 2A, we noted a dose-dependent binding of bIgG alone to the CD14$^+$ monocytes. However, the combination of bIgG and preF protein (bIgG: preF) showed a higher binding, especially at lower bIgG concentrations used, suggesting that multivalent ICs are formed and bound to the monocytes (Figure 2A). Subtraction of the bIgG signal from the MFI of the bIgG: preF combination (ΔMFI) resulted in a bell-shaped curve suggestive of immune complex binding (Figure 2B). The ΔMFI curve had a peak at 10 µg/mL and 50 µg/mL for bIgG and PreF protein, respectively, indicative of the optimal ratio for the formation of large ICs. We observed comparable findings for additional donors tested, with the bell-shaped curves peaking at 10 µg/mL of bIgG (Figure S6A–D) and the average maximum ΔMFI of about 17k B and Figure S6B,D). The data obtained for the three different donors were thus highly consistent.

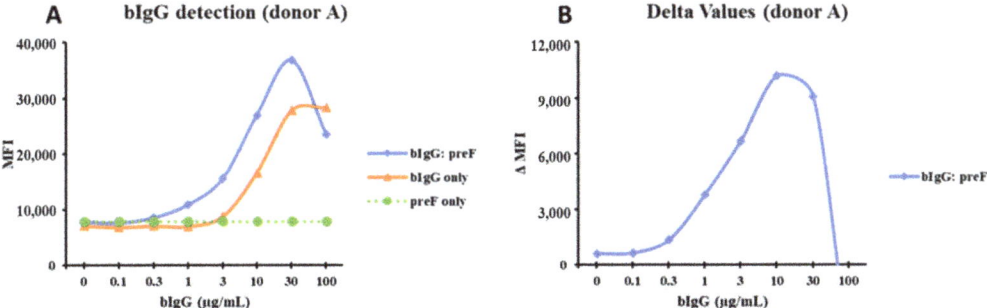

Figure 2. The curves drawn from MFI of the bIgG detection signal: CD14+ monocytes were exposed to bIgG only (0–100 μg/mL), preF protein only (50 μg/mL), and the bIgG: preF ICs in one representative donor (donor A); the MFI was used to generate the detection curve (**A**). The delta MFI (ΔMFI) was produced when the MFI of the bIgG only signal was deducted from the MFI of the bIgG: preF ICs signal (**B**).

As the window between the binding of bIgG: preF ICs and bIgG alone was relatively small, we tried a similar approach by using a monoclonal anti-bIgG (α-bIgG) in the hope that because of the high specificity, the peak of the binding would be at a lower bIgG concentration with even lower bIgG background binding. bIgG bound to human monocytes in a dose-dependent manner, while α-bIgG alone did not show any binding (Figure 3A). However, the combination of bIgG and α-bIgG showed a strong increase in binding to the monocytes suggesting IC formation (Figure 3A). This was true for both α-bIgG concentrations that were used (5 and 1 μg/mL). After subtracting the MFI of bIgG alone from the MFI of the ICs, we obtained bell-shaped curves with a peak at bIgG 3 μg/mL (Figure 3B). Similar results were found for additional donors with the bell-shaped curves, although these donors peaked at a slightly lower concentration of 1 μg/mL of bIgG (Figure S7A–D) and the average maximum ΔMFI of about 40k (Figures 3B and S7B,D). As the optimal concentrations for the formation of large ICs are at 3 and 5 μg/mL for bIgG and α-bIgG antibody, respectively, these concentrations were used in innate immune training experiments.

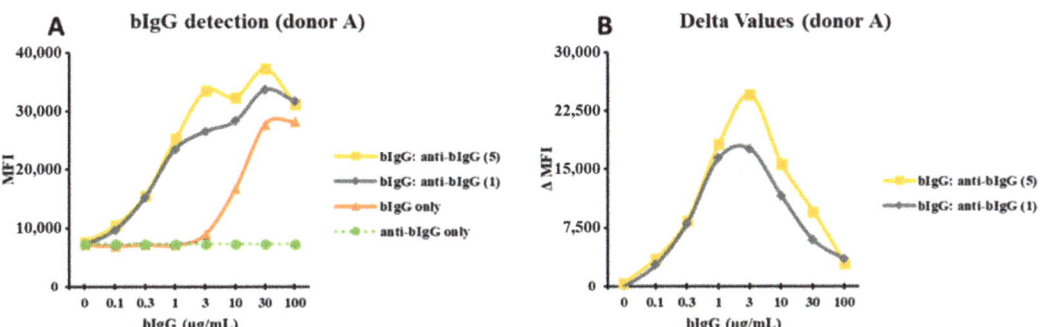

Figure 3. The curves drawn from MFI of the bIgG detection signal: the monocytes were exposed to bIgG only (0–100 μg/mL), α-bIgG (5 μg/mL) only, α-bIgG only (1 μg/mL), and the bIgG: α-bIgG ICs in one representative donor (donor A) (**A**). The delta MFI (ΔMFI) was produced when the MFI of the bIgG only signal was deducted from the MFI of the bIgG: α-bIgG ICs signal (**B**).

3.2. BIgG-Containing Immune Complexes and Innate Immune Training

Based on the above findings, we used the optimal ratios of bovine IgG to RSV preF protein or α-bIgG to study if these immune complexes could induce innate immune training in vitro at concentrations at which bIgG itself had no effect in this model. The generated

ICs were allowed to bind to freshly isolated CD14+ monocytes for 24 hrs, after which the training compounds were removed by washing and resting for 6 days. After this resting period, the cells were stimulated with TLR4 (LPS) or TLR7/8 (R848) ligands. Then, 24-h supernatants were collected, and the levels of IL-6 and TNF-α were measured by CBA.

Whole glucan particles (WGP) were used as a positive control for training, as described by Moerings et al. [44]. The cells trained with WGP produced a significantly higher amount of IL-6 and TNF-α in the culture supernatant upon re-stimulation with LPS (Figure 4A,B). We obtained similar results when stimulating the cells with R848, and the cells trained with WGP produced significantly more IL-6 (Figure 4C) and TNF-α (Figure 4D) than untrained cells.

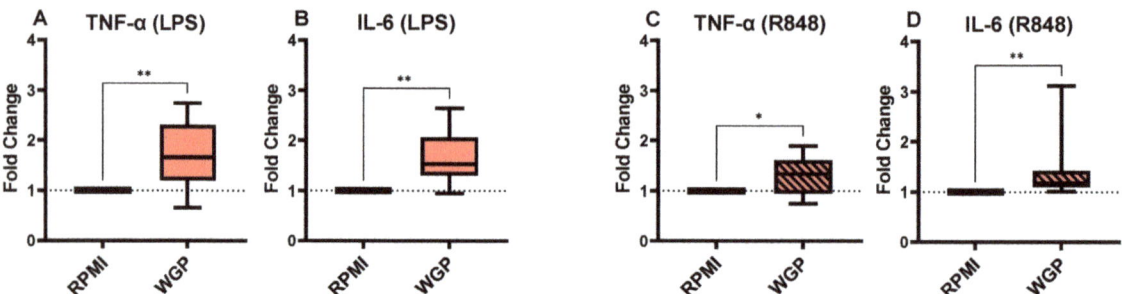

Figure 4. The fold changes in TNF-α (**A**) and IL-6 (**B**) production of the cells trained with WGP and stimulated with LPS in comparison to the untrained control. The TNF-α (**C**) and IL-6 (**D**) production fold changes for WGP-trained monocytes after stimulation with R848. The average (range) of cytokines in the RPMI controls of all 8 donors tested were 1805 (719–4825 pg/mL), 3181 (1044–7232 pg/mL), 3592 (1839–7434 pg/mL), and 9047 (3732–14230 pg/mL) for conditions A to D, respectively. The boxes represent 50% of the data, and the line is the median value where upper and lower whiskers present the upper and lower 25% of the data, respectively. The significance of differences is shown as p-value < 0.05 (*) and < 0.01 (**).

Similarly, IL-6 and TNF-α production levels were determined in the supernatants of restimulated monocytes that were trained with RSV preF protein only (50 µg/mL), bIgG only (10 µg/mL), or the ICs of the combination of these. The cells trained with bIgG: preF ICs showed significantly higher (3–4-fold) TNF-α levels compared to the untrained cells, both after stimulation with LPS (Figure 5A) and R848 (Figure 5C). TNF-α levels were not significantly increased in the cells trained with RSV preF protein only or bIgG alone, although some increase was seen in the preF protein group. Despite variation in the responses, all donors exposed to the ICs consistently produced higher levels of TNF-α compared to the untrained monocytes. Even though IL-6 levels were slightly increased after stimulation with the TLR4 ligand LPS (Figure 5B) or TLR7/8 ligand R848 (Figure 5D), this did not reach significance.

The same experimental setup was performed with bIgG: anti-bIgG ICs, evaluating the training potential of monoclonal anti-bIgG alone (5 µg/mL), bIgG alone (3 µg/mL), and the ICs resulted from combining both. As shown in Figure 6, contrary to the bIgG-RSV preF protein IC, no increases in IL-6 and TNF-a were noted. This holds true for stimulation with either LPS (Figure 6A) or R848 (Figure 6C). Similar to TNF-α, we did not observe any significant variation in the production of IL-6 in different conditions. Neither α-bIgG only, bIgG only, nor the ICs could enhance IL-6 production in monocytes after LPS (Figure 6B) or R848 (Figure 6D) stimulation.

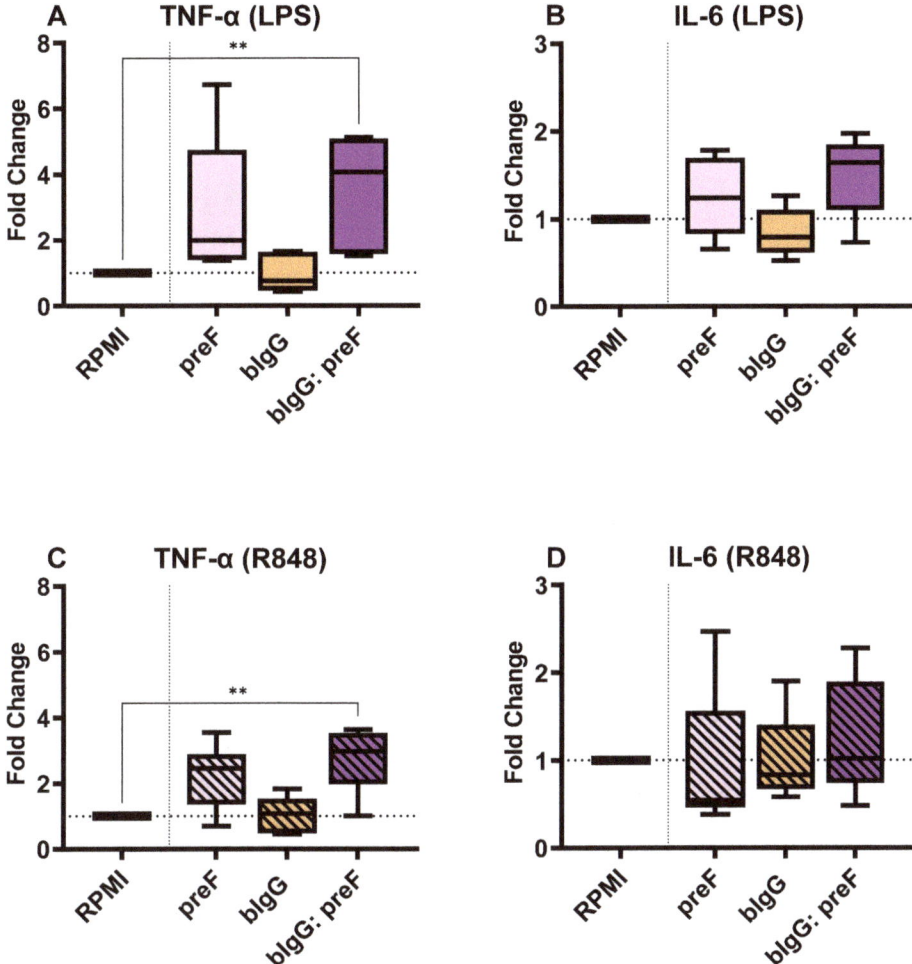

Figure 5. The fold changes in the TNF-α (**A**) and IL-6 (**B**) production in the cells trained with preF only (50 μg/mL) bIgG alone (10 μg/mL), or bIgG: preF ICs compared to untrained monocytes (RPMI) upon stimulation with LPS. Also, the TNF-α (**C**) and IL-6 (**D**) production fold changes compared to the RPMI control in the group of monocytes trained with single components or the bIgG: preF ICs after stimulation with and R848. The average (range) of cytokines in the RPMI controls of all 8 donors tested were 1791 (719–4825 pg/mL), 3522 (1044–7232 pg/mL), 3181 (1839–7434 pg/mL), and 9840 (3732–14,230 pg/mL) for conditions A to D, respectively. The boxes represent 50% of the data, and the line is the median value where upper and lower whiskers present the upper and lower 25% of the data, respectively. The significance of differences is shown as p-value < 0.01 (**).

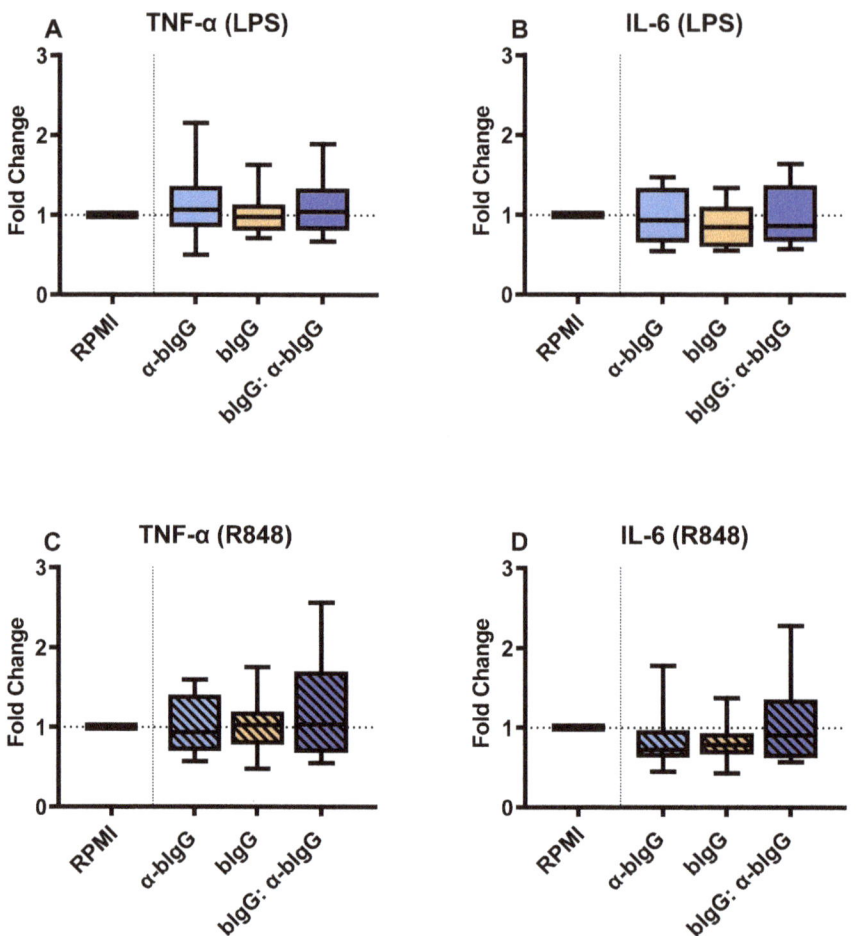

Figure 6. The fold changes in the production of TNF-α (**A**) and IL-6 (**B**) in the cells trained with α-bIgG only (5 μg/mL) only, bIgG alone (3 μg/mL), or bIgG: α-bIgG ICs compared to untrained monocytes (RPMI) upon stimulation with LPS and also TNF-α (**C**) and IL-6 (**D**) production after R848 stimulation. The average (range) of cytokines in the RPMI controls of all 8 donors tested were 1740 (719–4825 pg/mL), 3279 (1044–7232 pg/mL), 3508 (1839–7434 pg/mL), and 8961 (3732–14,230 pg/mL) for conditions A to D, respectively. The boxes represent 50% of the data, and the line is the median value where upper and lower whiskers present the upper and lower 25% of the data, respectively.

4. Discussions

Here, we show that immune complexes comprising bIgG and RSV preF protein can induce innate immune training in human CD14[+] monocytes, while bIgG monomers did not have the same effects. We established and optimized an experimental system for detecting the direct binding of ICs to human monocytes. Using that system, we determined the optimal antibody: antigen ratio for the formation of ICs between bIgG and RSV preF protein, as well as bIgG: α-bIgG, and tested them on the in vitro innate immune training model.

The FcγRII (CD32) family consisting of CD32a, CD32b, and CD32c are key IgG receptors expressed by various leukocytes. While CD32a and CD32c have a tyrosine-based activation motif (ITAM) on their C-terminal cytoplasmic tail mediating the activator signal,

CD32b contains a tyrosine-based inhibitory motif (ITIM) [23]. CD32 expression has been identified in monocytes, DCs, and B cells, as well as neutrophils, eosinophils, basophils, and mast cells [14,23]. Monocytes/macrophages and DCs eminently express CD32a with an ITAM motif, but also CD32b, while B cells exclusively possess the inhibitory CD32b [23]. The interplay between the activator and inhibitory signal regulates the antibody effector functions, including B cell IgG responses, APC maturation, and antigen presentation [45,46]. CD32 expression on monocytes and DCs is essential for their distinct functions, including ADCP for clearing the pathogens, also known as FcγRII-dependent phagocytosis [47,48]. Following the phagocytosis of antibody-opsonized targets, the capacity of DCs for activating naive T cells increases [49]. DCs present the antigen epitopes on major histocompatibility complex class II (MHC-II) molecules, upregulate the expression of costimulatory molecules such as CD80/86 to interact with their T cells counterpart (CD28), and produce cytokines to drive T cell differentiation [50]. However, monomeric forms of IgG do not bind to low-affinity receptors such as CD32. Binding to and crosslinking multiple neighboring CD32 is essential for both FcγR-mediated phagocytosis and initiating the signal via the receptors' ITAM motif [51]. In fact, signaling cascades are activated by immunoreceptor aggregation rather than ligand-induced changes in receptor conformation [51]. In other words, the size matters when it comes to the level of IC binding and interaction with the low-affinity FcγRs, and only large multivalent ICs can bind to CD32 and induce the effector function [20,52]. Large ICs can be formed when an optimal antibody: antigen ratio is present in the environment. When either the antibody or the antigen is in excess, large ICs are not formed, the interaction with CD32 does not occur, and hence, the antibody's effector function is weak [14]. As a result, the concentration-dependent binding of immune complexes to receptors typically results in a bell shaped curve, as confirmed in this paper.

RSV-specific IgG in breast milk was shown to correlate with protection against RSV acute respiratory infection in the first 6 months of life [31]. Bovine milk IgG (bIgG) binds to and can neutralize RSV, a major human pathogen associated with respiratory tract infections, in in vitro infection studies [13]. In addition, bIgG was shown to interact with the FcγRII on human immune cells, which is essential for exerting the antibody effector functions [13,28]. The interaction of bIgG with human immune cells conferred protection against experimental RSV infection in mice and also increased activation of RSV-specific human T cells [28]. The augmented T cell activity at low RSV preF protein levels is an effect resulting from the direct interaction of antigen-bound bIgG (ICs) with APCs. The interaction of IC with APCs enhances antigen presentation to RSV-specific T cells. However, the direct binding of bIgG ICs to APCs has not been shown before. In the current study, we succeeded in generating bIgG and RSV preF protein ICs and demonstrated their direct binding to $CD14^+$ monocytes (Figure 2). The bell-shaped curves on ΔMFI results indicate that large ICs were formed and bound to CD32 on monocytes. The findings are especially important since we show the binding of bIgG ICs to the APC, an intermediate step linking the previously shown bIgG and preF binding with the consequent enhanced T cell response.

The method described here can be applied in future studies as a proxy to identify the optimal bIgG: antigen ratio for IC formation for additional pathogenic molecules, and can also be used to detect IC binding on other immune cells, such as neutrophils and DCs. We selected monocytes to study bIgG ICs binding for a number of reasons. Monocytes and B cells both express a high level of CD32 and the results from $CD19^+$ B cells support the findings from $CD14^+$ cells on optimal bIgG: antigen ratios (data not shown). However, unlike B cells that only express inhibitory CD32b, monocytes eminently express CD32a, which is essential for studying the cell-activating properties of bIgG ICs. This includes the innate immune training model applied in this research, which also has been optimized for monocytes.

It should be noted that the study did not address the relevance of the FcRn receptor in bIgG binding to monocytes because the binding of bovine IgG to human monocytes was reported to be mainly CD32-dependent [13]. However, FcRn is expressed on monocytes, macrophages, and DCs [53], and its role in IgG IC-mediated antigen presentation has been demonstrated [26,27]. As blocking with anti-CD32/CD16 antibodies [13] or anti-CD16/32/64 [54] cannot completely block the binding of bIgG to monocytes and granulocytes, a role for FcRn cannot be excluded.

Concurrent engagement and crosstalk between FcγRs and pattern recognition receptors (PRRs) are critical for identifying and eliminating the pathogen [55,56]. TLRs and C-type lectin receptors (CLRs) are among the PRRs that were found to be involved in this crosstalk, which is necessary for the induction of inflammatory mediators such as IL-6 and TNF-α [55,56]. On the other hand, trained immunity is mediated by the involvement of CLRs, such as Dectin-1, as was demonstrated for β-1, 3-(D)-glucan derived from *Candida albicans* [37]. After training, the quality of cell responses improves, as evidenced by increased IL-6 and TNF-α production in response to TLR re-stimulation [57]. This trained immunity results in enhanced innate immune responses to a wide array of TLR signals, resulting in improved protection against infection. Given that bIgG has been demonstrated to possess training abilities and interact with FcγRs, we hypothesized that these receptors would play a role in monocyte training. Immune complexes internalized via the engagement of FcγRs can stimulate endosomal or cytoplasmic PRRs such as TLRs to further activate the cells [58–62]. If the assumption holds true, ICs may be more potent training-inducing components than bIgG alone.

Although the training effects of bIgG have been demonstrated previously [33,34], the relevance of ICs in the training effects has not been studied. CD64 receptors on monocytes freshly isolated from human blood are occupied by human serum IgG, leaving no room for bIgG monomers to bind. Monomeric forms of bIgG, on the other hand, do not interact with the low-affinity CD32. Therefore, if we assume that the training potential of bIgG is (partly) exerted via interacting with FcγRs, the engagement of bIgG ICs and CD32 is critical. The ICs can crosslink several receptors and induce a much stronger effector signal. Surprisingly, although no antigen was added to the bIgG preparations and, therefore, no ICs are expected, the training effects were still evident in the previous studies [33,34]. The explanation could be within the bIgG stock itself. IgG molecules tend towards aggregation, particularly after (long) storage in the freezer [63]. It is likely that the antibody aggregates present in the bIgG stock have mimicked IC properties and could be responsible for the previously observed training effects of bIgG alone, especially since they used high concentrations of the IgG.

We exposed monocytes to bIgG monomers and bIgG: preF ICs as the training agents to address this hypothesis. The experiment's positive control, WGP (a Dectin-1 agonist with an established training potential [44]), ensured the validity of the model system used. Interestingly, incubation with the ICs increased the TNF-α production in the cells upon TLR stimulation (Figure 5). Pair-wise comparisons showed that IC-trained cells produced 2–4 times higher TNF-α than the untrained cells upon LPS and R848 stimulation. Remarkably, the training effect was not seen for the monomeric forms of the bIgG. This is in line with the fact that the bIgG alone concentration used is too low to induce innate immune training.

Given the increased TNF-α response, it appears that there is a general increase in the vigilance of the monocytes. The heightened response was observed towards not only TLR7/8 activation with R848, but also LPS. The ICs contained RSV preF protein as a viral protein. Interestingly, higher TNF-α levels were also produced by IC-trained cells after stimulation of TLR4 with LPS, a compound found in the membrane of Gram-negative bacteria. A documented aspect of trained immunity is an increase in the responsiveness of the cells to the same but also homologous stimuli [64]. Nevertheless, further research on cells' epigenetic changes and metabolic pathways is required to substantiate this notion.

The monocytes trained with bIgG: preF ICs also produced a relatively higher IL-6 than the untrained cells in response to LPS stimulation (Figure 5B). However, the changes did not reach statistical significance, probably due to higher variation in the response of the donors. In fact, TNF-α was previously described as a better indicator of innate immune training by bIgG than IL-6 [34]. However, the RSV preF protein alone seemed to induce some increase in the production of TNF-a and IL-6 in these assays, although this did not reach significance. Interestingly, the preF protein was recently shown to bind to insulin-like growth factor 1 (IGFR1) for cellular entry [65]. IGF, the natural ligand for this receptor, has been shown to induce innate immune training [66], which can explain why the preF protein by itself has an effect on this model system as well. In addition, viruses and viral proteins may be internalized, given their antigenic nature, without the involvement of antibodies. When they are internalized, they can activate cytoplasmic or endosomal PRRs, inducing inflammatory responses. This fact could also partly explain why monocytes treated with RSV preF alone released more cytokines. More investigation is needed to determine what we described is the reason or whether a contaminant in the preparation caused the effect.

Contrary to our expectations, incubation with IC consisting of bIgG with a murine α-bIgG monoclonal antibody (mAb) did not induce monocyte training (Figure 6). The optimal ratio for bIgG and the α-bIgG antibody to form ICs was identified, and even the average of maximum ΔMFI for the α-bIgG ICs on the three donors tested was more than twice the level of the preF ICs (40k vs. 17k). This difference, in theory, should give a bigger window for the effects of α-bIgG ICs than preF ICs, which was not the case in practice. A possible explanation of these findings is that lower bIgG concentrations were used to generate ICs with α-bIgG than RSV preF protein (3 vs. 10 ug/mL). In addition, it is known that murine IgG does not bind efficiently to human CD32 [19]. This could result in ICs that consist of bIgG, of which the Fc region is mostly blocked by the murine mAb. As a result, in α-bIgG ICs, fewer bIgG molecules may be available to interact with CD32 on the monocytes, which may not result in efficient crosslinking and uptake of the IC. As the binding of the IC was detected with a polyclonal anti-bIgG, higher levels of binding were detected in the FACS analysis of these IC. Another highly likely explanation for no training effects could be the absence of the antigen. IgG bound to antigen likely sends a different signal via FcγRs than an antibody linked to another antibody, possibly due to different IgG Fc glycosylation patterns between the different antibodies used [16,67]. In addition, when the ICs that contain antigens are internalized, other endosomal or cytoplasmic PRRs, such as CLRs and TLRs, may become activated and synergistically complement the FcγRs signal, as discussed earlier. However, further investigation is necessary before ascertaining these claims.

In conclusion, we established a method for detecting the direct binding of bIgG-containing ICs to monocytes by flow cytometry. Our results also indicate that bIgG: preF ICs can induce monocyte training in vitro. The effects could be at least partly mediated by the interaction of bIgG ICs with the CD32 receptors on the monocytes, as this interaction was shown before. However, to formally prove the putative role of bIgG ICs in trained immunity, this has to be investigated with more antigen-bIgG ICs and should be extended to also include human IgG-antigen ICs.

Supplementary Materials: The following supporting information can be downloaded at: https://www.mdpi.com/article/10.3390/nu14214452/s1. Figure S1. The gating strategy to identify T- and B cells, monocytes, mDC, and pDCs. Afterward, CD16, CD32, and CD64 expression levels were determined within each cell population. Figure S2. The gating strategy for selecting the CD14$^+$ monocytes and quantifying the MFI of the bIgG signal. Figure S3. A schematic representation of the in vitro innate immune training model. CD14$^+$ monocytes were isolated from the buffy coats, exposed to the training compounds for 24 h, and rested for six days to differentiate into macrophages. Then the cells were stimulated for 24 h with TLR ligands (LPS and R848), and the production of IL-6 and TNF-α was quantified in the culture supernatant of the cells. Figure S4. Histograms showing the relative expression of CD16 (A), CD32 (B), and CD64 (C) on T- and B lymphocytes, monocytes, mDCs, and pDCs cells within the PBMC fraction. See Supplementary Figure S1 regarding the gating strategy for PBMC immunophenotyping. Figure S5. Native-PAGE gel from bIgG samples. The bIgG stock was spun down to remove the aggregates. Different concentrations (1000, 100, 10 μg/mL) of the stock itself, the supernatant after centrifugation, and the pellet were prepared in a non-reducing non-denaturing sample buffer (without SDS) and were loaded on the 4-15% 4–15% Mini-PROTEAN TGX Precast Protein Gel (Bio-RAD #456-1083). The gel was run at 110v for 75 min. The silver staining was used to stain the gel. Figure S6. The curves drawn from MFI of the bIgG detection signal:

The generation of bIgG detection curve for bIgG only, preF protein only, and the bIgG: preF ICs on monocytes of two selected donors (A & C). The delta MFI values resulted from the deduction of bIgG background values from the ICs curve (B & D). Figure S7. The curves drawn from MFI of the bIgG detection signal: bIgG detection curves were generated for bIgG only, α-bIgG (5 μg/mL) only, α-bIgG (1 μg/mL) only, and the ICs on monocytes of two selected donors (A & C). The delta MFI values resulted from the deduction of bIgG background values from the ICs curve (B & D).

Author Contributions: Conceptualization, R.J.J.v.N. and M.P.; methodology, M.P.; investigation, M.P.; writing—original draft preparation, M.P.; writing—review and editing, all authors; supervision, R.J.J.v.N. and M.T. All authors have read and agreed to the published version of the manuscript.

Funding: M.P. was funded by an unrestricted grant from FrieslandCampina.

Institutional Review Board Statement: Not applicable.

Informed Consent Statement: Not applicable.

Data Availability Statement: The data presented in this study are available on request from the corresponding author.

Conflicts of Interest: R.J.J.v.N. is employed by FrieslandCampina. All other authors have nothing to declare.

References

1. Wopereis, H.; Oozeer, R.; Knipping, K.; Belzer, C.; Knol, J. The first thousand days–Intestinal microbiology of early life: Establishing a symbiosis. *Pediatr. Allergy Immunol.* **2014**, *25*, 428–438. [CrossRef] [PubMed]
2. Alduraywish, S.A.; Lodge, C.J.; Campbell, B.; Allen, K.J.; Erbas, B.; Lowe, A.J.; Dharmage, S.C. The march from early life food sensitization to allergic disease: A systematic review and meta-analyses of birth cohort studies. *Allergy* **2016**, *71*, 77–89. [CrossRef] [PubMed]
3. Du Toit, G.; Sampson, H.A.; Plaut, M.; Burks, A.W.; Akdis, C.A.; Lack, G. Food allergy: Update on prevention and tolerance. *J. Allergy Clin. Immunol.* **2018**, *141*, 30–40. [CrossRef]
4. Chen, K.; Chai, L.; Li, H.; Zhang, Y.; Xie, H.-M.; Shang, J.; Tian, W.; Yang, P.; Jiang, A.C. Effect of bovine lactoferrin from iron-fortified formulas on diarrhea and respiratory tract infections of weaned infants in a randomized controlled trial. *Nutrition* **2016**, *32*, 222–227. [CrossRef]
5. Abbring, S.; Hols, G.; Garssen, J.; van Esch, B.C.A. Raw cow's milk consumption and allergic diseases—The potential role of bioactive whey proteins. *Eur. J. Pharmacol.* **2019**, *843*, 55–65. [CrossRef] [PubMed]
6. van Esch, B.C.A.M.; Porbahaie, M.; Abbring, S.; Garssen, J.; Potaczek, D.P.; Savelkoul, H.F.J.; van Neerven, R.J.J. The Impact of Milk and Its Components on Epigenetic Programming of Immune Function in Early Life and Beyond: Implications for Allergy and Asthma. *Front. Immunol.* **2020**, *11*, 2141. [CrossRef] [PubMed]
7. Ulfman, L.H.; Leusen, J.H.W.; Savelkoul, H.F.J.; Warner, J.O.; van Neerven, R.J.J. Effects of Bovine Immunoglobulins on Immune Function, Allergy, and Infection. *Front. Nutr.* **2018**, *5*, 52. [CrossRef]
8. van Neerven, R.J.J.; Knol, E.F.; Heck, J.M.L.; Savelkoul, H.F.J. Which factors in raw cow's milk contribute to protection against allergies? *J. Allergy Clin. Immunol.* **2012**, *130*, 853–858. [CrossRef]
9. Perdijk, O.; Van Splunter, M.; Savelkoul, H.F.J.; Brugman, S.; Van Neerven, R.J.J. Cow's Milk and Immune Function in the Respiratory Tract: Potential Mechanisms. *Front. Immunol.* **2018**, *9*, 143. [CrossRef]
10. van Neerven, J. The effects of milk and colostrum on allergy and infection: Mechanisms and implications. *Anim. Front.* **2014**, *4*, 16–22. [CrossRef]
11. van Kempen, M.J.P.; Rijkers, G.T.; van Cauwenberge, P.B. The Immune Response in Adenoids and Tonsils. *Int. Arch. Allergy Immunol.* **2000**, *122*, 8–19. [CrossRef] [PubMed]
12. Govers, C.; Calder, P.C.; Savelkoul, H.F.J.; Albers, R.; van Neerven, R.J.J. Ingestion, Immunity, and Infection: Nutrition and Viral Respiratory Tract Infections. *Front. Immunol.* **2022**, *13*, 841532. [CrossRef] [PubMed]
13. Hartog, G.D.; Jacobino, S.; Bont, L.; Cox, L.; Ulfman, L.H.; Leusen, J.H.W.; van Neerven, R.J.J. Specificity and Effector Functions of Human RSV-Specific IgG from Bovine Milk. *PLoS ONE* **2014**, *9*, e112047. [CrossRef]
14. Lu, L.L.; Suscovich, T.J.; Fortune, S.M.; Alter, G. Beyond binding: Antibody effector functions in infectious diseases. *Nat. Rev. Immunol.* **2017**, *18*, 46. [CrossRef]
15. Bournazos, S.; Gupta, A.; Ravetch, J.V. The role of IgG Fc receptors in antibody-dependent enhancement. *Nat. Rev. Immunol.* **2020**, *20*, 633–643. [CrossRef] [PubMed]
16. Hayes, J.M.; Wormald, M.R.; Rudd, P.M.; Davey, G.P. Fc gamma receptors: Glycobiology and therapeutic prospects. *J. Inflamm. Res.* **2016**, *9*, 209–219. [CrossRef] [PubMed]
17. Nimmerjahn, F.; Ravetch, J.V. Fcγ receptors as regulators of immune responses. *Nat. Rev. Immunol.* **2008**, *8*, 34. [CrossRef]

18. Swisher, J.F.A.; Feldman, G.M. The many faces of FcγRI: Implications for therapeutic antibody function. *Immunol. Rev.* **2015**, *268*, 160–174. [CrossRef]
19. Bruhns, P. Properties of mouse and human IgG receptors and their contribution to disease models. *Blood* **2012**, *119*, 5640–5649. [CrossRef]
20. Bruhns, P.; Iannascoli, B.; England, P.; Mancardi, D.A.; Fernandez, N.; Jorieux, S.; Daëron, M. Specificity and affinity of human Fcγ receptors and their polymorphic variants for human IgG subclasses. *Blood* **2009**, *113*, 3716–3725. [CrossRef]
21. Chen, X.; Song, X.; Li, K.; Zhang, T. FcγR-Binding Is an Important Functional Attribute for Immune Checkpoint Antibodies in Cancer Immunotherapy. *Front. Immunol.* **2019**, *10*, 292. [CrossRef] [PubMed]
22. Holgado, M.P.; Sananez, I.; Raiden, S.; Geffner, J.R.; Arruvito, L. CD32 Ligation Promotes the Activation of CD4+ T Cells. *Front. Immunol.* **2018**, *9*, 2814. [CrossRef] [PubMed]
23. Anania, J.C.; Chenoweth, A.M.; Wines, B.D.; Hogarth, P.M. The Human FcγRII (CD32) Family of Leukocyte FcR in Health and Disease. *Front. Immunol.* **2019**, *10*, 464. [CrossRef] [PubMed]
24. Simister, N.E. Placental transport of immunoglobulin G. *Vaccine* **2003**, *21*, 3365–3369. [CrossRef]
25. Ober, R.J.; Martinez, C.; Vaccaro, C.; Zhou, J.; Ward, E.S. Visualizing the Site and Dynamics of IgG Salvage by the MHC Class I-Related Receptor, FcRn. *J. Immunol.* **2004**, *172*, 2021–2029. [CrossRef] [PubMed]
26. Qiao, S.-W.; Kobayashi, K.; Johansen, F.-E.; Sollid, L.M.; Andersen, J.T.; Milford, E.; Roopenian, D.C.; Lencer, W.I.; Blumberg, R.S. Dependence of antibody-mediated presentation of antigen on FcRn. *Proc. Natl. Acad. Sci. USA* **2008**, *105*, 9337–9342. [CrossRef]
27. Weflen, A.W.; Baier, N.; Tang, Q.-J.; Hof, M.V.D.; Blumberg, R.S.; Lencer, W.I.; Massol, R.H. Multivalent immune complexes divert FcRn to lysosomes by exclusion from recycling sorting tubules. *Mol. Biol. Cell* **2013**, *24*, 2398–2405. [CrossRef]
28. Nederend, M.; Van Stigt, A.H.; Jansen, J.H.M.; Jacobino, S.R.; Brugman, S.; De Haan, C.A.M.; Bont, L.J.; Van Neerven, R.J.J.; Leusen, J.H.W. Bovine IgG Prevents Experimental Infection With RSV and Facilitates Human T Cell Responses to RSV. *Front. Immunol.* **2020**, *11*, 1701. [CrossRef]
29. Mohapatra, S.S.; Boyapalle, S. Epidemiologic, Experimental, and Clinical Links between Respiratory Syncytial Virus Infection and Asthma. *Clin. Microbiol. Rev.* **2008**, *21*, 495–504. [CrossRef]
30. Régnier, S.A.; Huels, J. Association Between Respiratory Syncytial Virus Hospitalizations in Infants and Respiratory Sequelae: Systematic Review and Meta-analysis. *Pediatr. Infect. Dis. J.* **2013**, *32*, 820–826. [CrossRef]
31. Mazur, N.I.; Horsley, N.M.; A Englund, J.; Nederend, M.; Magaret, A.; Kumar, A.; Jacobino, S.R.; Haan, C.A.M.D.; Khatry, S.K.; LeClerq, S.C.; et al. Breast Milk Prefusion F Immunoglobulin G as a Correlate of Protection Against Respiratory Syncytial Virus Acute Respiratory Illness. *J. Infect. Dis.* **2018**, *219*, 59–67. [CrossRef] [PubMed]
32. Xu, M.L.; Kim, H.J.; Wi, G.R.; Kim, H.-J. The effect of dietary bovine colostrum on respiratory syncytial virus infection and immune responses following the infection in the mouse. *J. Microbiol.* **2015**, *53*, 661–666. [CrossRef] [PubMed]
33. van Splunter, M.; van Osch, T.L.J.; Brugman, S.; Savelkoul, H.F.J.; Joosten, L.A.B.; Netea, M.G.; van Neerven, R.J.J. Induction of Trained Innate Immunity in Human Monocytes by Bovine Milk and Milk-Derived Immunoglobulin G. *Nutrients* **2018**, *10*, 1378. [CrossRef] [PubMed]
34. Hellinga, A.H.; Tsallis, T.; Eshuis, T.; Triantis, V.; Ulfman, L.H.; Van Neerven, R.J.J. In Vitro Induction of Trained Innate Immunity by bIgG and Whey Protein Extracts. *Int. J. Mol. Sci.* **2020**, *21*, 9077. [CrossRef]
35. Netea, M.G.; Joosten, L.A.B.; Latz, E.; Mills, K.H.G.; Natoli, G.; Stunnenberg, H.G.; O'Neill, L.A.J.; Xavier, R.J. Trained immunity: A program of innate immune memory in health and disease. *Science* **2016**, *352*, 6284. [CrossRef]
36. Divangahi, M.; Aaby, P.; Khader, S.A.; Barreiro, L.B.; Bekkering, S.; Chavakis, T.; van Crevel, R.; Curtis, N.; DiNardo, A.R.; Dominguez-Andres, J.; et al. Trained immunity, tolerance, priming and differentiation: Distinct immunological processes. *Nat. Immunol.* **2021**, *22*, 2–6. [CrossRef]
37. Quintin, J.; Saeed, S.; Martens, J.H.A.; Giamarellos-Bourboulis, E.J.; Ifrim, D.C.; Logie, C.; Jacobs, L.; Jansen, T.; Kullberg, B.J.; Wijmenga, C.; et al. Candida albicans infection affords protection against reinfection via functional reprogramming of monocytes. *Cell Host Microbe* **2012**, *12*, 223–232. [CrossRef]
38. Domínguez-Andrés, J.; Joosten, L.A.B.; Netea, M.G. Induction of innate immune memory: The role of cellular metabolism. *Curr. Opin. Immunol.* **2019**, *56*, 10–16. [CrossRef]
39. Miyake, Y.; Toyonaga, K.; Mori, D.; Kakuta, S.; Hoshino, Y.; Oyamada, A.; Yamada, H.; Ono, K.-I.; Suyama, M.; Iwakura, Y.; et al. C-type Lectin MCL Is an FcRγ-Coupled Receptor that Mediates the Adjuvanticity of Mycobacterial Cord Factor. *Immunity* **2013**, *38*, 1050–1062. [CrossRef]
40. Cheng, S.-C.; Quintin, J.; Cramer, R.A.; Shepardson, K.M.; Saeed, S.; Kumar, V.; Giamarellos-Bourboulis, E.J.; Martens, J.H.A.; Rao, N.A.; Aghajanirefah, A.; et al. mTOR- and HIF-1α-mediated aerobic glycolysis as metabolic basis for trained immunity. *Science* **2014**, *345*, 1250684. [CrossRef]
41. McLellan, J.S.; Chen, M.; Joyce, M.G.; Sastry, M.; Stewart-Jones, G.B.E.; Yang, Y.; Zhang, B.; Chen, L.; Srivatsan, S.; Zheng, A.; et al. Structure-Based Design of a Fusion Glycoprotein Vaccine for Respiratory Syncytial Virus. *Science* **2013**, *342*, 592–598. [CrossRef] [PubMed]
42. Widjaja, I.; Wicht, O.; Luytjes, W.; Leenhouts, K.; Rottier, P.J.M.; van Kuppeveld, F.J.M.; Haijema, B.J.; de Haan, C.A.M. Characterization of Epitope-Specific Anti-Respiratory Syncytial Virus (Anti-RSV) Antibody Responses after Natural Infection and after Vaccination with Formalin-Inactivated RSV. *J. Virol.* **2016**, *90*, 5965–5977. [CrossRef] [PubMed]

43. Domínguez-Andrés, J.; Arts, R.J.; Bekkering, S.; Bahrar, H.; Blok, B.A.; de Bree, L.C.J.; Bruno, M.; Bulut, Ö.; Debisarun, P.A.; Dijkstra, H.; et al. In vitro induction of trained immunity in adherent human monocytes. *STAR Protoc.* **2021**, *2*, 100365. [CrossRef] [PubMed]
44. Moerings, B.G.J.; de Graaff, P.; Furber, M.; Witkamp, R.F.; Debets, R.; Mes, J.J.; van Bergenhenegouwen, J.; Govers, C. Continuous Exposure to Non-Soluble β-Glucans Induces Trained Immunity in M-CSF-Differentiated Macrophages. *Front. Immunol.* **2021**, *12*, 672796. [CrossRef] [PubMed]
45. Hjelm, F.; Carlsson, F.; Getahun, A.; Heyman, B. Antibody-Mediated Regulation of the Immune Response. *Scand. J. Immunol.* **2006**, *64*, 177–184. [CrossRef]
46. van Erp, E.A.; Luytjes, W.; Ferwerda, G.; van Kasteren, P.B. Fc-Mediated Antibody Effector Functions During Respiratory Syncytial Virus Infection and Disease. *Front. Immunol.* **2019**, *10*, 548. [CrossRef]
47. Tay, M.Z.; Wiehe, K.; Pollara, J. Antibody-Dependent Cellular Phagocytosis in Antiviral Immune Responses. *Front. Immunol.* **2019**, *10*, 332. [CrossRef]
48. Underhill, D.M.; Goodridge, H.S. Goodridge, Information processing during phagocytosis. Nature reviews. *Immunology* **2012**, *12*, 492–502.
49. Boross, P.; van Montfoort, N.; Stapels, D.A.C.; van der Poel, C.E.; Bertens, B.; Meeldijk, J.; Jansen, J.H.M.; Verbeek, J.S.; Ossendorp, F.; Wubbolts, R.; et al. FcRγ-chain ITAM signaling is critically required for cross-presentation of soluble antibody-antigen complexes by dendritic cells. *J. Immunol.* **2014**, *193*, 5506–5514. [CrossRef]
50. Pennock, N.; White, J.T.; Cross, E.W.; Cheney, E.E.; Tamburini, B.A.; Kedl, R.M. T cell responses: Naive to memory and everything in between. *Adv. Physiol. Educ.* **2013**, *37*, 273–283. [CrossRef]
51. Jaumouillé, V.; Grinstein, S. Receptor mobility, the cytoskeleton, and particle binding during phagocytosis. *Curr. Opin. Cell Biol.* **2011**, *23*, 22–29. [CrossRef] [PubMed]
52. Lux, A.; Yu, X.; Scanlan, C.N.; Nimmerjahn, F. Impact of Immune Complex Size and Glycosylation on IgG Binding to Human FcγRs. *J. Immunol.* **2013**, *190*, 4315. [CrossRef] [PubMed]
53. Zhu, X.; Meng, G.; Dickinson, B.L.; Li, X.; Mizoguchi, E.; Miao, L.; Wang, Y.; Robert, C.; Wu, B.; Smith, P.D.; et al. MHC class I-related neonatal Fc receptor for IgG is functionally expressed in monocytes, intestinal macrophages, and dendritic cells. *J. Immunol.* **2001**, *166*, 3266–3276. [CrossRef] [PubMed]
54. Kramski, M.; Lichtfuss, G.; Navis, M.; Isitman, G.; Wren, L.; Rawlin, G.; Center, R.J.; Jaworowski, A.; Kent, S.J.; Purcell, D.F.J. Anti-HIV-1 antibody-dependent cellular cytotoxicity mediated by hyperimmune bovine colostrum IgG. *Eur. J. Immunol.* **2012**, *42*, 2771–2781. [CrossRef]
55. van Egmond, M.; Vidarsson, G.; Bakema, J.E. Cross-talk between pathogen recognizing Toll-like receptors and immunoglobulin Fc receptors in immunity. *Immunol. Rev.* **2015**, *268*, 311–327. [CrossRef]
56. Rittirsch, D.; Flierl, M.A.; Day, D.E.; Nadeau, B.A.; Zetoune, F.S.; Sarma, J.V.; Werner, C.M.; Wanner, G.A.; Simmen, H.-P.; Huber-Lang, M.S.; et al. Cross-Talk between TLR4 and FcγReceptorIII (CD16) Pathways. *PLOS Pathog.* **2009**, *5*, e1000464. [CrossRef]
57. Saeed, S.; Quintin, J.; Kerstens, H.H.D.; Rao, N.A.; Aghajanirefah, A.; Matarese, F.; Cheng, S.-C.; Ratter, J.; Berentsen, K.; van der Ent, M.A.; et al. Epigenetic programming of monocyte-to-macrophage differentiation and trained innate immunity. *Science* **2014**, *345*, 1251086. [CrossRef]
58. Means, T.K.; Latz, E.; Hayashi, F.; Murali, M.R.; Golenbock, D.T.; Luster, A.D. Human lupus autoantibody-DNA complexes activate DCs through cooperation of CD32 and TLR9. *J. Clin. Investig.* **2005**, *115*, 407–417. [CrossRef]
59. Bunk, S.; Sigel, S.; Metzdorf, D.; Sharif, O.; Triantafilou, K.; Triantafilou, M.; Hartung, T.; Knapp, S.; von Aulock, S. Internalization and Coreceptor Expression Are Critical for TLR2-Mediated Recognition of Lipoteichoic Acid in Human Peripheral Blood. *J. Immunol.* **2010**, *185*, 3708–3717. [CrossRef]
60. Parcina, M.; Wendt, C.; Goetz, F.; Zawatzky, R.; Zähringer, U.; Heeg, K.; Bekeredjian-Ding, I. *Staphylococcus aureus*-Induced Plasmacytoid Dendritic Cell Activation Is Based on an IgG-Mediated Memory Response. *J. Immunol.* **2008**, *181*, 3823–3833. [CrossRef]
61. Boulé, M.W.; Broughton, C.; Mackay, F.; Akira, S.; Marshak-Rothstein, A.; Rifkin, I.R. Toll-like receptor 9-dependent and -independent dendritic cell activation by chromatin-immunoglobulin G complexes. *J. Exp. Med.* **2004**, *199*, 1631–1640. [CrossRef] [PubMed]
62. Lovgren, T. Induction of interferon-alpha by immune complexes or liposomes containing systemic lupus erythematosus autoantigen-and Sjogren's syndrome autoantigen-associated RNA. *Arthritis Rheumatol.* **2006**, *54*, 1917–1927. [CrossRef] [PubMed]
63. Miller, M.A.; Rodrigues, M.A.; Glass, M.A.; Singh, S.K.; Johnston, K.P.; Maynard, J.A. Frozen-State Storage Stability of a Monoclonal Antibody: Aggregation is Impacted by Freezing Rate and Solute Distribution. *J. Pharm. Sci.* **2013**, *102*, 1194–1208. [CrossRef] [PubMed]
64. Netea, M.G.; van der Meer, J.W.M. Trained Immunity: An Ancient Way of Remembering. *Cell Host Microbe* **2017**, *21*, 297–300. [CrossRef]
65. Griffiths, C.D.; Bilawchuk, L.M.; McDonough, J.E.; Jamieson, K.C.; Elawar, F.; Cen, Y.; Duan, W.; Lin, C.; Song, H.; Casanova, J.-L.; et al. IGF1R is an entry receptor for respiratory syncytial virus. *Nature* **2020**, *583*, 615–619. [CrossRef]

66. Bekkering, S.; Arts, R.J.; Novakovic, B.; Kourtzelis, I.; van der Heijden, C.D.; Li, Y.; Popa, C.D.; ter Horst, R.; van Tuijl, J.; Netea-Maier, R.T.; et al. Metabolic Induction of Trained Immunity through the Mevalonate Pathway. *Cell* **2018**, *172*, 135–146.e9. [CrossRef]
67. Lux, A.; Nimmerjahn, F. *Impact of Differential Glycosylation on IgG Activity*; Springer: New York, NY, USA, 2011.

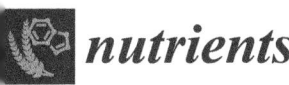

Article

Proposal to Screen for Zinc and Selenium in Patients with IgA Deficiency

Soraya Regina Abu Jamra [1], Camila Gomes Komatsu [2], Fernando Barbosa, Jr. [3], Persio Roxo-Junior [1,*] and Anderson Marliere Navarro [4]

1. Department of Pediatrics, Ribeirão Preto Medical School—University of São Paulo—FMRP/USP, Sao Paulo 05508-090, Brazil; sajamra@hcrp.usp.br
2. Department of Food and Nutrition, Faculty of Pharmaceutical Sciences, São Paulo State University UNESP, Araraquara 14800-060, Brazil; camila_komatsu@yahoo.com.br
3. Laboratory of Toxicology and Metal Essentiality, Faculty of Pharmaceutical Sciences of Ribeirão Preto, University of São Paulo—USP, Sao Paulo 05508-090, Brazil; fbarbosa@fcfrp.usp.br
4. Department of Health Sciences, Division of Nutrition and Metabolism, Ribeirão Preto Medical School—University of São Paulo—FMRP/USP, Sao Paulo 05508-090, Brazil; navarro@fmrp.usp.br
* Correspondence: persiorj@fmrp.usp.br

Abstract: The increase in life expectancy can be a consequence of the world's socioeconomic, sanitary and nutritional conditions. Some studies have demonstrated that individuals with a satisfactory diet variety score present a lower risk of malnutrition and better health status. Zinc and selenium are important micronutrients that play a role in many biochemical and physiological processes of the immune system. Deficient individuals can present both innate and adaptive immunity abnormalities and increased susceptibility to infections. Primary immunodeficiency diseases, also known as inborn errors of immunity, are genetic disorders classically characterized by an increased susceptibility to infection and/or dysregulation of a specific immunologic pathway. IgA deficiency (IgAD) is the most common primary antibody deficiency. This disease is defined as serum IgA levels lower than 7 mg/dL and normal IgG and IgM levels in individuals older than four years. Although many patients are asymptomatic, selected patients suffer from different clinical complications, such as pulmonary infections, allergies, autoimmune diseases, gastrointestinal disorders and malignancy. Knowing the nutritional status as well as the risk of zinc and selenium deficiency could be helpful for the management of IgAD patients. Objectives: to investigate the anthropometric, biochemical, and nutritional profiles and the status of zinc and selenium in patients with IgAD. Methods: in this descriptive study, we screened 16 IgAD patients for anthropometric and dietary data, biochemical evaluation and determination of plasma and erythrocyte levels of zinc and selenium. Results: dietary intake of zinc and selenium was adequate in 75% and 86% of the patients, respectively. These results were consistent with the plasma levels (adequate levels of zinc in all patients and selenium in 50% of children, 25% of adolescents and 100% of adults). However, erythrocyte levels were low for both micronutrients (deficiency for both in 100% of children, 75% of adolescents and 25% of adults). Conclusion: our results highlight the elevated prevalence of erythrocyte zinc and selenium deficiency in patients with IgAD, and the need for investigation of these micronutrients in their follow-up.

Keywords: IgA deficiency; selenium deficiency; zinc deficiency; recommended dietary allowances; immune system

1. Introduction

Growth varies during life and it is recognized as a good indicator of a child's health [1]. Robust evidence has shown the important role of diet in the maintenance of human health, as approximately one in five deaths around the world due to chronic cardiovascular and neoplastic diseases can be attributed to an unhealthy diet [2]. Therefore, to empower people to choose healthy foods and to create healthy environments has become one of the main global objectives of health policies [3].

Optimal nutrition plays a fundamental role in the adequate performance of the immune system. An adequate supply of nutrients is essential for immune cells proliferation and biosynthesis of several immune factors [4]. Micronutrients participate and support every stage of the response against pathogens, and have specific antibacterial and anti-viral functions. Micronutrients also act as substrates for the intestinal microbiota, regulate the immune cell metabolism, protect from oxidative and inflammatory stress and contribute to the production of proteins (antibodies, cytokines, receptors) and new cells [5]. It is well known that proper nutrition can help support optimal immune function, reducing the frequency and severity of infectious diseases. Inadequate dietary intake of some nutrients and malnutrition of a child or an adult can cause chronic inflammation due to dysregulation of the immune response and recurrent infections as a consequence of secondary immunodeficiency [5,6]. Childs et al. [7] have shown that malnourished individuals can present impaired phagocytosis and decreased cytokine production. On the other hand, chronic infection can lead to nutrient deficiencies through reduced appetite, greater consumption and reduced nutrient absorption, resulting in a vicious cycle of malnutrition and infection [8]. Moreover, according to the World Health Organization, there is a synergistic relationship between malnutrition and infection, in which the immune response exacerbates a poor nutritional state and causes an increase in the demand for micronutrients [9]. As a similar form, the hidden hunger, defined as an inadequate micronutrient intake, in contrast to an adequate or even excessive energy consumption, can also compromise the immune response [10]. Thus, an adequate dietary intake rich in some nutrients like protein, copper, iron, selenium and zinc has a significant role in immune health improving the quality of life [4].

Zinc (Zn) is one of the most abundant micronutrients in the human body. As a component of several enzymes and transcription factors, Zn is involved in many biochemical and physiological processes at the molecular, cellular and systemic levels. Zn participates in cell membrane repair, cell proliferation, inflammation, DNA damage response and antioxidant defenses [11]. Deficiency of Zn is related to the pathophysiology of many human conditions, ranging from cancer to neurological disorders, impairment in cognitive function, aging, diabetes, growth retardation and infection [12,13]. Zn also has antioxidant functions and plays a significant role in the maintenance of immune homeostasis. In the innate immune system, Zn is important for phagocytosis; it affects the production of cytokines, the maturation of dendritic cells and the activity of the complement system [14]. Regarding adaptive immunity, Zn influences the formation and function of T cells, as well as the maturation of B cells, and consequently antibody production. Zn is also crucial for the balance between the different T-cell subsets, since its deficiency decreases the production of Th1 cytokines (IFN-γ, IL-2 and TNF-α) that are essential for the adequate response against pathogens [14,15].

Selenium (Se) is present in 25 human selenoproteins involved in a variety of essential biological functions, ranging from the regulation of reactive oxygen species (ROS) to the biosynthesis of hormones [16]. Selenoprotein-mediated biochemical mechanisms play an important role in the clinical outcome of diseases that include cancer, diabetes, viral infections (including SARS-CoV-2 and HIV) and neurological disorders. Se can affect both the adaptive and innate immune systems. Neutrophils, macrophages and natural killer cells (NKs) need Se to function effectively [17]. Se also plays a role as a NF-κB inhibitor, with consequent immune-modulation and anti-inflammatory action [18]. Se deficiency affects the activation and functions of T and B-lymphocytes, as T lymphocytes may be unable to proliferate in response to mitogens, and B lymphocytes may be ineffective to produce IgM and IgG [19]. An appropriate intake of Se might help alleviate oxidative stress and inflammation, and also reduce bacterial and viral infections [17].

The immune system is composed of two parts: the innate (epithelial barriers, lysozyme, interferon, complement, toll-like receptors, NK cells and phagocytes) and the adaptive (T and B lymphocytes and immunoglobulin) responses, which are integrated and cooperate with each other [20].

B-cells are responsible for the humoral immunity, also known as antibody-mediated immunity, through the differentiation into plasma cells that play a role in producing immunoglobulins. B lymphocytes undergo genetic modifications of their immunoglobulin genes to produce highly specific antibodies and five different immunoglobulin isotypes (IgG, IgM, IgA, IgE and IgD) [21]. Two thirds of all immunoglobulin produced by the body is IgA, which has an important influence in both humoral and mucosal immunity [22]. IgA exists in two forms: the monomeric form is free and dominant in the serum, while the dimeric form is wrapped by the secretory component and plays a fundamental role in mucosal immunity. Secretory IgA is more resistant to the proteolytic activity of bacteria, has an anti-inflammatory effect and protects against infectious agents and allergen sensitization, serving as an interface between the body and the microbiome [23].

Primary immunodeficiencies, also known as inborn errors of immunity, are a large and heterogeneous group of genetic diseases that impair the immune system. More than 400 diseases have been described [24]. In general, patients with primary immunodeficiencies are at risk for recurrent, prolonged, and sometimes life-threatening infections caused by several kind of pathogens, including opportunistic agents, autoimmunity, failure to thrive and malignancies [25,26]. An international expert committee composed of pediatric and adult clinical immunologists under the auspices of the International Union of Immunological Societies has provided the clinical and genetic classification of the inborn errors of immunity since 1970. Thus, these diseases are currently categorized into 10 groups, as follows: combined immunodeficiencies; combined immunodeficiencies with syndromic features; predominantly antibody deficiencies; diseases of immune dysregulation; congenital defects of phagocytes; defects in intrinsic and innate immunity; autoinflammatory diseases; complement deficiencies; bone marrow failure; and phenocopies of inborn errors of immunity [24].

Selective IgA deficiency (IgAD) is part of the predominantly antibody deficiencies group. IgAD is the most prevalent inborn error of immunity, with prevalence from about 1:3000 to even 1:150, depending on the population. According to the European Society for Immunodeficiency (ESID), the definition of primary IgAD was established as serum IgA levels less than 7 mg/dL, normal IgG and IgM and the exclusion of other causes of hypogammaglobulinemia in individuals aged over 4 years [27]. Many patients are oligosymptomatic, but less frequently they can present increased susceptibility for recurrent infections, and predisposition for allergies, gastrointestinal, endocrine and autoimmune disorders [22]. IgAD has been associated with lactase deficiency, celiac and Crohn's disease, type 1 diabetes mellitus and rheumatoid arthritis. Allergies are present in 56% of individuals with IgAD, and asthma in 29.8%. Between 25.5 and 31.7% of individuals with IgAD develop systemic lupus erythematosus [22]. An increased risk for infections has been widely reported in individuals with IgAD. The most common infections are upper respiratory tract infections (40–90%), mainly viral, while bacterial infections are less frequent. Gastrointestinal tract infections are also common and include intermittent or chronic diarrhea due to Giardia lamblia [23]. There is no specific treatment for the disease, and management is directed to the clinical manifestations that may arise.

Our hypothesis is that patients with IgAD may have Zn and Se deficiency. Considering the importance of Zn and Se for several functions of the immune system, and the scarcity of previous studies that evaluated this association, the present study aimed to evaluate the nutritional status and the plasma and erythrocyte levels of these micronutrients in patients with IgAD. This assessment may be important for the implementation of changes in dietary behaviors and the possible supplementation of these micronutrients in order to modulate the immune system response and to reduce the susceptibility to infections.

2. Methods

2.1. Study Design

A cross-sectional, retrospective and descriptive study was conducted to evaluate some nutritional aspects of IgAD patients at the Clinics Hospital of Ribeirão Preto Medical School, University of São Paulo, Brazil.

2.2. Participants

Patients aged more than 4 years old with a confirmed diagnosis of selective IgAD, according to the ESID, were included. Age range was defined according to the recommendations of the World Health Organization, whereby children are individuals aged up to 10 years and adolescents are individuals between 10 and 20 years old [28]. Patients were selected among those who attended the Pediatric Allergy Outpatient Clinics at our hospital.

Individuals less than 4 years old, pregnant women, transitory or secondary IgAD, other secondary or primary immunodeficiencies, and the use of immunosuppressants or Zn and Se supplements were excluded.

This study was approved by the Ethics Committee of Clinics Hospital and patients were included after signing the consent and assent term to participate in the research (Protocol HCRP no 14444/2010).

2.3. Dietary Intake

All participants fulfilled a three days form with a detailed description of the ingested quantity and type of foods (food record). Forms were delivered to the participants or their parents. The form was returned during the next routine visit at the Outpatient Clinic. "Programa de apoio a Nutrição da Universidade Paulista de São Paulo "Nut Win" and "Tabela Brasileira de Composição de Alimentos da Universidade de Campinas (TACO-UNICAMP)" were used to estimate the daily intake of Zn and Se, according to the recommendations of the Reference Daily Intake (DRI).

2.4. Anthropometric Evaluation

Weight, height, measurement of triceps, biceps and subscapular skinfold thickness and mid upper arm circumference were performed in all patients. The nutritional status was based according to the classification of body mass index for age (BMI/age) for children and adolescents [29] and to BMI for adults [30]. The measurements of triceps skinfold thickness (TSF) and midarm muscle circumference (MAMC) were standardized according to Lohman [31] and classified according to Frisancho [32].

2.5. Laboratory Evaluation

Immunoglobulin measures were determined by automated nephelometry and repeated three times in different periods to confirm the values.

Zn and Se were measured in plasma and erythrocytes. Whole blood was collected in the morning in metal free tubes after 12 h of fasting.

The micronutrients concentration in plasma and erythrocytes was determined using a plasma couple mass spectrometer equipped with a reaction cell (DRC-ICP-MS ELAN DRCII, Perkin Elmer, Sciex, Norwalk, CT, USA) operating with high purity (99.999%) argon (Praxaair, Brazil). Each sample was diluted in 15 mL Falcon® polypropylene tubes (Becton Dickison) at a 1:50 proportion with a solution containing 0.01%Triton X-100 (v/v), 0.5% HNO3 (v/v) and 10 $\mu g/L^{-1}$ Rh of the internal standard Rh. The analytical calibration standards were prepared at a concentration ranging from 0 to 50 µg/L in the same diluent.

The quality control of the analyses was insured by the analysis of reference materials of the National Public Health Institute of Quebec, Canada. The analyses were carried out in the Laboratory of Toxicology and Essentiality of Metals, Faculty of Pharmaceutical Sciences of Ribeirão Preto, University of São Paulo.

The laboratory tests were carried out in the Central Laboratory of HCFMRP-USP according to standardized methods routinely used in the Institution. Total proteins and fractions were analyzed with the Konelab instrument (Wiener-lab®) and blood count and white cell count were performed using the ABX Pentra DX 120 instrument (HORIBA)®.

2.6. Statistical Analysis

The Shapiro Wilk test was used to assess data normality in the case of continuous variables, and the Kolmogorov Smirnoff test was used to determine the presence of possible associations between the variables of interest. When the normality was not rejected, parametric tests were used (Pearson correlation coefficient), and when there was no normality, nonparametric tests were used (Spearman correlation coefficient) [33].

p-value of less than 0.05 was considered significant. All the statistical analyses were performed with the SPSS (version. 22.0) and R (version. R-3.5.1) software.

3. Results

The study included 16 patients (9M:7F), 4 adults, 8 adolescents and 4 children with a confirmed diagnosis of IgAD. All patients presented at least one infection in the last 12 months and sinusitis was the most common infection. Table 1 shows the baseline demographic characteristics of the 16 patients.

Table 1. Demographic characteristics of the patients.

Variables	n (%)
Sex	
Male	9 (56)
Female	7 (44)
Age Distribution	
Children	4 (25)
Adolescent	8 (50)
Adult	4 (25)
Outpatient infections in the last 12 months	
Acute otitis media	3 (19)
Sinusitis	8 (50)
Diarrhea	5 (31)
Pneumonia	2 (12)
Other	7 (44)

Table 2 shows daily intake of nutrients in means and standard deviation (SD). All patients had an adequate intake of macronutrients according to the DRIs.

Table 2. Daily intake of nutrients of the patients.

	4–10 Years Mean ± SD	11–19 Years Mean ± SD	20–25 Years Mean ± SD
Energy (kcal/day)	1533.3 ± 338.6	1852.5 ± 865.1	2304.1 ± 379.9
DRI (kcal/day)	1759.5 ± 171.5	2272.6 ± 588.5	3193.87 ± 634.3
Protein (g/day)	65.4 ± 20.5	74.8 ± 21.9	100.11 ± 22.6
DRI (g/day)	20.7 ± 4.6	37.9 ± 11.4	58.2 ± 8.3
Protein (%)	16.8 ± 1.9	16.6 ± 4.7	16.6 ± 1.9
DRI (%)	10–35	10–35	10–35
Carbohydrates (%)	57.2 ± 4.9	57.6 ± 5.9	61.3 ± 7.2
DRI (%)	45–65	45–65	45–65
Lipids (%)	26.9 ± 3.1	26.0 ± 1.2	22.5 ± 5.6
DRI (%)	25–35	25–35	20–35
Zn (mg/day)	8.2 ± 2.7	9.8 ± 3.2	11.3 ± 2.6
DRI (mg/day)	4–7 (EAR)	7–8.5 (EAR)	6.8–9.4 (EAR)
Se (µg/day)	64.5 ± 26.1	69.7 ± 21.4	96.7 ± 14.4
DRI (µg/day)	23–35 (EAR)	35–45 (EAR)	45 (EAR)

DRI: Dietary Reference Intake.

As observed in Table 2, 1 child, 2 adolescents and 1 adult had an inadequate intake of Zn, and only 1 adolescent had inadequate intake of Se.

Regarding the nutritional status, 75% of the children had an adequate BMI. Overweight and obesity were observed in 25% and 12,5% of the adolescents, respectively. All adults were classified as overweight or obese (Table 3).

Table 3. Nutritional status of the patients.

Nutritional Status	Groups		
	Children * n (%)	Adolescents * n (%)	Adults ** n (%)
Low weight	1 (25)	-	-
Eutrophy	3 (75)	5 (62)	-
Overweight	-	2 (25)	2 (50)
Obesity	-	1 (12)	2 (50)

* Eutrophic: BMI/age between 3rd and 85th percentile. Low weight: BMI/age below 3rd percentile. Overweight: BMI/age between 85th and 97th percentile. Obesity: BMI/age above 97th percentile (WHO [29]). ** Eutrophic: BMI between 18.5 and 25 kg/m². Low weight: BMI bellow 18.5 kg/m². Overweight: BMI between 25 and 30 kg/m². Obesity: BMI above 30 kg/m² (WHO [30]).

Midarm muscle circumference (MAMC) and TSF were adequate for the majority of the patients. However, adults and adolescents would be classified as obese if only TSF was considered in the evaluation (152% and 189%, respectively).

Zn levels were evaluated for all patients in plasma and erythrocytes, as shown in Table 4.

Table 4. Zinc concentration in plasma (μg/dL) and erythrocytes (μg/dL) of the patients.

Zn	Children		Adolescents		Adults	
	Plasma	Erythrocytes	Plasma	Erythrocytes	Plasma	Erythrocytes
Recommendation *	70–110	10–14	70–110	10–14	70–110	10–14
Mean	195	8	189	9	225	11
Below Normal	0	100%	0	75%	0	25%
Normal	100%	0	100%	25%	100%	75%

* Based on Mafra et al. [34].

We found normal levels of plasma Zn for the entire sample. However, all children, 75% of adolescents and 25% of adults had low levels of erythrocyte Zn.

Figures 1 and 2 demonstrate the concentration of plasma (μg/dL) and erythrocyte Zn (μg/dL), respectively. There was a moderate correlation between plasma and erythrocyte Zn levels ($r^2 = 0.547$, $p = 0.028$).

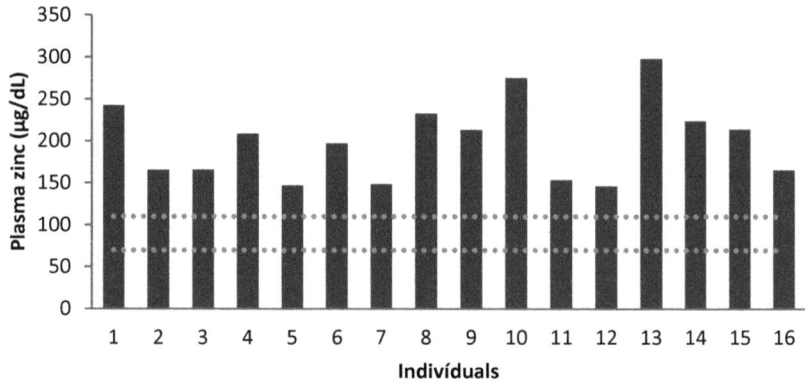

Figure 1. Plasma zinc concentration (μg/dL) of the patients (dotted lines correspond to the reference values, according to Mafra et al. [34]). Age group: patients 1 to 4: 7–9 years old; patients 5 to 12: 10–17 years old; patients 13 to 16: 19–25 years old.

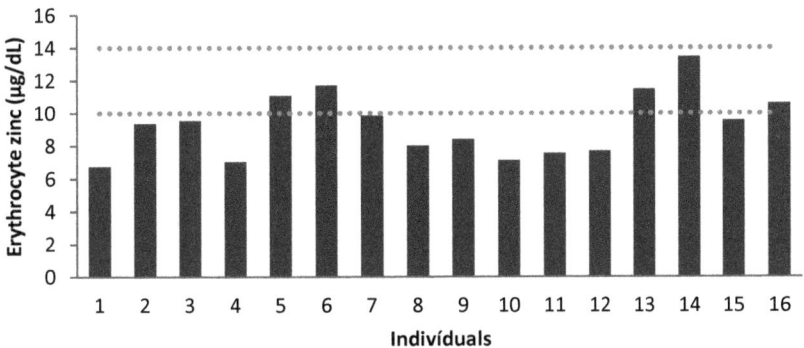

Figure 2. Erythrocyte zinc concentration (μg/dL) of the patients (dotted lines correspond to the reference values, according to Mafra et al. [34]). Age group: patients 1 to 4: 7–9 years old; patients 5 to 12: 10–17 years old; patients 13 to 16: 19–25 years old.

No correlation was found between erythrocyte or plasma zinc and BMI, nutritional status or Zn intake.

Se levels were evaluated for all patients in plasma and erythrocytes. Plasma levels were higher than erythrocyte levels. All patients had low erythrocyte levels, as shown in Table 5.

Table 5. Selenium concentration in plasma (μg/L) and erythrocytes (μg/L) of the patients.

Se	Children		Adolescents		Adults	
	Plasma	Erythrocytes	Plasma	Erythrocytes	Plasma	Erythrocytes
Recommendation *	84–100	>90	84–100	>90	84–100	>90
Mean	95.86	66.70	81.03	61.43	111.96	68.57
Below Normal	50%	100%	75%	100%	0	100%
Normal	50%	0	25%	0%	100%	0%

* Based on Millán Adame et al. [35].

Figures 3 and 4 show the concentration of plasma (μg/L) and erythrocyte Se (μg/L), respectively.

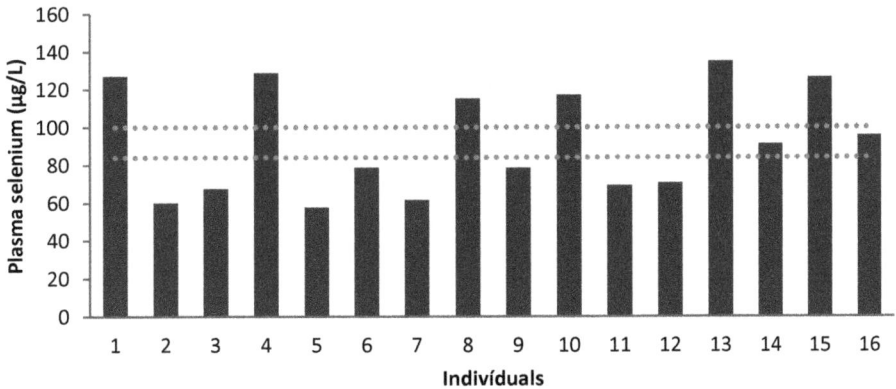

Figure 3. Plasma selenium concentration (μg/L) of the patients (dotted lines correspond to the reference values, according to Millán Adame et al. [35]). Age group: patients 1 to 4: 7–9 years old; patients 5 to 12: 10–17 years old; patients 13 to 16: 19–25 years old.

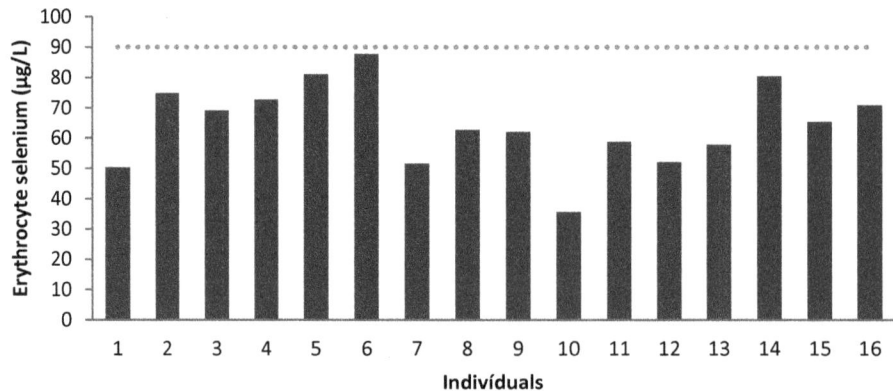

Figure 4. Erythrocyte selenium concentration (µg/L) of the patients (levels above the dotted line correspond to the reference value, according to Millán Adame et al. [35]). Age group: patients 1 to 4: 7–9 years old; patients 5 to 12: 10–17 years old; patients 13 to 16: 19–25 years old.

There was no correlation between Se levels and BMI, nutritional status or Se intake.

As for other relevant laboratory findings, all patients had normal levels of albumin and only 1 patient presented a mild reduction of the lymphocyte count.

Blood count, white cell count, albumin and total protein data are listed in Table 6. Albumin levels were within reference values for all patients. Another relevant biochemical indicator was total leukocyte count, since it evaluates immunological competence. Only one patient (6%) presented mild lymphocyte depletion, whereas all other subjects were within normal limits.

Table 6. Laboratory parameters of the patients with IgAD.

	Children		Adolescents		Adults	
	Mean	SD	Mean	SD	Mean	SD
Hemoglobin (g/dL)	13.28	0.83	12.94	0.52	16.23	2.09
Hematocrit (%)	40.50	2.65	38.88	1.36	48.75	6.50
MCV (µ/mm^3)	79.75	10.53	87.75	6.09	90.75	5.68
MCH (pg)	26.28	3.59	29.15	1.93	30.40	1.79
Leukocytes (cells × 10^3/mm^3)	8.42	4.36	7.72	2.62	7.82	0.95
Total lymphocytes (cells × 10^3/mm^3)	2.35	0.97	2.54	0.78	2.14	0.8.5
Total proteins (g/dL)	7.35	0.29	7.55	0.41	7.16	0.73
Albumin (g/dL)	4.27	0.44	4.21	0.40	4.13	0.51

SD: standard deviation; MCV: Mean corpuscular volume; MCH: Mean corpuscular hemoglobin.

4. Discussion

Proper nutrition and adequate Zn and Se levels can help to maintain optimal immune function, reducing the impact of infections and other comorbidities. Accessibility to a proper amount of quality food is essential to maintain adequate body composition and immune function, especially for patients with inborn errors of immunity. The objective measurement of "enough food or nutrients" can be done by measuring the status of specific nutrients in the body, and is expressed in terms of their adequacy or deficiency [36].

In this cross-sectional and retrospective study, we assessed some biochemical parameters, the nutritional profile and the status of plasma and erythrocyte Zn and Se in patients with IgAD. We found a high proportion of patients that presented very low levels of Zn and Se in the erythrocytes. To our knowledge, this is the first study that investigated the plasma and erythrocyte status of Zn and Se in IgAD patients. Therefore, we highlight the relevance of the present study for the nutritional health of these patients.

Dos Santos-Valente et al. [37] evaluated 17 patients with common variable immunodeficiency, a severe inborn error of immunity, and 17.65% of the patients were considered malnourished and the serum and erythrocyte Zn levels were below normal. Kouhkan et al. [9] found different results. Approximately 3% of patients with different types of immunodeficiency, including IgAD, presented obesity, and 21% of patients presented with nutritional deficiency, according to the BMI. Also in this study, 86.8% of patients showed adequate levels of Zn in serum. On the other hand, Mariz et al. [38] evaluated adults with HIV infection and found a higher occurrence of overweight and obesity, similar to our study.

A high proportion of our patients had respiratory and intestinal infections in the last 12 months. Respiratory infections are an important cause of morbidity and mortality worldwide, and the importance of public health practices to reduce their spread is well established [39]. Zn has anti-infectious properties and a relevant role in defense against respiratory infections and regulating of the immune response in the respiratory tract [40].

Analyzing food consumption, Zn intake was considered adequate for the majority of patients, as only 4 individuals had intake inferior to the recommendation of DRI. However, Zn levels in the erythrocytes were deficient in 100% of children, 75% of adolescents and 25% of adults. Adequate Zn intake and homeostasis are essential for a healthy life, as Zn deficiency is associated with several immune disorders, metabolic and chronic diseases, as well as recurrent respiratory infections, malaria, HIV and tuberculosis [41]. On the other hand, the data intake was obtained by patient's reports. Thus, these data may be underestimated or overestimated, depending on the quality of the reported information. As there is no storage compartment for these micronutrients in the human body, the micronutrients should be ingested daily in sufficient amounts [41].

The difference found between plasma and erythrocyte Zn concentration might be explained by changes in the erythrocyte levels according to several chronic conditions. Despite being the most used Zn biomarker, plasma level has low specificity and sensitivity as it can be influenced by recent changes in diet [41]. Erythrocyte Zn does not reflect these changes and can be considered a long-term biomarker [34]. This can justify why all patients evaluated in our study had both adequate intake and plasma levels, although erythrocytes levels were reduced. Zn supplementation may be more effective in children with deficient levels as compared to children with normal levels [42].

With respect to Se, almost all patients had an adequate intake. Se is acquired through food sources like nuts, breads, cereals, meat, fish, milk and dairy products [43]. Although some of these foods were adequately consumed by our sample, the data intake was obtained by patient's reports, as for Zn.

Regarding the plasma and erythrocyte Se levels, our results were even more striking, as 100% of the patients had low erythrocyte levels, while 50% of children and 75% of adolescents had inadequate plasma levels. However, as for Zn, the plasma levels of Se can be considered an appropriate indicator of nutritional status in the short term, while erythrocytes levels may indicate a long-term nutritional status [35,44] Therefore, lower erythrocyte Se levels found in our patients might reflect a chronic deficiency state. Al Fify et al. [45] investigated patients with systemic inflammatory conditions and pointed out that erythrocytes measurements of certain micronutrients may be more reliable than plasma measurements.

Kouhkan et al. [9] had also demonstrated that Se deficiency was present in 37.5% of children with primary antibody immunodeficiency. When Se and Zn were evaluated in vegetarian adults, plasma levels were also higher compared to erythrocyte levels [46].

Further studies are necessary to evaluate if the normal range of Zn and Se levels in IgAD patients can be considered the same as in immunocompetent patients. This step would be important to assess if appropriate supplementation could reduce the recurrent infections.

Al Fify et al. [45] defined new standards to prevent the misdiagnosis and inadequate treatment of micronutrient deficiencies. They demonstrated that erythrocyte measurements can overcome the limitations of plasma measurements in patients with chronic inflammatory diseases.

Zn has an important role in the formation, maturation and function of T and B cells. Moreover, Zn deficiency can cause reduced maturation of these cells, resulting in reduced antibody production. Adequate Se levels are also fundamental for immune system function, since selenoproteins can regulate inflammation and immunity [15]. Patients with inborn errors of immunity, including IgAD, are at risk for infections and autoimmunity. Therefore, it is essential to evaluate their nutritional status for seeking possible mineral deficiencies that may be supplemented in order to guarantee a more effective functioning of the immune system.

The main strength of this study is that Zn and Se were measured in erythrocytes for all patients who were evaluated by the same investigator throughout the study.

We can point to some limitations of this study. The low number of patients, despite IgAD being considered an inborn error of immunity and therefore being included in the rare diseases group. This was a retrospective study. The lack of a control group.

Micronutrient deficiencies are frequently found in clinical practice, in both children and adults. However, these deficiencies are often underrecognized. Therefore, clinicians should be aware of the risk factors and act properly [44]. Further studies should explore the impact of specific micronutrient supplementation for patients with IgAD and other inborn errors of immunity.

5. Conclusions

The erythrocyte levels of Zn and Se were low in IgAD patients, as compared with the reference values by age range. Our findings suggest the need for monitoring both the intake and erythrocyte levels of these micronutrients in this group of patients.

Author Contributions: S.R.A.J.—writing of the manuscript; C.G.K.—study design, data collecting and writing of the manuscript; F.B.J.—lab work; P.R.-J.—study design, data analysis and writing of the manuscript; A.M.N.—study design, data analysis and writing of the manuscript. All authors have read and agreed to the published version of the manuscript.

Funding: Coordenação de Aperfeiçoamento de Pessoal de Nível Superior (CAPES).

Institutional Review Board Statement: The study was approved by the Ethics Committee from the Clinics Hospital, Ribeirão Preto Medical School, University of São Paulo (Protocol HCRP n° 14444/2010) on 11 May 2011.

Informed Consent Statement: Informed consent was obtained from all subjects involved in the study.

Data Availability Statement: The data presented in this study are available on request from the corresponding author.

Conflicts of Interest: The authors declare no conflict of interest.

References

1. Inzaghi, E.; Pampanini, V.; Deodati, A.; Cianfarani, S. The Effects of Nutrition on Linear Growth. *Nutrients* **2022**, *14*, 1752. [CrossRef] [PubMed]
2. The Global Burden of Disease Diet Collaborators. Health effects of dietary risks in 195 countries, 1990–2017: A systematic analysis for the Global Burden of Disease Study 2017. *Lancet* **2019**, *393*, 1958–1972. [CrossRef] [PubMed]
3. Visiolia, F.; Marangonic, F.; Polic, A.; Ghisellid, A.; Martini, D. Nutrition and health or nutrients and health? *Int. J. Food Sci. Nutr.* **2022**, *73*, 141–148. [CrossRef] [PubMed]
4. Chen, O.; Mah, E.; Dioum, E.; Marwaha, A.; Shanmugam, S.; Malleshi, N.; Sudha, V.; Gayathri, R.; Unnikrishnan, R.; Anjana, R.M.; et al. The Role of Oat Nutrients in the Immune System: A Narrative Review. *Nutrients* **2021**, *13*, 1048. [CrossRef] [PubMed]
5. Calder, P.C. Nutrition and immunity: Lessons for COVID-19. *Eur. J. Clin. Nutr.* **2021**, *75*, 1309–1318. [CrossRef] [PubMed]
6. Verduci, E.; Köglmeier, J. Immunomodulation in Children: The Role of the Diet. *J. Pediatr. Gastroenterol. Nutr.* **2021**, *73*, 293–298. [CrossRef]
7. Childs, C.E.; Calder, P.C.; Miles, E.A. Diet and Immune Function. *Nutrients* **2019**, *11*, 1933. [CrossRef]
8. Katona, P.; Katona-Apte, J. The interaction between nutrition and infection. *Clin. Infect. Dis.* **2008**, *46*, 1582–1588. [CrossRef]

9. Kouhkan, A.; Pourpak, Z.; Moin, M.; Dorosty, A.R.; Safaralizadeh, R.; Teimorian, S.; Farhoudi, A.; Aghamohammadi, A.; Mesdaghi, M.; Kazemnejad, A. A study of malnutrition in Iranian patients with primary antibody deficiency. *Iran. J. Allergy Asthma Immunol.* **2004**, *3*, 189–196.
10. Eggersdorfer, M.; Akobundu, U.; Bailey, R.L.; Shlisky, J.; Beaudreault, A.R.; Bergeron, G.; Blancato, R.B.; Blumberg, J.B.; Bourassa, M.W.; Gomes, F.; et al. Hidden Hunger: Solutions for America's Aging Populations. *Nutrients* **2018**, *10*, 1210. [CrossRef]
11. Costa, M.I.; Sarmento-Ribeiro, A.B.; Gonçalves, A.C. Zinc: From Biological Functions to Therapeutic Potential. *Int. J. Mol. Sci.* **2023**, *24*, 4822. [CrossRef] [PubMed]
12. Hussain, A.; Jiang, W.; Wang, X.; Shahid, S.; Saba, N.; Ahmad, M.; Dar, A.; Masood, S.U.; Imran, M.; Mustafa, A. Mechanistic Impact of Zinc Deficiency in Human Development. *Rev. Front. Nutr.* **2022**, *9*, 717064. [CrossRef] [PubMed]
13. Salgueiro, M.J.; Zubillaga, M.B.; Lysionek, A.E.; Caro, R.A.; Weill, R.; Boccio, J.R. The Role of Zinc in the Growth and Development of Children. *Nutrition* **2002**, *18*, 510–519. [CrossRef] [PubMed]
14. Bonaventura, P.; Benedetti, G.; Albarède, F.; Miossec, P. Zinc and its role in immunity and inflammation. *Autoimmun. Rev.* **2015**, *14*, 277–285. [CrossRef] [PubMed]
15. Weyh, C.; Krüger, K.; Peeling, P.; Castell, L. The Role of Minerals in the Optimal Functioning of the Immune System. *Nutrients* **2022**, *14*, 644. [CrossRef]
16. Hoffmann, P.R.; Berry, M.J. The influence of selenium on immune responses. *Mol. Nutr. Food Res.* **2008**, *52*, 1273–1280. [CrossRef]
17. Xia, X.; Zhang, X.; Liu, M.; Duan, M.; Zhang, S.; Wei, X.; Liu, X. Toward improved human health: Efficacy of dietary selenium on immunity at the cellular level. *Food Funct.* **2021**, *12*, 976–989. [CrossRef]
18. Barchielli, G.; Capperucci, A.; Tanini, D. The Role of Selenium in Pathologies: An Updated Review. *Antioxidants* **2022**, *11*, 251. [CrossRef]
19. Razaghi, A.; Poorebrahim, M.; Sarhan, D.; Björnstedt, M. Selenium stimulates the antitumour immunity: Insights to future research. *Eur. J. Cancer* **2021**, *155*, 256–267. [CrossRef]
20. Delves, P.J.; Roitt, I.M. The immune system. First of two parts. *N. Engl. J. Med.* **2000**, *343*, 37–49. [CrossRef]
21. Bruzeau, C.; Cook-Moreau, J.; Pinaud, E.; Le Noir, S. Contribution of Immunoglobulin Enhancers to B Cell Nuclear Organization. *Front. Immunol.* **2022**, *13*, 877930. [CrossRef]
22. Odineal, D.D.; Gershwin, M.E. The Epidemiology and Clinical Manifestations of Autoimmunity in Selective IgA Deficiency. *Clin. Rev. Allergy Immunol.* **2020**, *58*, 107–133. [CrossRef] [PubMed]
23. Morawska, I.; Kurkowska, S.; Bębnowska, D.; Hrynkiewicz, R.; Becht, R.; Michalski, A.; Piwowarska-Bilska, H.; Birkenfeld, B.; Załuska-Ogryzek, K.; Grywalska, E.; et al. The Epidemiology and Clinical Presentations of Atopic Diseases in Selective IgA Deficiency. *J. Clin. Med.* **2021**, *10*, 3809. [CrossRef] [PubMed]
24. Tangye, S.G.; Al-Herz, W.; Bousfiha, A.; Cunningham-Rundles, C.; Franco, J.L.; Holland, S.M.; Klein, C.; Morio, T.; Oksenhendler, E.; Picard, C.; et al. Human Inborn Errors of Immunity: 2022 Update on the Classification from the International Union of Immunological Societies Expert Committee. *J. Clin. Immunol.* **2022**, *42*, 1473–1507. [CrossRef] [PubMed]
25. Reust, C.E. Evaluation of primary immunodeficiency disease in children. *Am. Fam. Physician* **2013**, *87*, 773–778. [PubMed]
26. Elsink, K.; van Montfrans, J.M.; van Gijn, M.E.; Blom, M.; van Hagen, P.M.; Kuijpers, T.W.; Frederix, G.W.J. Cost and impact of early diagnosis in primary immunodeficiency disease: A literature review. *Clin. Immunol.* **2020**, *213*, 108359. [CrossRef] [PubMed]
27. Yel, L. Selective IgA Deficiency. *J. Clin. Immunol.* **2010**, *30*, 10–16. [CrossRef] [PubMed]
28. WHO. WHO Child Growth Standards. 2007. Available online: http://www.who.int/childgrowth/en/index.html (accessed on 15 January 2023).
29. *WHO Child Growth Standards: Length/Height-for-Age, Weight-for-Age, Weight-for-Length, Weight-for-Height and Body Mass Index-for-Age. Methods and Development*; WHO: Geneva, Switzerland, 2006.
30. *Obesity: Preventing and Managing the Global Epidemic: Report of a WHO Consultation on Obesity; WHO Technical Report Series n. 894*; WHO: Geneva, Switzerland, 2000.
31. Lohman, G.L.; Roche, A.F.; Martorell, R. *Anthropometric Standardization Reference Manual*; Human Kinetics Books: Champaign, IL, USA, 1988.
32. Frisancho, A. *Anthropometric Standards for the Assessment of Growth and Nutritional Status*; University of Michigan: Ann Arbor, MI, USA, 1990.
33. Lee, S.W. Methods for testing statistical differences between groups in medical research: Statistical standard and guideline of Life Cycle Committee. *Life Cycle* **2022**, *2*, e1. [CrossRef]
34. Mafra, D.; Maria, S.; Cozzolino, F. The importance of zinc in human nutrition. *Rev. Nutr. Campinas* **2004**, *17*, 79–87. [CrossRef]
35. Millán Adame, E.; Florea, D.; Sáez Pérez, L.; Molina López, J.; López-González, B.; Pérez de la Cruz, A.; Planells del Pozo, E. Deficient selenium status of a healthy adult Spanish population. *Nutr. Hosp.* **2012**, *27*, 524–528. [CrossRef]
36. Ghosh, S.; Kurpad, A.V.; Sachdev, H.S.; Thomas, T. A risk-based approach to measuring population micronutrient status from blood biomarker concentrations. *Front. Nutr.* **2022**, *9*, 991707. [CrossRef] [PubMed]
37. dos Santos-Valente, E.C.; da Silva, R.; de Moraes-Pinto, M.I.; Sarni, R.O.; Costa-Carvalho, B.T. Assessment of nutritional status: Vitamin A and zinc in patients with common variable immunodeficiency. *J. Investig. Allergol. Clin. Immunol.* **2012**, *22*, 427–431. [PubMed]

38. Mariz, C.A.; de Albuquerque, M.F.P.M.; Ximenes, R.A.A.; de Melo, H.R.L.M.; Bandeira, F.; Braga e Oliveira, T.G.; de Carvalho, E.H.; da Silva, A.P.; Miranda Filho, D.B. Body mass index in individuals with HIV infection and factors associated with thinness and overweight/obesity. *Cad. Saude Publica* **2011**, *27*. [CrossRef] [PubMed]
39. Pecora, F.; Persico, F.; Argentiero, A.; Neglia, C.; Esposito, S. The Role of Micronutrients in Support of the Immune Response against Viral Infections. *Nutrients* **2020**, *12*, 3198. [CrossRef]
40. Sadeghsoltani, F.; Mohammadzadeh, I.; Safari, M.M.; Hassanpour, P.; Izadpanah, M.; Qujeq, D.; Moein, S.; Vaghari-Tabari, M. Zinc and Respiratory Viral Infections: Important Trace Element in Anti-viral Response and Immune Regulation. *Biol. Trace Elem. Res.* **2022**, *200*, 2556–2571. [CrossRef]
41. Maywald, M.; Rink, L. Zinc in Human Health and Infectious Diseases. *Biomolecules* **2022**, *12*, 1748. [CrossRef]
42. Vlieg-Boerstra, B.; de Jong, N.; Meyer, R.; Agostoni, C.; De Cosmi, V.; Grimshaw, K.; Milani, G.P.; Muraro, A.; Oude Elberink, H.; Pali-Schöl, I.; et al. Nutrient supplementation for prevention of viral respiratory tract infections in healthy subjects: A systematic review and meta-analysis. *Allergy* **2022**, *77*, 1373–1388. [CrossRef]
43. Hariharan, S.; Dharmaraj, S. Selenium and selenoproteins: It's role in regulation of inflammation. *Inflammopharmacology* **2020**, *28*, 667–695. [CrossRef]
44. Zemrani, B.; Bines, J.E. Recent insights into trace element deficiencies: Causes, recognition and correction. *Curr. Opin. Gastroenterol.* **2020**, *36*, 110–117. [CrossRef]
45. Al Fify, M.; Nichols, B.; Arailoudi Alexiadou, L.; Stefanowicz, F.; Armstrong, J.; Russell, R.K.; Raudaschl, A.; Pinto, N.; Duncan, A.; Catchpole, A.; et al. Development of age-dependent micronutrient centile charts and their utility in children with chronic gastrointestinal conditions at risk of deficiencies: A proof-of-concept study. *Clin. Nutr.* **2022**, *41*, 931–936. [CrossRef]
46. de Bortoli, M.C.; Cozzolino, S.M.F. Zinc and selenium nutritional status in vegetarians. *Biol. Trace Elem. Res.* **2009**, *127*, 228–233. [CrossRef] [PubMed]

Disclaimer/Publisher's Note: The statements, opinions and data contained in all publications are solely those of the individual author(s) and contributor(s) and not of MDPI and/or the editor(s). MDPI and/or the editor(s) disclaim responsibility for any injury to people or property resulting from any ideas, methods, instructions or products referred to in the content.

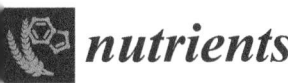

Article

Milk Allergen Micro-Array (MAMA) for Refined Detection of Cow's-Milk-Specific IgE Sensitization

Victoria Garib [1,2], Daria Trifonova [1,3], Raphaela Freidl [1], Birgit Linhart [1], Thomas Schlederer [1], Nikolaos Douladiris [4], Alexander Pampura [5], Daria Dolotova [6], Tatiana Lepeshkova [7], Maia Gotua [8], Evgeniy Varlamov [5], Evgeny Beltyukov [7], Veronika Naumova [7], Styliani Taka [4], Alina Kiyamova [2], Stefani Katsamaki [2], Alexander Karaulov [3] and Rudolf Valenta [1,3,9,10,*]

[1] Center for Pathophysiology, Infectiology and Immunology, Institute of Pathophysiology and Allergy Research, Medical University of Vienna, 1090 Vienna, Austria; viktoriya.garib@meduniwien.ac.at (V.G.)
[2] International Center of Molecular Allergology, Ministry of Innovation Development, Tashkent 100174, Uzbekistan
[3] Laboratory of Immunopathology, Department of Clinical Immunology and Allergy, Sechenov First Moscow State Medical University, 119991 Moscow, Russia
[4] Allergy Department, 2nd Pediatric Clinic, National & Kapodistrian University of Athens, 11527 Athens, Greece
[5] Department of Allergology and Clinical Immunology, Research and Clinical Institute for Pediatrics Named after Yuri Veltischev at the Pirogov Russian National Research Medical University of the Russian Ministry of Health, 117997 Moscow, Russia; anpampura1@gmail.com (A.P.); ev4832525@gmail.com (E.V.)
[6] Department of Bioinformatics, Department of Pediatric Surgery, Pirogov Russian National Research Medical University of the Russian Ministry of Health, 117997 Moscow, Russia
[7] Department of Faculty Therapy, Endocrinology, Allergology and Immunology, Ural State Medical University, 620028 Ekaterinburg, Russia
[8] Center of Allergy and Immunology, 123182 Tbilisi, Georgia
[9] NRC Institute of Immunology FMBA of Russia, 115478 Moscow, Russia
[10] Karl Landsteiner University for Health Sciences, 3500 Krems, Austria
* Correspondence: rudolf.valenta@meduniwien.ac.at; Tel.: +43-1-40400-50420

Citation: Garib, V.; Trifonova, D.; Freidl, R.; Linhart, B.; Schlederer, T.; Douladiris, N.; Pampura, A.; Dolotova, D.; Lepeshkova, T.; Gotua, M.; et al. Milk Allergen Micro-Array (MAMA) for Refined Detection of Cow's-Milk-Specific IgE Sensitization. *Nutrients* 2023, 15, 2401. https://doi.org/10.3390/nu15102401

Academic Editor: Eva Untersmayr

Received: 18 April 2023
Revised: 4 May 2023
Accepted: 11 May 2023
Published: 21 May 2023

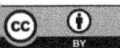

Copyright: © 2023 by the authors. Licensee MDPI, Basel, Switzerland. This article is an open access article distributed under the terms and conditions of the Creative Commons Attribution (CC BY) license (https://creativecommons.org/licenses/by/4.0/).

Abstract: Background: Immunoglobulin-E(IgE)-mediated hypersensitivity to cow's milk allergens is a frequent cause of severe and life-threatening anaphylactic reactions. Besides case histories and controlled food challenges, the detection of the IgE antibodies specific to cow's milk allergens is important for the diagnosis of cow-milk-specific IgE sensitization. cow's milk allergen molecules provide useful information for the refined detection of cow-milk-specific IgE sensitization. Methods: A micro-array based on ImmunoCAP ISAC technology was developed and designated milk allergen micro-array (MAMA), containing a complete panel of purified natural and recombinant cow's milk allergens (caseins, α-lactalbumin, β-lactoglobulin, bovine serum albumin-BSA and lactoferrin), recombinant BSA fragments, and α-casein-, α-lactalbumin- and β-lactoglobulin-derived synthetic peptides. Sera from 80 children with confirmed symptoms related to cow's milk intake (without anaphylaxis: $n = 39$; anaphylaxis with a Sampson grade of 1–3: $n = 21$; and anaphylaxis with a Sampson grade of 4–5: $n = 20$) were studied. The alterations in the specific IgE levels were analyzed in a subgroup of eleven patients, i.e., five who did not and six who did acquire natural tolerance. Results: The use of MAMA allowed a component-resolved diagnosis of IgE sensitization in each of the children suffering from cow's-milk-related anaphylaxis according to Sampson grades 1–5 requiring only 20–30 microliters of serum. IgE sensitization to caseins and casein-derived peptides was found in each of the children with Sampson grades of 4–5. Among the grade 1–3 patients, nine patients showed negative reactivity to caseins but showed IgE reactivity to alpha-lactalbumin ($n = 7$) or beta-lactoglobulin ($n = 2$). For certain children, an IgE sensitization to cryptic peptide epitopes without detectable allergen-specific IgE was found. Twenty-four children with cow-milk-specific anaphylaxis showed additional IgE sensitizations to BSA, but they were all sensitized to either caseins, alpha-lactalbumin, or beta-lactoglobulin. A total of 17 of the 39 children without anaphylaxis lacked specific IgE reactivity to any of the tested components. The children developing tolerance showed a reduction in allergen and/or peptide-specific IgE levels, whereas those remaining sensitive did not.

Conclusions: The use of MAMA allows for the detection, using only a few microliters of serum, of IgE sensitization to multiple cow's milk allergens and allergen-derived peptides in cow-milk-allergic children with cow-milk-related anaphylaxis.

Keywords: cow's milk allergy; allergen molecules; milk allergen micro-array; peptides; anaphylaxis; milk tolerance; diagnosis; IgE sensitization; children

1. Introduction

An intolerance to cow's milk is particularly common. In most cases, it is due to lactose intolerance and can be avoided by the consumption of lactose-free milk products. Immunoglobulin-E-(IgE)-mediated cow's milk allergy (CMA) is more rare and affects approximately 3% of the population [1,2]. CMA occurs very early in childhood when children are exposed to cow's milk (CM) in their diet. Despite the relatively low number of sensitized patients, CMA is especially important to diagnose because it can cause severe and life-threatening anaphylaxis, which may lead to death upon the consumption of CM [3,4]. The cornerstone for a diagnosis of IgE-mediated CMA is a well-documented case history documenting immediate occurrences of allergic symptoms that can be unambiguously attributed to the consumption of CM [5,6]. Whenever possible, it is important to confirm CMA via a controlled food challenge in a safe clinical setting [4,7]. IgE sensitization to CM allergens should be confirmed by the detection of allergen-specific IgE antibodies with serological measurements. Furthermore, skin testing and basophil activation tests are useful for demonstrating the allergenic activity of CM in a given patient; however, the basophil activation test is mainly used for research [4,8,9].

Traditionally, the serological detection of CM-allergen-specific IgE antibodies is performed with the use of CM allergen extracts, of which some are able to help quantify CM-allergen-specific IgE levels [10]. Interestingly, the quantification of CM-allergen-specific IgE antibodies has turned out to be useful for the prediction of the severity of CM-related allergic symptoms; however, the cut-off levels are not sharp and have been found to vary in different populations [10,11]. Similar to many other allergen sources, it has become possible to purify the individual allergen molecules in cow's milk to produce them as recombinant allergen molecules and to synthesize CM-allergen-derived peptides for the mapping of the IgE, IgG and T-cell epitopes that are recognized by CM-allergic patients [11–13]. Purified allergen molecules and the peptides derived thereof have brought forward another era in allergy diagnosis, one which is commonly referred to as component-resolved allergy diagnosis or molecular allergy diagnosis [13–16]. Cow's milk contains different amounts of allergen molecules that show different resistances against heating and digestion, and which, accordingly, have been suggested to be associated with very severe forms, as well as severe and mild forms of CMA. In addition, some compounds such as BSA do not seem to cause the relevant symptoms of CMA [9,15,17,18]. Individual CM allergens became available in the form of single allergen components, which allow for the measurement of IgE levels that are specific for certain allergens. In parallel to this, multiplex allergen tests have been developed, which allow for the simultaneous measurement of IgE levels for several allergens and/or allergen peptides by macro-, micro-array technology, or by bead-based assays [16,17,19–22]. In using such tests, interesting information was obtained regarding IgE reactivity profiles, as well as regarding IgE levels to certain allergens and/or allergen-derived peptides, such as biomarkers for different phenotypes, the severities of CM allergy, the outgrowth of CM allergy and the monitoring of allergen-specific immunotherapy [10,13,21–25].

In this study, we present a novel milk allergen micro-array (MAMA) that allows one to measure, with only a few microliters of serum, the IgE levels of to all known CM allergens and certain CM-allergen-derived peptides. In addition, MAMA was also used for the high-resolution mapping of allergen- and peptide-specific IgE reactivity profiles in a cohort of clinically well-defined CM-allergic children. Our study not only provides a multiplex assay that allows a hitherto unmatched detailed survey of CM allergen- and peptide-specific IgE reactivity profiles, but it also appears to be useful for the reliable detection of CM-allergen-specific IgE reactivity in patients with anaphylactic reactions to CM, as well as for monitoring the development of patient tolerance following an elimination diet.

2. Materials and Methods

2.1. Cow-Milk-Allergic Patients, Sera and PBMC Samples

Children suffering from CMA (Table 1) were observed in the Allergy Department, 2nd Pediatric Clinic University of Athens, Greece; in the Center of Allergy and Immunology, Tbilisi, Georgia; in the Department of Allergology and Clinical Immunology, Research and Clinical Institute for Pediatrics named after Yuri Veltischev at the Pirogov Russian National Research Medical University, Moscow, Russia; and in the Department of Faculty Therapy, Endocrinology, Allergology and Immunology, Ural State Medical University, Ekaterinburg, Russia. For patients with anaphylactic reactions to CM, the diagnosis of CMA was based on specific criteria [26], including the presence of clinical symptoms of an immediate type of CMA (which could only be unambiguously attributed to CM) and a clear-cut history of anaphylaxis following milk consumption, in accordance with published guidelines [27]. Skin prick testing with CM allergen extracts and/or the measurement of IgE levels specific for CM allergen extracts obtained with ImmunoCAP (Thermo Fisher Scientific, Uppsala, Sweden) was performed in the study population (Table 1).

Table 1. Demographic, clinical and serological characterizations of CM-allergic patients.

Patients	Number	Gender	Age	CM-Related Symptoms	SPT CM	Total IgE	sIgE to CM	Other Allergy
	n % of total	f/m (%)	Years [Q_1–Q_3] (min–max)	Type: n	n	kU/L [Q_1–Q_3] (min–max), n	kUA/L [Q_1–Q_3] (min–max), n	Type: n
Total CM allergic	80 100%	28/52 (35/65%)	MV: 3.1 [2.0–5.5] (0.5–12)	Skin: 62 GI: 42 Sys: 41	pos: 27 neg: 6 nd: 46	MV: 99 [34.1–649] (6.7–7372) n = 67	MV: 4.6 [0.9–24.3] (0–100) n = 57	BA: 18 AR: 28 FA: 52
With anaphylaxis	41 51.25%	14/27 (34.2/65.8%)	MV: 5.0 [2.9–8.5] (1–12)	Skin: 29 GI: 20 Sys: 41	pos: 16 neg: 1 nd: 24	MV: 212 [45.9–705] (6.7–7372) n = 36	MV: 20.4 [8–93.9] (0.12–100) n = 26	BA: 12 AR: 18 FA: 29
A4-5 Sampson score 4-5	20 25%	7/13 (35/65%)	MV: 4.9 [2.9–8.8] (2.3–12)	Skin: 14 GI: 9 Sys: 20	pos: 3 neg: 0 nd: 17	MV: 257.5 [95–791.3] (6.7–7372) n = 18	MV: 46.6 [20–98] (6–100) n = 12	BA: 8 AR: 9 FA: 15
A1-3 Sampson score 1-3	21 26.25%	7/14 (33.3/66.7%)	MV: 5.0 [2.5–8.5] (1–11.2)	Skin: 15 GI: 11 Sys: 21	pos: 13 neg: 1 nd: 7	MV: 95 [43.3–699.3] (20.2–4030) n = 18	MV: 13.3 [2.1–46.1] (0.12–100) n = 14	BA: 4 AR: 9 FA: 14
NA Without anaphylaxis	39 48.75%	14/25 (35.9/64.1%)	MV: 2.5 [1.3–3.9] (0.5–6)	Skin: 33 GI: 22 Sys: 0	pos: 11 neg: 5 nd: 22	MV: 68.5 [23.3–311] (7.5–1661) n = 31	MV: 1.3 [0.4–3.6] (0–100) n = 31	BA: 6 AR: 10 FA: 23

Abbreviations: f, female; m, male; CM, cow's milk; n, numbers; MV, median value; Skin, skin symptoms; GI, gastrointestinal symptoms; Sys, systemic reactions; SPT, skin prick test; BA, bronchial asthma; AR, allergic rhinitis; FA, food allergy; nd, not done.

The CM-related allergic symptoms of patients were ranked as non-anaphylactic and anaphylactic. Anaphylactic reactions were graded as grades 1–5 according to Sampson [28]. The majority of CM-allergic patients (i.e., 52/80) were also sensitized to other food allergen sources such as egg, peanut, wheat, nuts, soy, cereals, fish and caviar.

A subset of 11 children (Table 2) were subjected to a milk elimination diet, (#1, 11, 25, 30, 32, 36, 38, 70) or a milk modification diet (i.e., they received only baked milk) (#65–67).

Table 2. Demographic, clinical and immunological characterizations of CM-allergic patients who underwent CM diet for different durations.

Patient ID	Gender	Age (Months)	Time Difference (Months)	Tolerance Development	Tolerance to Milk	Symptoms Severity	Symptoms Other	Eosinophils %	Eosinophils ×10⁹/L	Total IgE (kU/L)
1	f	34	18		no	5	BA, AR, GI	8	0.68	440
1a		52		no	no	5	BA, AR, GI	5	0.6	440
25	m	44	18		no	3	AD, BA	5	0.4	39.5
25a		62		no	no	3	AD, BA	5	0.4	39.5
65	m	72	9		baked	0	AD, AR, GI	6.3	0.42	nd
65a		81		no	baked	0	AD, AR, GI	6.3	0.42	nd
66	m	16	18		baked	0	AD, AR, GI	2	0.02	248.7
66a		34		no	baked	0	AD, AR, GI	2	0.13	127.8
11	m	58	11		no	4	AD, AR, GI	8	0.67	nd
11a		69		no	no	4	AD, AR, GI	5	0.4	nd
36	f	35	18		no	2	AR, GI	3.6	0.3	32.3
36a		53		yes	baked	0	AR	3.6	0.3	32.3
32	m	134	9		no	2	AR, GI	3.7	0.3	48.1
32a		143		yes	baked	0	0	nd	nd	nd
38	f	88	18		no	2	AD, AR, GI	3	0.2	82.5
38a		106		yes	baked	0	0	nd	nd	nd
67	m	30	18		baked	0	AD, GI	4	0.24	78.8
67a		48		yes	fermented	0	AD	4.6	0.3	58.6
70	m	67	12		baked	0	AD, BA, AR, GI	8.8	1	nd
70a		79		yes	fermented	0	BA, AR	11.6	1.27	nd
30	m	21	8		no	3	AD, GI	8	0.68	nd
30a		29		yes	baked	0	AD	3.2	0.3	nd

Abbreviations: f, female; m, male; CM, cow's milk; GI, gastrointestinal symptoms; BA, bronchial asthma; AR, allergic rhinitis; AD, atopic dermatitis; nd, not done.

Episodes of anaphylaxis due to accidental intake of cow's milk were recorded by the treating physicians.

The development of clinical tolerance in the form of baked, fermented, or whole milk when re-introduced into the diet under controlled conditions was monitored also by the treating physicians. No controlled challenges were performed in the clinics.

Written informed consent was obtained from the parents or legal guardians of the children in order to obtain blood samples and immunological analysis (these were also approved by the corresponding local ethics committees in Greece, Georgia and Russia). The analysis of the pseudonymized samples with MAMA was conducted with approval from the Ethics Committee of the Medical University of Vienna, Austria (EK1641/2014).

2.2. ImmunoCAP ISAC Measurements

Allergen-specific IgE antibodies were measured in certain serum samples with ImmunoCAP ISAC micro-arrays containing 112 allergens, and this was conducted according to the manufacturer's recommendations (Thermo Fisher, Uppsala, Sweden) with permission from the Ethics Committee of the Medical University of Vienna (EK1641/2014).

2.3. Milk Allergen Micro-Array (MAMA)

The natural and recombinant milk allergens, recombinant BSA fragments and milk-allergen-derived synthetic peptides are summarized and characterized in Table S1 in the Supplementary Materials. The spotting of proteins and peptides was performed as described in [29]. However, in more detail, the glass slides containing six microarrays were surrounded by an epoxy frame (Paul Marienfeld GmbH & Co. KG, Lauda-Königshofen, Germany) and were coated with an amine-reactive complex organic polymer, MCP-2 (Lucidant Polymers, Sunnyvale, CA, USA). This surface was meant to facilitate the immobilization of the proteins and peptides. The spotting conditions, buffers and concentrations in the pilot experiments to obtain round-shaped and compact spots of comparable size were optimized for each protein/peptide. During the final printing stage, milk allergens were spotted, in triplicates, in concentrations of 0.5–1 mg/mL in phosphate buffer (75 mM Na_2HPO_4, pH = 8.4) with a SciFlexArrayer S12 (Scienion AG, Berlin, Germany).

IgE reactivity and IgE levels specific for micro-arrayed proteins and peptides were measured as follows: The microarrays were washed for 5 min with phosphate-buffered saline containing 0.5% Tween 20 (PBST) and were dried via centrifugation with a Sigma 2-7 centrifuge and MTP-11113 rotor (both Sigma Laborzentrifugen GmbH, Osterode am Harz, Germany). Subsequently, 35 µL of undiluted serum sample was added per array and incubated for 2 h at 22 °C. After another washing step, the bound IgE antibodies were detected as described in [30]. The slides were again washed, dried and subsequently scanned with a confocal laser scanner (Tecan, Männedorf, Switzerland).

Image analysis was performed via MAPIX microarray image acquisition and analysis software version 8.5.0 (Innopsys, Carbonne, France), and through a conversion of measured fluorescence units to ISAC standardized units (ISU), which was performed as described in [31].

2.4. Statistical Analyses

Given the small number of patients in the studied groups, the median and the interquartile range (Me [Q1; Q3]) were used in the description of the variable distributions. The pairwise comparison of groups was performed with a Mann–Whitney U test. Considering the problem of multiple hypothesis testing, the significance threshold was Holm-corrected to 0.000385 [32].

The graphical representation included box and whisker diagrams that demonstrated the median (a horizontal line inside the "box"), the first and third quartiles (upper and lower bounds of the "box") and the minimum and maximum ("whiskers"). Additionally, the distribution of allergen values within the ranges of [0.3; 1), [1; 15) and ≥ 15 was illustrated using different color codes.

The analysis was performed using IBM SPSS Statistics 20.0 (New York, NY, USA).

The graphical representation was performed using GraphPad Prism 6 software (GraphPad Software, La Jolla, CA, USA), RStudio software 2022.11.4-20 and Microsoft Office Excel 2010. Correlations of allergen-specific IgE levels determined by MAMA and ImmunoCAP ISAC were assessed by Spearman's rank correlation coefficient. p values of <0.05 were considered as significant.

3. Results
3.1. Characterization of CM-Allergic Patients

In this study, we investigated 80 subjects (28 females, 52 males, age range 0.5–12 years, median age 3.1 years) with allergic symptoms that could be clearly attributed to the consumption of CM (Table 1). In total, 60 of the children showed skin symptoms, 42 showed gastrointestinal symptoms and 41 showed systemic reactions (Table 1). Among the 41 children with systemic reactions, 21 presented reactions at grades 1–3 (according to Sampson [24]) and 20 presented grade 4–5 reactions (Table 1). Mild symptoms (skin reactions, gastrointestinal reactions, etc.) without systemic reactions were found in 39 patients (Table 1). The results from skin prick testing and from the measurements of specific IgE to CM allergen extracts were available for 46 and 41 of the 80 CM-allergic patients, respectively (Table 1).

Table 2 shows the characteristics of patients (n = 11) who were prescribed a CM elimination or modification diet. The duration of the prescribed diet was from 8 to 18 months. Two children suffered from CM-related anaphylaxis at grade 4–5, five from anaphylaxis grade 1–3 and four had mild symptoms (Table 2). Five of the children (#1: grade 5; #25: grade 3; #65: grade 0; #66: grade 0; and #11: grade 4) did not develop a tolerance, whereas six developed a tolerance (i.e., #36: grade 2; #32: grade 2; #38: grade 2; #67: grade: 0;

#70: grade: 0; #30: grade 3) and the rest developed some form of tolerance (Table 2). The duration of the elimination diet was not associated with the development of tolerance.

3.2. Creation of MAMA

Each of the glass slides (i.e., chips) contained six milk allergen micro-arrays (MAMAs), which were surrounded by a frame to avoid an overflow of serum (Figure 1A). The MAMA comprised triplicate spots of each allergen and allergen-derived peptides together with four guide dot triplicates (red), as is indicated in Figure 1A. The MAMA contained purified natural CM allergens, recombinant CM allergens, recombinant BSA fragments and allergen-derived peptides, as is indicated in Figure 1A,B. The sources and characteristics of the proteins and peptides, together with the key references [9,33,34] describing the recombinant proteins and peptides are summarized in Table S1. The MAMA allowed the testing of antibody reactivity against 44 components with a volume of approximately 30 microliters of serum, plasma or other body fluids. Hence, it is especially suitable for the analysis of samples from children and when it is difficult to obtain larger volumes of test substances.

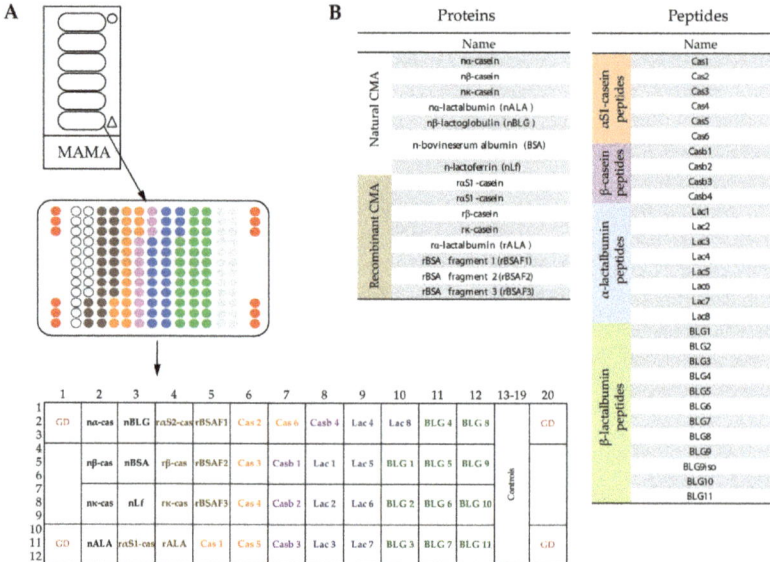

Figure 1. The layout and composition of the milk allergen micro-array (MAMA). (**A**) Glass slides containing six micro-arrays surrounded by an epoxy frame, magnification of one micro-array showing the order of dots (triplicates), and further magnification showing guide dots (GD), positions of cow's milk (CM) allergens and peptides in boxes. (**B**) Lists of the natural CM allergens, recombinant CM allergens and CM-derived peptides according to Table S1.

3.3. MAMA, but Not ImmunoCAP, or Skin Testing with CM Extracts Identifies all Patients with CMA According to a Sampson Score of 1–5

Figure 2A,B show the levels of IgE that are specific for CM allergens, recombinant BSA fragments and CM-allergen-derived peptides in the study population with and without CM-related anaphylaxis (Figure 2A,B; Table 1). We found that each of the patients with anaphylactic reactions to CM, in Sampson grades of 1–5 (n = 41), showed an IgE reactivity to at least one of the CM-allergen components. The heat map indicates already that patients with Sampson grades of 4–5 exhibited higher specific IgE levels than patients with anaphylaxis grades of 1–3 (Figure 2A,B).

Figure 2. *Cont.*

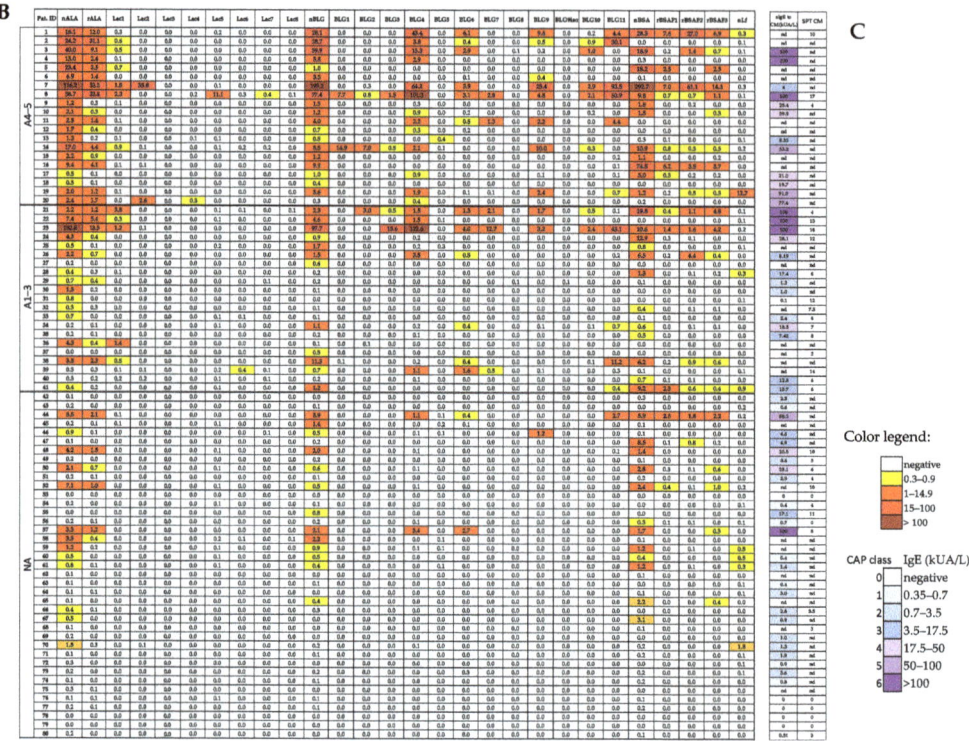

Figure 2. Heat map of the IgE levels specific for caseins and casein-derived peptides (**A**), other milk allergen proteins and peptides thereof (**B**), and milk allergen extract-specific IgE levels and SPT results (**C**) in patients suffering from different intensities of CMA (A4–5, milk-related anaphylaxis with a Sampson grade of 4–5; A1–3, milk-related anaphylaxis with a Sampson grade of 1–3; and NA, without anaphylaxis). The IgE (ISU-E, kUA/L) levels are shown with a color code.

In total, 17 out of 41 patients with anaphylactic reactions to CM had been tested via SPT for CM allergen extracts (Table 1). Moreover, 1 of the 17 patients with grades 1–3 tested negative via skin testing with CM allergen extracts (Table 1). Furthermore, 26 of the 41 patients with anaphylactic reactions and CM-allergen-specific IgE levels to CM allergen extracts were assessed via ImmunoCAP testing. One of the patients (i.e., patients #31) with an anaphylactic reaction of grade 1–3 showed CM-allergen-extract-specific IgE levels 0.12 kUA/L, which is CAP class 0, according to the established cut-off 0.35 kUA/L, despite the fact that the technical cut-off for ImmunoCAP is 0.1 kUA/L. Thus, 2 out of 29 patients who had been tested with conventional allergen-extract-based methods (i.e., either SPT and/or ImmunoCAP) tested negative, whereas CM-allergen-specific IgE levels could be detected in all 41 patients with anaphylactic reactions to CM with the use of a MAMA.

3.4. All CM-Allergic Patients with a Sampson Grade of 4–5 (but Bot Those with a Score of 1–3) Show Casein-Specific IgE Reactivity

When comparing the IgE reactivity profiles and the levels of patients with anaphylactic reactions with CM grades of 1–3 with the patients who had grade 4–5 reactions, we found that all patients who had grade 4–5 reactions showed IgE reactivity to at least one of the caseins (particularly alpha-casein (Figure 2A)). By contrast, only 12 out of 21 grade 1–3 patients showed IgE reactivity to caseins, 10 to alpha-casein, 1 to beta-casein (i.e., patient 40) and 1 to kappa-casein (i.e., patient 34) (Figure 2A). Interestingly, patient 34 showed IgE levels above the cut-off threshold (i.e., 0.3 ISU) of the alpha-casein-derived peptide Cas4 but not of the complete alpha-casein molecule (Figure 2A).

The nine patients with a grade of 1–3 who were negative to caseins showed IgE reactivity to alpha-lactalbumin ($n = 7$) or beta-lactoglobulin ($n = 2$). Of note, all seven alpha-lactalbumin-positive patients were negative to caseins and beta-lactoglobulin but showed grade 1–3 reactions. However, BSA was also recognized in casein-negative patients, but these patients were positive to alpha-lactalbumin and/or beta-lactoglobulin (Figure 2A,B).

3.5. The Use of MAMA Reveals IgE Reactivity to Cryptic Milk-Allergen-Derived Peptides

We made an interesting observation when comparing the IgE reactivities to the complete allergens and allergen-derived peptides in our study population. In general, IgE reactivity and specific IgE levels to allergen-derived peptides were lower than those for complete allergens. However, we found six patients who showed IgE reactivity to cryptic allergen-derived peptides without exhibiting allergen-specific IgE reactivity. Patients #30, #34, #37 and #69 showed IgE reactivity to alpha-casein-derived peptides but not to alpha-casein (Figure 2A). Furthermore, patient #39 showed IgE reactivity to the alpha-lactalbumin peptide Lac6 but not to the complete allergen, and patient #20 showed IgE levels against the beta-lactoglobulin peptide BLG4 but not against beta-lactoglobulin (Figure 2B).

3.6. IgE Levels to CM Allergens and Allergen-Derived Peptides Are Higher in Patients with Anaphylactic Reactions to CM than in Patients without Anaphylactic Symptoms

Figure 3 shows, in patients with and without anaphylactic reactions, the frequencies of IgE reactivity, as well as the specific IgE levels for the individual CM allergens and CM-allergen-derived peptides. The frequency of the IgE recognition of caseins and casein-derived peptides was approximately twice as high in patients with a grade of 4–5 when compared to patients with a grade of 1–3 and those without anaphylactic reactions (Figure 3). Importantly, grade 4–5 patients showed higher IgE levels to caseins and casein-derived peptides than grade 1–3 patients and those patients without anaphylaxis (Figures 3 and 4A).

3.7. CM-Allergic Patients Who Develop Tolerance after an Elimination Diet Show a Drop of Allergen-Specific IgE When Using MAMA

For 11 of the patients (Table 2), 7 were with and 4 were without anaphylactic reactions to CM. We had the chance to compare the allergen- and peptide-specific IgE levels before and after an elimination diet with the use of a MAMA (Table 2, Figure 5). A total of six of the patients developed partial tolerance to CM because they were able to eat baked or fermented milk products after an elimination diet (Table 2). The patients who developed tolerances were the grade 1–3 patients or those patients without CM-related anaphylactic reactions. Each of the six patients who developed tolerance showed a decline in allergen- and/or peptide-specific IgE, whereas no relevant decline in specific IgE levels was noted for the five patients who did not develop tolerance (Figure 5). Further, two out of the five patients who did not develop tolerance were grade 4–5 patients. No relevant differences regarding the duration of the time of the elimination diet were noted among the tolerant or intolerant patients (Table 2).

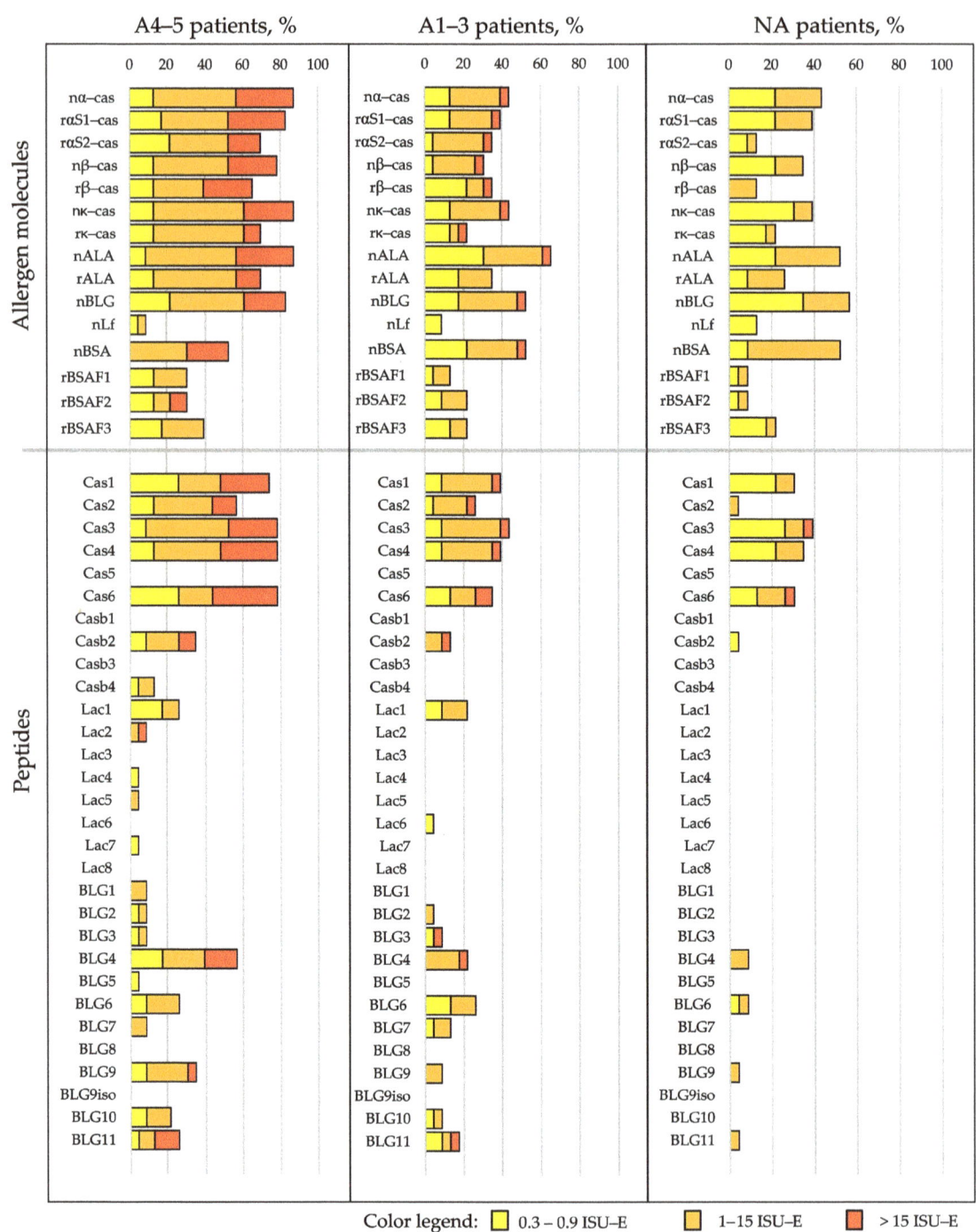

Figure 3. Frequencies and intensities of IgE recognition (the percentages of reactive sera and IgE levels according to a color code) of milk allergen proteins and peptides in patients with anaphylaxis according to Sampson criteria of 4–5 (A4–5 patients), with anaphylaxis according to Sampson criteria of 1–3 (A1–3 patients) and without anaphylaxis (NA patients).

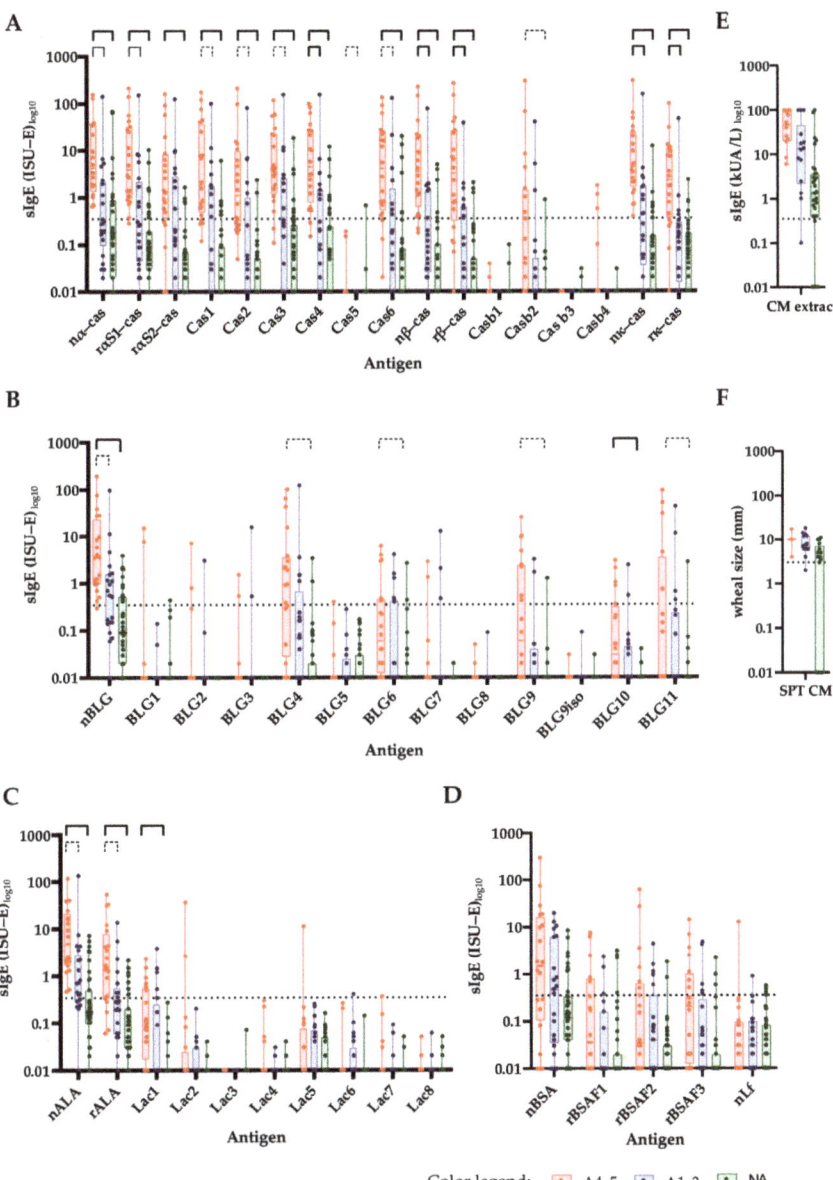

Figure 4. The IgE levels of CM-allergic patients to micro-arrayed milk proteins and peptides. The specific IgE levels (y-axes: ISU-E or kUA/L log10, box and whisker diagrams showing the first and third quartiles, as well as the minima and maxima, i.e., whiskers) toward (**A**) caseins and casein-derived peptides (**B**); β-lactoglobulins and β-lactoglobulin-derived peptides (**C**); α-lactalbumin and α-lactalbumin-derived peptides (**D**); BSA recombinant BSA fragments and lactoferrin, (**E**) cow's milk allergen extract and (**F**) SPT results (mean wheal diameters in mm) in patients with a Sampson grade of 4–5 (A4–5: red), a Sampson grade of 1–3 (A1–3: blue) and those without anaphylaxis (NA: green) are shown. Statistically significant differences between the groups are shown by a capped line as in the above, p-value << 0.001 (Holm-corrected to 0.000385; continuous bold line), p-value < 0.001 (continuous line) and p-value < 0.01 (dotted line).

	Continued intolerance										Tolerance development											
Allergen	1	1a	25	25a	65	65a	66	66a	11	11a	36	36a	32	32a	38	38a	67	67a	70	70a	30	30a
nα-cas	22.4	15.8	2.4	2.5	0.7	1.0	0.0	0.2	0.7	0.6	0.0	0.0	0.1	0.1	2.0	0.2	0.0	0.0	0.1	0.1	0.2	0.0
rαS1-cas	28.6	16.0	2.6	2.4	0.8	1.1	0.0	0.2	1.1	0.7	0.0	0.0	0.0	0.0	1.7	0.1	0.0	0.0	0.1	0.1	0.1	0.0
rαS2-cas	19.7	21.0	2.3	1.5	0.2	0.2	0.0	0.0	0,6	0.3	0.0	0.0	0.1	0.1	4.3	0.0	0.0	0.0	0.1	0.0	0.0	0.0
Cas1	8.0	8.7	1.2	0.7	1.3	0.6	0,1	0.8	0.8	0.5	0.0	0.0	0.1	0.0	1.9	0.0	0.0	0.0	0.0	0.0	0.0	0.0
Cas2	14.1	7.4	0.8	0.4	0.0	0.0	0.0	0.0	0.2	0.2	0.0	0.0	0.0	0.0	2.1	0.0	0.0	0.0	0.0	0.0	0.0	0.0
Cas3	22.3	20.3	2.6	1.6	1.0	1.9	0.0	0.0	1.5	1.3	0.0	0.0	0.0	0.0	2.0	0.0	0.0	0.0	0.2	0.1	0.0	0.0
Cas4	62.5	26.0	1.5	1.7	0.7	0.4	0.0	0.0	0.6	0.6	0.0	0.0	0.0	0.0	1.9	0.0	0.0	0.0	0.0	0.0	0.0	0.0
Cas5	0.0	0.0	0.0	0.0	0.0	0.0	0.0	0.0	0.0	0.0	0.0	0.0	0.0	0.0	0.0	0.0	0.0	0.0	0.0	0.0	0.0	0.0
Cas6	62.0	23.3	2.3	4.1	0.1	0.0	0.0	0.0	0.5	0.3	0.0	0.0	0.0	0.0	0.2	0.1	0.0	0.0	0.0	0.0	0.6	0.1
nβ-cas	18.3	10.2	2.0	1.8	0.3	0.5	0.0	0.0	1.2	1.0	0.0	0.0	0.0	0.0	2.0	0.0	0.0	0.0	0.1	0.0	0.0	0.0
rβ-cas	23.5	16.7	0.7	1.5	0.1	0.0	0.0	0.0	0.8	0.4	0.0	0.0	0.1	0.1	0.4	0.0	0.0	0.0	0.0	0.0	0.0	0.0
Casb1	0.0	0.0	0.0	0.0	0.0	0.0	0.0	0.0	0.0	0.0	0.0	0.0	0.0	0.0	0.0	0.0	0.0	0.0	0.0	0.0	0.0	0.0
Casb2	4.3	4.4	0.1	0.0	0.0	0.0	0.0	0.0	0.1	0.1	0.1	0.0	0.0	0.0	0.0	0.0	0.0	0.0	0.0	0.0	0.0	0.0
Casb3	0.0	0.0	0.0	0.0	0.0	0.0	0.0	0.0	0.0	0.0	0.0	0.0	0.0	0.0	0.0	0.0	0.0	0.0	0.0	0.0	0.0	0.0
Casb4	0.0	0.0	0.0	0.0	0.0	0.0	0.0	0.0	0.0	0.0	0.0	0.0	0.0	0.0	0.0	0.0	0.0	0.0	0.0	0.0	0.0	0.0
nκ-cas	24.7	10.2	1.7	1.8	0.5	0.7	0.0	0.0	2.5	2.2	0.0	0.0	0.1	0.0	4.2	0.0	0.0	0.0	0.2	0.1	0.0	0.0
rκ-cas	11.2	3.3	0.4	0.6	0.3	0.2	0.0	0.0	1.7	1.6	0.0	0.0	0.2	0.1	0.2	0.0	0.0	0.0	0.2	0.1	0.1	0.1
nALA	16.1	17.6	0.5	0.6	0.1	0.2	0.4	0.6	2.5	2.7	4.3	3.6	0.3	0.1	3.5	0.2	0.5	0.1	1.5	0.4	1.3	0.2
rALA	12.0	9.1	0.1	0.2	0.0	0.0	0.1	0.0	1.4	1.1	0.4	2.0	0,3	0.1	2.3	0.2	0.0	0.0	0.3	0.1	0.2	0.1
Lac1	0.2	0.1	0.0	0.0	0.0	0.0	0.0	0.0	0.1	0.3	1.4	0.0	0.0	0.0	0.5	0.0	0.0	0.0	0.0	0.0	0.0	0.0
Lac2	0.0	0.0	0.0	0.0	0.0	0.0	0.0	0.0	0.0	0.0	0.0	0.0	0.0	0.0	0.0	0.0	0.0	0.0	0.1	0.0	0.0	0.0
Lac3	0.0	0.0	0.0	0.0	0.0	0.0	0.0	0.0	0.0	0.0	0.0	0.0	0.0	0.0	0.0	0.0	0.0	0.0	0.0	0.0	0.0	0.0
Lac4	0.0	0.0	0.0	0.0	0.0	0.0	0.0	0.0	0.0	0.0	0.0	0.0	0.0	0.0	0.0	0.0	0.0	0.0	0.0	0.0	0.0	0.0
Lac5	0.2	1.0	0.2	0.4	0.0	0.0	0.0	0.0	0.0	0.0	0.0	0.0	0.0	0.0	0.0	0.0	0.0	0.0	0.0	0.0	0.0	0.0
Lac6	0.0	0.0	0.0	0.0	0.0	0.0	0.0	0.0	0.0	0.0	0.0	0.0	0.0	0.0	0.0	0.0	0.0	0.0	0.0	0.0	0.0	0.0
Lac7	0.0	0.0	0.0	0.0	0.0	0.0	0.0	0.0	0.0	0.0	0.0	0.0	0.0	0.0	0.0	0.0	0.0	0.0	0.0	0.0	0.0	0.0
Lac8	0.0	0.0	0.0	0.0	0.0	0.0	0.0	0.0	0.0	0.0	0.0	0.0	0.0	0.0	0.0	0.0	0.0	0.0	0.0	0.0	0.0	0.0
nBLG	28.1	21.5	1.7	2.1	0.4	0.3	0.2	0.1	4.0	3.8	0.1	0.0	0.1	0.1	11.3	0.2	0.0	0.0	0.2	0.1	0.1	0.1
BLG1	0.0	0.1	0.0	0.0	0.0	0.0	0.0	0.0	0.0	0.0	0.0	0.0	0.0	0.0	0.1	0.0	0.0	0.0	0.0	0.0	0,0	0,0
BLG2	0.0	0.0	0.0	0.0	0.0	0.0	0.0	0.0	0.0	0.0	0.1	0.0	0.0	0.0	0.0	0.0	0.0	0.0	0.0	0.0	0.0	0.0
BLG3	0.0	0.0	0.0	0.0	0.0	0.0	0.0	0.0	0.0	0.0	0.0	0.0	0.0	0.0	0.0	0.0	0.0	0.0	0.0	0.0	0.0	0.0
BLG4	43.4	36.1	0.2	0.3	0.0	0.0	0.0	0.0	2.2	1.5	0.0	0.0	0.0	0.0	0.2	0.0	0.0	0.0	0.1	0.0	0.0	0.0
BLG5	0.0	0.0	0.2	0.2	0.0	0.0	0.0	0.0	0.0	0.0	0.0	0.0	0.0	0.0	0.0	0.0	0.0	0.0	0.0	0.0	0.0	0.0
BLG6	6.1	20.9	0.0	0.0	0.0	0.0	0.0	0.0	0.5	0.2	0.0	0.0	0.0	0.0	0.4	0,0	0.0	0.0	0.0	0.0	0.0	0.0
BLG7	0.0	0.0	0.0	0.0	0.0	0.0	0.0	0.0	1.3	1.1	0.0	0.0	0.0	0.0	0.0	0.0	0.0	0.0	0.0	0.0	0.0	0.0
BLG8	0.0	0.1	0.0	0.0	0.0	0.0	0.0	0.0	0.0	0.0	0.0	0.0	0.0	0.0	0.0	0.0	0.0	0.0	0.0	0.0	0.0	0.0
BLG9	9.6	0.6	0.0	0.1	0.0	0.0	0.0	0.0	2.2	1.3	0.0	0.0	0.0	0.0	0.0	0.0	0.0	0.0	0.0	0.0	0.0	0.0
BLG9iso	0.0	0,0	0.0	0.0	0.0	0.0	0.0	0.0	0.0	0.0	0.0	0.0	0.0	0.0	0.0	0.0	0.0	0.0	0.0	0.0	0.0	0.0
BLG10	0.2	0.2	0.0	0.0	0.0	0.0	0.0	0.0	0.0	0.0	0.0	0.0	0.0	0.0	0.1	0.0	0.0	0.0	0.0	0.0	0.0	0.0
BLG11	4.4	1.7	0.0	0.0	0.0	0.0	0.0	0.0	4.4	2.3	0.0	0.0	0.0	0.0	11.2	0.0	0.0	0.0	0.0	0.0	0.0	0.0
nBSA	28.3	25.4	0.8	1.2	2.2	1.7	0.0	0.0	0.0	0.0	0.0	0.0	0.4	0.2	6.2	1.0	3.1	1.6	0.2	0.1	0.0	0.1
rBSAF1	7.6	5.1	0.0	0.0	0.0	0.0	0.0	0.0	0.0	0.0	0.0	0.0	0.0	0.0	0.2	0.0	0.0	0.0	0.0	0.0	0.0	0.0
rBSAF2	27.0	14.1	0.0	0.1	0.0	0.0	0.0	0.0	0.0	0.0	0.0	0.0	0.1	0.1	0.9	0.0	0.0	0.0	0.0	0.0	0.0	0.0
rBSAF3	6.9	4.1	0.0	0.0	0.4	0.3	0.0	0.0	0.0	0.0	0.0	0.0	0.1	0.0	0.6	0.1	0.0	0.0	0.0	0.0	0.0	0.0
nLf	0.3	0.3	0.1	0.2	0.0	0.0	0.0	0.0	0.0	0.0	0.0	0.0	0.0	0.0	0.0	0.4	0.0	0.0	1.8	0.7	0.0	0.0

Color legend:

negative
0.3–0.9
1–14.9
> 15
new reactivity

Figure 5. Heat map of the IgE levels specific for caseins and casein-derived peptides and other milk allergen proteins and peptides thereof in the sera of patients with continued intolerance and those developing tolerance before and after elimination (a). The IgE (ISU-E) levels are shown with a color code.

4. Discussion

Different mechanisms may be responsible for CM intolerance, and among them are lactose intolerance, IgE-mediated allergy and others [3]. In order to confirm the diagnosis of an IgE-mediated allergy, the detection of CM-allergen-specific IgE antibodies is crucial [4,5]. Serological tests for the detection of CM-allergen-specific IgE antibodies based on allergen extracts do not allow one to discriminate between the molecular IgE sensitization profiles [13]. For example, IgE sensitization to BSA is usually not associated with severe allergic reactions to CM exposure and can be a result of primary respiratory sensitization to albumins from pets [18]. On the other hand, IgE sensitization to caseins, beta-lactoglobulin and alpha-lactalbumin is often associated with anaphylactic symptoms [13]. Accordingly, multi-allergen tests containing different milk allergen molecules or CM-allergen-derived peptides have been developed [19–22]. These tests have been useful methods through which to establish molecular IgE sensitization profiles, monitor the effects of CM AIT and establish the development of tolerance to CM [21–25].

The milk allergen micro-array (MAMA) developed by us is unique and different from published and currently available multi-allergen tests for measuring CM-specific IgE antibodies (which either contain only purified CM allergen molecules [19] or only peptides and fragments from certain cow's milk allergens [20–22]). By contrast, the MAMA used in this study contains each of the milk allergens (i.e., caseins, alpha-lactalbumin, beta-lactoglobulin, BSA and lactoferrin), as well as the CM-allergen-derived peptides. According to the results obtained in our cohort of patients with anaphylactic symptoms to CM, all patients with IgE-mediated anaphylactic reactions were identified through the use of the MAMA, whereas this was not the case when using established methods for the quantification of CM-allergen-specific IgE (i.e., ImmunoCAP) or when in vivo testing (i.e., SPT) with CM allergen extracts was performed. Thus, the use of the MAMA appears to be superior to the latter allergen-extract-based methods for detecting IgE-mediated sensitization in CM-specific anaphylactic patients. However, although there was a good concordance between IgE positivity measured by MAMA and allergen extract-based ImmunoCAP and SPT, concordance was not complete for all children with non-anaphylactic reactions to cow's milk (Figure 2). Similar results have been reported by other authors for micro-array-based diagnostics [35,36]. Another limitation of our study was that we have not tested sera from non-allergic subjects with MAMA. Yet, there are advantages of using MAMA over traditional ImmunoCAP detection methods of CM-allergen-specific IgE: With the use of a MAMA, IgE sensitization to multiple allergens and allergen-derived peptides can be detected with an incredibly small amount of serum, whereas almost twice the volume is needed for one ImmunoCAP determination. This advantage is particularly important for measuring specific IgE sensitization in small children from whom it may be difficult to obtain large amounts of serum. When using MAMA, a capillary blood sample is sufficient. It should be also mentioned that we found an excellent correlation of allergen-specific IgE levels determined by MAMA and the approved ImmunoCAP ISAC micro-array (Figure S1), although some discordances were noted which may be attributed to some differences regarding technology and allergen preparations.

Yet another important aspect of MAMA should be mentioned, which may become more relevant if MAMA is further refined for routine diagnosis. In fact, the production costs of MAMA are relatively low; thus, it may be possible to provide MAMA for the large-scale screening of IgE sensitization to milk in children.

The testing of IgE reactivity profiles to allergen molecules and allergen-derived peptides with MAMA revealed certain interesting and notable findings. For example, we found that certain CM-allergic children reacted only to allergen-derived peptides, so-called "cryptic epitopes", which seem to be hidden in the intact allergen molecules and may become exposed only after digestion and/or the denaturation of the allergens. On the other hand, many CM-allergic patients suffering from CM-related anaphylaxis reacted only with intact allergen molecules; thus, this diagnosis would have escaped the diagnostic tests that are based only on allergen-derived peptides [20–22].

Furthermore, the use of MAMA appeared to be useful for monitoring the development of CM tolerance following an elimination diet, although tolerance was not assessed by controlled challenges in the clinic. In fact, we found that those patients who developed some form of CM tolerance upon the reintroduction of milk in the diet showed a reduction in allergen-specific IgE levels, whereas this was not observed for patients who did not develop signs of clinical tolerance.

In our study, we were not able to investigate patients who underwent AIT or OIT with CM allergens and therefore we do not have data regarding the development of allergen-specific IgG. However, the technology used by us for generating the MAMA is based on the well-established printing of allergens or peptides on pre-activated glass slides, which has been shown to also be useful for measuring allergen-specific IgG (IgG_1, IgG_4) responses [30]. Although not investigated in this study, it is known that under the given amounts of immobilized antigens in MAMA, one would expect that the blocking effect of AIT-induced IgG can be visualized via the competition with IgE binding by blocking the

IgG antibodies that can be visualized by a reduction in allergen-specific IgE binding as a surrogate biomarker for the effects of AIT [30,37,38].

Although we were able to test a relatively large number of sera from CM-allergic children from different centers, it may be considered a limitation of our study that no double-blind, placebo-controlled food challenges had been performed in our patients. However, clinicians were able to provide a meticulous clinical characterization of the milk-allergic children, and this corresponded with the requirements set by international guidelines [26], including the presence of the clinical symptoms of immediate types of CMA that could be unambiguously attributed to CM and that had a clear-cut history of anaphylaxis following milk consumption [27].

In conclusion, we developed MAMA, containing milk allergens and allergen-derived peptides, as a useful research tool for the detection of IgE sensitization to multiple allergen molecules and allergen-derived peptides in CM-allergic patients, particularly for children that requires only small amounts of serum samples.

Supplementary Materials: The following supporting information can be downloaded at https://www.mdpi.com/article/10.3390/nu15102401/s1, Table S1: Sources, sequences and characteristics of the allergens and peptides of MAMA; Table S2: Detailed statistical analysis of the differences in median IgE levels specific for CM allergens and CM-allergen-derived peptides in patients with anaphylaxis according Sampson criteria 4–5 (A4–5 patients), with anaphylaxis according to Sampson criteria 1–3 (A1–3 patients) and those without anaphylaxis (NA patients); Figure S1: Heat map (A) and correlation (B) of IgE levels (ISU-E) specific for cow's milk allergen molecules (na-cas, nAla, nBLG, nBSA) as determined by MAMA (x-axes) versus ImmunoCAP ISAC (y-axes).

Author Contributions: V.G., investigation, software, validation, analysis, writing—original draft preparation, review and editing; D.T., validation, analysis, writing—original draft preparation, review and editing; R.F., investigation, software, validation, analysis, review and editing; B.L., validation, analysis, review and editing; B.L. validation, analysis, review and editing; T.S., investigation, software, validation, analysis, review and editing; N.D., A.P., D.D., T.L., M.G., E.V., E.B., V.N., S.T., A.K. (Alina Kiyamova), A.K. (Alexander Karaulov) and S.K., investigation, software, validation, analysis, review and editing; A.K. (Alexander Karaulov), project administration, funding acquisition, review and editing; R.V., conceptualization, writing—original draft preparation, analysis, review and editing. All authors have read and agreed to the published version of the manuscript.

Funding: This research was funded by HVD Biotech, Vienna, Austria; the Medical University of Vienna, Austria; and the Danube Allergy Research Cluster program of the Country of Lower Austria. The data analysis and their summary in the form of a structured paper were supported by a grant from the Russian Science Foundation (project no.: 23-75-30016: "Allergen micro-array-based assessment of allergic sensitization profiles in the Russian Federation as basis for personalized treatment and prevention of allergy (AllergochipRUS)").

Institutional Review Board Statement: This study was conducted in accordance with the guidelines detailed in the Declaration of Helsinki, and was approved by the ethics committees of different clinical centers and of the Medical University of Vienna, Austria (EK1641/2014).

Informed Consent Statement: Written informed consent to obtain blood samples and immunological analysis was obtained from the parents or legal guardians of all the children.

Data Availability Statement: All data are available upon reasonable request. Furthermore, the MAMA will be made available as a research tool upon reasonable request for others to use in the course of collaborative research projects.

Conflicts of Interest: A.P. received personnel fees from LLC "Nutricia" and Friesland Campina. R.V. received research grants from HiPP GmbH & Co. Vertrieb KG, Pfaffenhofen, Germany; Worg Pharmaceuticals, Hangzhou, China; HVD Biotech, Vienna, Austria; and Viravaxx, Vienna, Austria. He serves as a consultant for Viravaxx and Worg. The other authors declare no conflicts of interest. The funders had no role in the design of the study; in the collection, analyses, or interpretation of data; or in the decision to publish the results.

Abbreviations

MAMA	Milk allergen micro-array
CM	cow's milk
CMA	Cow's milk allergy
BSA	Bovine serum albumin
HSA	Human serum albumin
AIT	Allergen-specific immunotherapy
OIT	Oral immunotherapy
GI	Gastrointestinal symptoms
BA	Bronchial asthma
AR	Allergic rhinitis
AD	Atopic dermatitis
FA	Food allergy
SPT	Skin prick test
MV	Median value
ISU	ISAC standardized units
ISU-E	IgE level presented in ISAC standardized units
A4–5	Patients with milk-related anaphylaxis with a Sampson score of 4–5
A1–3	Patients with milk-related anaphylaxis with a Sampson score of 1–3
NA	Patients without anaphylaxis
na-cas	natural alpha casein
nALA	natural alpha lactalbumin
nBLG	natural betalagtoglobulin

References

1. Arasi, S.; Cafarotti, A.; Fiocchi, A. Cow's milk allergy. *Curr. Opin. Allergy Clin. Immunol.* **2022**, *22*, 181–187. [CrossRef]
2. Östblom, E.; Lilja, G.; Pershagen, G.; van Hage, M.; Wickman, M. Phenotypes of food hypersensitivity and development of allergic diseases during the first 8 years of life. *Clin. Exp. Allergy* **2008**, *38*, 1325–1332. [CrossRef]
3. Valenta, R.; Hochwallner, H.; Linhart, B.; Pahr, S. Food Allergies: The Basics. *Gastroenterology* **2015**, *148*, 1120–1131.e4. [CrossRef] [PubMed]
4. Fiocchi, A.; Brozek, J.; Schünemann, H.; Bahna, S.L.; von Berg, A.; Beyer, K.; Bozzola, M.; Bradsher, J.; Compalati, E.; Ebisawa, M.; et al. World Allergy Organization (WAO) Diagnosis and Rationale for Action against Cow's Milk Allergy (DRACMA) Guidelines. *World Allergy Organ. J.* **2010**, *3*, 57–161. [CrossRef] [PubMed]
5. Canani, R.B.; Ruotolo, S.; Discepolo, V.; Troncone, R. The diagnosis of food allergy in children. *Curr. Opin. Pediatr.* **2008**, *20*, 584–589. [CrossRef] [PubMed]
6. Lieberman, J.A.; Sicherer, S.H. Diagnosis of Food Allergy: Epicutaneous Skin Tests, In Vitro Tests, and Oral Food Challenge. *Curr. Allergy Asthma Rep.* **2011**, *11*, 58–64. [CrossRef] [PubMed]
7. Perry, T.T.; Matsui, E.C.; Conover-Walker, M.K.; Wood, R.A. Risk of oral food challenges. *J. Allergy Clin. Immunol.* **2004**, *114*, 1164–1168. [CrossRef]
8. Sporik, R.; Hill, D.J.; Hosking, C.S. Specificity of allergen skin testing in predicting positive open food challenges to milk, egg and peanut in children. *Clin. Exp. Allergy* **2000**, *30*, 1541–1546. [CrossRef]
9. Hochwallner, H.; Schulmeister, U.; Swoboda, I.; Balic, N.; Geller, B.; Nystrand, M.; Harlin, A.; Thalhamer, J.; Scheiblhofer, S.; Niggemann, B.; et al. Microarray and allergenic activity assessment of milk allergens. *Clin. Exp. Allergy* **2010**, *40*, 1809–1818. [CrossRef]
10. Sampson, H.A.; Ho, D.G. Relationship between food-specific IgE concentrations and the risk of positive food challenges in children and adolescents. *J. Allergy Clin. Immunol.* **1997**, *100*, 444–451. [CrossRef]
11. Cuomo, B.; Indirli, G.C.; Bianchi, A.; Arasi, S.; Caimmi, D.; Dondi, A.; La Grutta, S.; Panetta, V.; Verga, M.C.; Calvani, M. Specific IgE and skin prick tests to diagnose allergy to fresh and baked cow's milk according to age: A systematic review. *Ital. J. Pediatr.* **2017**, *43*, 93. [CrossRef] [PubMed]
12. Hochwallner, H.; Schulmeister, U.; Swoboda, I.; Spitzauer, S.; Valenta, R. Cow's milk allergy: From allergens to new forms of diagnosis, therapy and prevention. *Methods* **2014**, *66*, 22–33. [CrossRef] [PubMed]
13. Matricardi, P.M.; Kleine-Tebbe, J.; Hoffmann, H.J.; Valenta, R.; Hilger, C.; Hofmaier, S.; Aalberse, R.C.; Agache, I.; Asero, R.; Ballmer-Weber, B.; et al. EAACI Molecular Allergology User's Guide. *Pediatr. Allergy Immunol.* **2016**, *27*, S23. [CrossRef] [PubMed]
14. Valenta, R.; Lidholm, J.; Niederberger, V.; Hayek, B.; Kraft, D.; Grönlund, H. The recombinant allergen-based concept of component-resolved diagnostics and immunotherapy (CRD and CRIT). *Clin. Exp. Allergy* **1999**, *29*, 896–904. [CrossRef] [PubMed]
15. Linhart, B.; Freidl, R.; Elisyutina, O.; Khaitov, M.; Karaulov, A.; Valenta, R. Molecular Approaches for Diagnosis, Therapy and Prevention of Cow's Milk Allergy. *Nutrients* **2019**, *11*, 1492. [CrossRef] [PubMed]

16. Cerecedo, I.; Zamora, J.; Shreffler, W.G.; Lin, J.; Bardina, L.; Dieguez, M.C.; Wang, J.; Muriel, A.; de la Hoz, B.; Sampson, H.A. Mapping of the IgE and IgG4 sequential epitopes of milk allergens with a peptide microarray–based immunoassay. *J. Allergy Clin. Immunol.* **2008**, *122*, 589–594. [CrossRef] [PubMed]
17. Savilahti, E.; Kuitunen, M. Allergenicity of cow milk proteins. *J. Pediatr.* **1992**, *121*, S12–S20. [CrossRef]
18. Karsonova, A.V.; Riabova, K.A.; Khaitov, M.R.; Elisyutina, O.G.; Ilina, N.; Fedenko, E.S.; Fomina, D.S.; Beltyukov, E.; Bondarenko, N.L.; Evsegneeva, I.V.; et al. Milk-Specific IgE Reactivity Without Symptoms in Albumin-Sensitized Cat Allergic Patients. *Allergy Asthma Immunol. Res.* **2021**, *13*, 668–670. [CrossRef]
19. Ansotegui, I.J.; Melioli, G.; Canonica, G.W.; Gómez, R.M.; Jensen-Jarolim, E.; Ebisawa, M.; Luengo, O.; Caraballo, L.; Passalacqua, G.; Poulsen, L.K.; et al. A WAO—ARIA—GA2LEN consensus document on molecular-based allergy diagnosis (PAMD@): Update 2020. *World Allergy Organ. J.* **2020**, *13*, 100091. [CrossRef]
20. Lin, J.; Bardina, L.; Shreffler, W.G.; Andreae, D.A.; Ge, Y.; Wang, J.; Bruni, F.M.; Fu, Z.; Han, Y.; Sampson, H.A. Development of a novel peptide microarray for large-scale epitope mapping of food allergens. *J. Allergy Clin. Immunol.* **2009**, *124*, 315–322.e3. [CrossRef]
21. Beyer, K.; Jarvinen, K.-M.; Bardina, L.; Mishoe, M.; Turjanmaa, K.; Niggemann, B.; Ahlstedt, S.; Venemalm, L.; Sampson, H.A. IgE-binding peptides coupled to a commercial matrix as a diagnostic instrument for persistent cow's milk allergy. *J. Allergy Clin. Immunol.* **2005**, *116*, 704–705. [CrossRef] [PubMed]
22. Sackesen, C.; Suárez-Fariñas, M.; Silva, R.; Lin, J.; Schmidt, S.; Getts, R.; Gimenez, G.; Yilmaz, E.A.; Cavkaytar, O.; Buyuktiryaki, B.; et al. A new Luminex-based peptide assay to identify reactivity to baked, fermented, and whole milk. *Allergy* **2019**, *74*, 327–336. [CrossRef] [PubMed]
23. Savilahti, E.M.; Rantanen, V.; Lin, J.S.; Karinen, S.; Saarinen, K.M.; Goldis, M.; Mäkelä, M.J.; Hautaniemi, S.; Savilahti, E.; Sampson, H.A. Early recovery from cow's milk allergy is associated with decreasing IgE and increasing IgG4 binding to cow's milk epitopes. *J. Allergy Clin. Immunol.* **2010**, *125*, 1315–1321.e9. [CrossRef] [PubMed]
24. Caubet, J.-C.; Nowak-Wegrzyn, A.; Moshier, E.; Godbold, J.; Wang, J.; Sampson, H.A. Utility of casein-specific IgE levels in predicting reactivity to baked milk. *J. Allergy Clin. Immunol.* **2013**, *131*, 222–224.e4. [CrossRef] [PubMed]
25. Wang, J.; Lin, J.; Bardina, L.; Goldis, M.; Nowak-Wegrzyn, A.; Shreffler, W.G.; Sampson, H.A. Correlation of IgE/IgG4 milk epitopes and affinity of milk-specific IgE antibodies with different phenotypes of clinical milk allergy. *J. Allergy Clin. Immunol.* **2010**, *125*, 695–702. [CrossRef] [PubMed]
26. Sicherer, S.H.; A Sampson, H. 9. Food allergy. *J. Allergy Clin. Immunol.* **2006**, *117*, 470–475. [CrossRef]
27. Muraro, A.; Roberts, G.; Clark, A.; Eigenmann, P.; Halken, S.; Lack, G.; Moneret-Vautrin, A.; Niggemann, B.; Rancé, F.; EAACI Task Force on Anaphylaxis in Children. The management of anaphylaxis in childhood: Position paper of the European academy of allergology and clinical immunology. *Allergy* **2007**, *62*, 857–871. [CrossRef]
28. Dribin, T.E.; Schnadower, D.; Spergel, J.M.; Campbell, R.L.; Shaker, M.; Neuman, M.I.; Michelson, K.A.; Capucilli, P.S.; Camargo, C.A., Jr.; Brousseau, D.C.; et al. Severity grading system for acute allergic reactions: A multidisciplinary Delphi study. *J. Allergy Clin. Immunol.* **2021**, *148*, 173–181. [CrossRef]
29. Gattinger, P.; Niespodziana, K.; Stiasny, K.; Sahanic, S.; Tulaeva, I.; Borochova, K.; Dorofeeva, Y.; Schlederer, T.; Sonnweber, T.; Hofer, G.; et al. Neutralization of SARS-CoV-2 requires antibodies against conformational receptor-binding domain epitopes. *Allergy* **2022**, *77*, 230–242. [CrossRef]
30. Lupinek, C.; Wollmann, E.; Baar, A.; Banerjee, S.; Breiteneder, H.; Broecker, B.M.; Bublin, M.; Curin, M.; Flicker, S.; Garmatiuk, T.; et al. Advances in allergen-microarray technology for diagnosis and monitoring of allergy: The MeDALL allergen-chip. *Methods* **2014**, *66*, 106–119. [CrossRef]
31. Niespodziana, K.; Stenberg-Hammar, K.; Megremis, S.; Cabauatan, C.R.; Napora-Wijata, K.; Vacal, P.C.; Gallerano, D.; Lupinek, C.; Ebner, D.; Schlederer, T.; et al. PreDicta chip-based high resolution diagnosis of rhinovirus-induced wheeze. *Nat. Commun.* **2018**, *9*, 2382. [CrossRef]
32. Holm, S. A simple sequentially rejective multiple test procedure. *Scand. J. Stat.* **1979**, *6*, 65–70.
33. Schulmeister, U.; Hochwallner, H.; Swoboda, I.; Focke-Tejkl, M.; Geller, B.; Nystrand, M.; Härlin, A.; Thalhamer, J.; Scheiblhofer, S.; Keller, W.; et al. Cloning, Expression, and Mapping of Allergenic Determinants of αS1-Casein, a Major Cow's Milk Allergen. *J. Immunol.* **2009**, *182*, 7019–7029. [CrossRef] [PubMed]
34. Hochwallner, H.; Schulmeister, U.; Swoboda, I.; Focke-Tejkl, M.; Civaj, V.; Balic, N.; Nystrand, M.; Härlin, A.; Thalhamer, J.; Scheiblhofer, S.; et al. Visualization of clustered IgE epitopes on α-lactalbumin. *J. Allergy Clin. Immunol.* **2010**, *125*, 1279–1285.e9. [CrossRef] [PubMed]
35. Ahrens, B.; De Oliveira, L.C.L.; Grabenhenrich, L.; Schulz, G.; Niggemann, B.; Wahn, U.; Beyer, K. Individual cow's milk allergens as prognostic markers for tolerance development? *Clin. Exp. Allergy* **2012**, *42*, 1630–1637. [CrossRef] [PubMed]
36. Wilson, J.; Workman, L.; Schuyler, A.J.; Rifas-Shiman, S.L.; McGowan, E.C.; Oken, E.; Gold, D.R.; Hamilton, R.G.; Platts-Mills, T.A. Allergen sensitization in a birth cohort at midchildhood: Focus on food component IgE and IgG4 responses. *J. Allergy Clin. Immunol.* **2018**, *141*, 419–423.e5. [CrossRef] [PubMed]

37. Lupinek, C.; Wollmann, E.; Valenta, R. Monitoring Allergen Immunotherapy Effects by Microarray. *Curr. Treat. Options Allergy* **2016**, *3*, 189–203. [CrossRef]
38. van Hage, M.; Hamsten, C.; Valenta, R. ImmunoCAP assays: Pros and cons in allergology. *J. Allergy Clin. Immunol.* **2017**, *140*, 974–977. [CrossRef]

Disclaimer/Publisher's Note: The statements, opinions and data contained in all publications are solely those of the individual author(s) and contributor(s) and not of MDPI and/or the editor(s). MDPI and/or the editor(s) disclaim responsibility for any injury to people or property resulting from any ideas, methods, instructions or products referred to in the content.

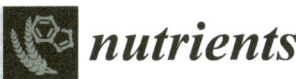

Correction

Correction: Quake et al. Early Introduction of Multi-Allergen Mixture for Prevention of Food Allergy: Pilot Study. *Nutrients* 2022, *14*, 737

Antonia Zoe Quake, Taryn Audrey Liu, Rachel D'Souza, Katherine G. Jackson, Margaret Woch, Afua Tetteh, Vanitha Sampath, Kari C. Nadeau *, Sayantani Sindher, R. Sharon Chinthrajah and Shu Cao

Department of Medicine, Division of Pulmonary, Allergy and Critical Care Medicine, Sean N. Parker Center for Allergy and Asthma Research at Stanford University, Stanford, CA 94304, USA
* Correspondence: knadeau@stanford.edu

1. Error in Figure 1

In the original publication [1], there was an error in **Figure 1**. **Change food challenge N = 15 for control to N = 45**. The corrected **Figure 1** appears below.

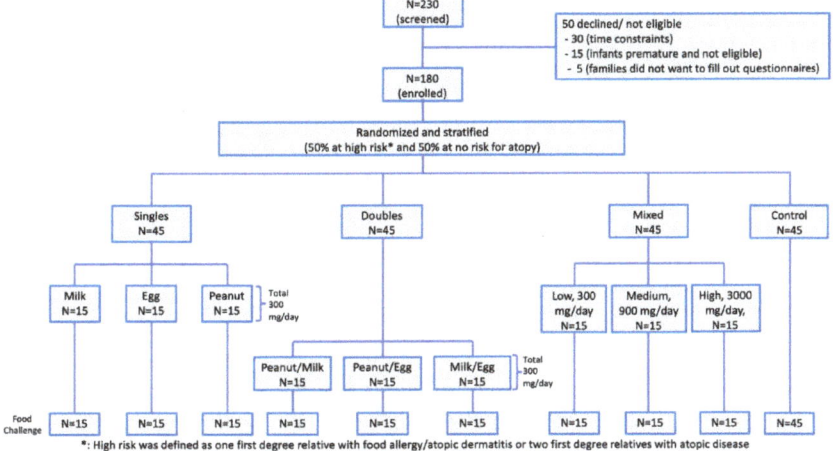

Figure 1. Consort diagram. 180 participants were randomized into three active and one control group. The active phase of the study was for one year and there were no dropouts. Single foods (milk, egg, or peanut); two foods (milk/egg, egg/peanut, milk/peanut), Mixed (milk/egg/peanut/cashew/almond/shrimp/walnut/wheat/salmon/hazelnut at low, medium, or high doses).

2. Error in Figure 2

In the original publication, there was an error in **Figure 2**. **Change the numbers of the sample sizes and Q value**. The corrected **Figure 2** appears below.

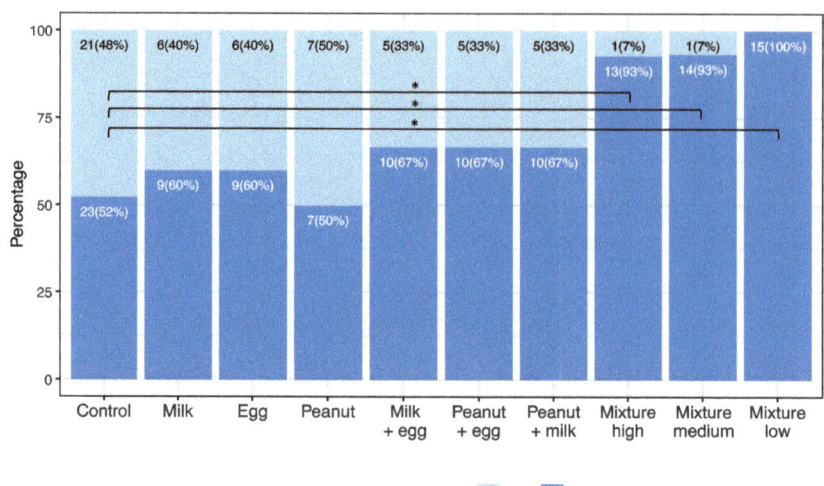

Figure 2. Oral Food Challenges: Food challenge outcome in active (singles, doubles, and mixtures) and control groups 2–4 years after start of study. Oral food challenges (up to 8 g of total protein from the 10-food allergen mixture) were conducted between 2–4 years after the start of the study in a facility with trained personnel with staged, monitored standard methods. Each food challenge consisted of several escalating doses of the food protein in flour or powder form concealed in an appropriate vehicle, such as applesauce or pudding, ingested by the participant every 15 min as tolerated. Typically challenges started with 2 mg and escalated upto a max of 8 g of total food protein as per our validated methods [26–28].

3. Text Correction

There was an error in the original publication. **The percent of participants able to consume 8 g of protein was significantly higher in all mixed protein groups compared to controls (q < 0.01)**.

A correction has been made to **Results**, **page 8**:

The percent of participants able to consume 8 g of protein was significantly higher in all mixed protein groups compared to the controls (q < 0.05). There were 44, 14, and 14 participants who had available OFC outcomes in the control, peanut, and mixture high groups, respectively.

The authors apologize for any inconvenience caused and state that the scientific conclusions are unaffected. This correction was approved by the Academic Editor. The original publication has also been updated.

Reference

1. Quake, A.Z.; Liu, T.A.; D'Souza, R.; Jackson, K.G.; Woch, M.; Tetteh, A.; Sampath, V.; Nadeau, K.C.; Sindher, S.; Chinthrajah, R.S.; et al. Early Introduction of Multi-Allergen Mixture for Prevention of Food Allergy: Pilot Study. *Nutrients* **2022**, *14*, 737. [CrossRef] [PubMed]

Disclaimer/Publisher's Note: The statements, opinions and data contained in all publications are solely those of the individual author(s) and contributor(s) and not of MDPI and/or the editor(s). MDPI and/or the editor(s) disclaim responsibility for any injury to people or property resulting from any ideas, methods, instructions or products referred to in the content.

MDPI
St. Alban-Anlage 66
4052 Basel
Switzerland
www.mdpi.com

Nutrients Editorial Office
E-mail: nutrients@mdpi.com
www.mdpi.com/journal/nutrients

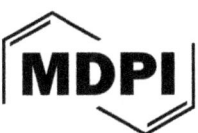

Disclaimer/Publisher's Note: The statements, opinions and data contained in all publications are solely those of the individual author(s) and contributor(s) and not of MDPI and/or the editor(s). MDPI and/or the editor(s) disclaim responsibility for any injury to people or property resulting from any ideas, methods, instructions or products referred to in the content.

www.ingramcontent.com/pod-product-compliance
Lightning Source LLC
LaVergne TN
LVHW070358100526
838202LV00014B/1342